Midwifery in Scotland:
A History

Lindsay Reid

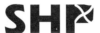

Scottish History Press

Scottish History Press is an imprint of Kea Publishing

Published in 2011 by
Scottish History Press
14 Flures Crescent
Erskine
Renfrewshire PA8 7DJ
Scotland
www.keapublishing.com

British Library Cataloguing in Publication Data

Reid, Lindsay.
   Midwifery in Scotland : a history.
   1. Midwifery--Scotland--History--20th century.
   2. Midwives--Scotland--History--20th century.
   3. Midwives--Legal status, laws, etc.--Scotland.
   4. Midwifery--Scotland--History--21st century.
   5. Midwives--Scotland--History--21st century.
   I. Title
   618.2'0233'09411'0904-dc22

   ISBN-13: 9780956447708

Typeset in Scotland by Delta Mac Artwork, Email: deltamacartwork@btinternet.com

Printed in Scotland by Kestrel Press (Irvine) Ltd, 25 Whittle Place, Irvine, Ayrshire
KA11 4HR

Midwifery in Scotland:
A History

To

Scotland's howdies and midwives

Contents

Abbreviations

AfC	Agenda for Change
AIMS	Association for the Improvement in Maternity Services
AMH	Aberdeen Maternity Hospital
ARM	Artificial rupture of membranes
ARM	Association of Radical Midwives
BHBC	*Better Health, Better Care*
BMA	British Medical Association
BNA	British Nurses Association
CMB Éire	Central Midwives Board for Éire
CMBE&W	Central Midwives Board for England and Wales
CMBS	Central Midwives Board for Scotland
CMU	Community Maternity Unit
CNO	Chief Nursing Officer
CRAG	Clinical Resource and Audit Group
DH	Department of Health [England]
DHS	Department of Health for Scotland [1929-1999]
DHSS	Department of Health and Social Security
DOMINO	Domiciliary 'in and out'
DRI	Dundee Royal Infirmary
DVT	Deep venous thrombosis
EAG	Educational Advisory Group
EBP	Evidence-based practice
EEC	European Economic Community
EGAMS	Expert Group on Maternity Services
EMS	Emergency Medical Services
EN	Enrolled Nurse
EOS	Edinburgh Obstetrical Society
GMC	General Medical Council
GP	General Practitioner
GRMH	Glasgow Royal Maternity Hospital
GRO(S)	General Register Office for Scotland
GUL	Glasgow University Library
HIMS	Highlands and Islands Medical Service
ICM	International Confederation of Midwives
IM	Independent Midwife
IMR	Infant Mortality Rate
IMUK	Independent Midwives UK
IOL	Induction of Labour
IOM	Inspector of Midwives
JNMCNI	Joint Nursing and Midwives Council Northern Ireland
KCND	Keeping Childbirth Natural and Dynamic
LA	Local Authority

LGBS	Local Government Board for Scotland
LHA	Local Health Authority
LSA	Local Supervising Authority
MCWP	Maternity Care Working Party
MDU	Midwifery Development Unit
MH	Ministry of Health
MIDIRS	Midwives' Information Retrieval Source
MLC	Midwifery Liaison Committee
MMR	Maternal Mortality Rate
MNC	Modernising Nursing Careers
MOH	Medical Officer of Health
MP	Member of Parliament
MSAG	Maternity Services Action Group
MTD	Midwife Teachers Diploma
NAS	National Archives of Scotland
NBS	National Board for Scotland (Nursing, Midwifery and Health Visiting), [1980-2002]
NHS	National Health Service
NHS QIS	NHS Quality Improvement Scotland
NICNM	Northern Ireland Council of Nursing and Midwifery
NICU	Neonatal Intensive Care Unit
NHS QIS	NHS Quality Improvement Scotland
NMC	Nursing and Midwifery Council
NMR	Neonatal Mortality Rate
PCT	Primary Care Trust
PID	Project Initiation Document [of Midwifery 2020]
PII	Professional Indemnity/Insurance
PMR	Perinatal Mortality Rate
PPH	Post partum haemorrhage
QAIMNS	Queen Alexandra's Imperial Military Nursing Service
QARANC	Queen Alexandra's Royal Army Nursing Corps
QIDNS	Queen's Institute for District Nursing in Scotland
QIS	NHS Quality Improvement Scotland
QVJIN	Queen Victoria Jubilee Institute for Nurses
RAMC	Royal Army Medical Corps
RCM	Royal College of Midwives
RCOG	Royal College of Obstetricians and Gynaecologists
RCS Ed.	Royal College of Surgeons of Edinburgh
RFN	Registered Fever Nurse
RGN	Registered General Nurse
RJCC	Refugees' Joint Consultative Committee.
RSCN	Registered Sick Children's Nurse
SBH	Scottish Board of Health (1919-1929)
SCBU	Special Care Baby Unit
SCM	State Certified Midwife

SCOTMEG	Scottish Management Executive Group
SEHD	Scottish Executive Health Department
SEN	State Enrolled Nurse (England and Wales)
SHHD	Scottish Home and Health Department
SMA	Scottish Midwives Association
SMMDP	Scottish Multi-professional Maternity Development Programme
SMMP	Simpson Memorial Maternity Pavilion, Edinburgh
SOHHD	Scottish Office Home and Health Department
SOM	Supervisor of Midwives
SOS	Secretary of State for Scotland
SOM	Supervisor of Midwives
SPCERH	Scottish Programme for Clinical Effectiveness in Reproductive Health
UKCC	United Kingdom Central Council [1983-2002]
VOL	Vale of Leven Hospital
WHO	World Health Organisation
WRHB	Western Regional Hospital Board

Glossary of Terms

Anent	(Scots), concerning, about.
Blue Book	Pupil midwife's case book required by the CMBS for Part 2 midwifery.
Caul	Term used to describe the fetal membranes when surrounding the baby at birth, e.g. 'The baby was born in the caul.' It is considered to be very lucky and it is said that babies who are born in the caul will never drown.
DOMINO	Domiciliary in and out: community midwife care for a hospital delivery and home six hours later.
Dunny	(Scots), dungeon, area under a tenement.
Gàidhealtachd	In this context, the area of Scotland mostly in the north and west where Gaelic is spoken.
Gallipot	Metal sterilisable bowl-shaped container.
Green Lady	Glasgow Municipal Midwife, called 'Green Lady' because of the green uniform. Glasgow health visitors also wore green and were also known as Green Ladies. However, for the purpose of this book, 'Green Lady' refers to midwife.
Howdie	Uncertified midwife.
Infant Mortality Rate	The IMR is defined as the number of infants dying within one year of birth per 1000 live births per year.[1]
Lochia	The term used to describe the discharges from the uterus during the puerperium.
Maternal Mortality Rate	The MMR is defined as the number of deaths due to pregnancy and childbirth per 1,000 total births (live and still) per year.[2]
Neonatal Mortality Rate	The NMR is defined as the number of infants dying within twenty-eight days of birth per 1,000 live births per year.[3]
Para	In this context, describing the number of babies a woman has given birth to, for example, 'para 1' means 'had one baby'.
Parous	Describing a woman who has had a baby previously.
Peerie body	(Shetland), a small person.
Perineal area/Perineum	Area of the body situated between the vagina and the rectum.
Perinatal Mortality Rate	The PMR is defined as the number of stillbirths and babies who die in the first week of life per 1,000 total births (live and still) per year.[4]

Prim/Primigravida	A mother who is pregnant for the first time.
Puerperium	The period from birth until six weeks after the baby is born.[5]
Rooming in	System of care in a maternity unit where babies stay with the mothers all the time.
Rottenrow	Glasgow Royal Maternity Hospital – it was located on a street named 'Rottenrow'.
Slunge/Slungeing	Terms used, mainly in hospitals, to describe work done in the sluice area of a ward.
Syntocinon	Artificial oxytocin used intravenously to induce or augment labour.
Syntometrine	A drug comprising syntocinon and ergometrine used to assist and speed up the third stage of labour.
Ticking	A strong cotton fabric, (sometimes striped) which was used as a mattress cover or, as a layer of material between the mattress and bed-springs.
Ventouse birth	An assisted birth where the cup of a vacuum extractor is placed on a baby's head and traction applied. It is used to assist maternal effort.
Vernix caseosa	A white sticky substance present on the baby's skin at birth, thought to have a protective function in utero.

1.   Educational Advisory Group of the Scottish Board of the Royal College of Midwives, *Social and Statistical Facts for Student Midwives*, (London: Pitman Books, 1982), p 83.
2.   *Ibid*, p 79.
3.   *Ibid*, p 82.
4.   *Ibid*, p 81.
5.   See Chapter 8, endnote 3.

Acknowledgements

I would like to thank all who helped in so many ways with the gestation and making of this book. These include those who listened and encouraged, telephoned, emailed, surfed the web for answers to queries, searched libraries and archives, negotiated on my behalf, accessed photographs, and gave permission for photographs and documents to be published. I am grateful to them all for their generosity of spirit, time and sharing of ideas and knowledge.

It is difficult to mention everyone involved, but the following list of names gives an indication of the level of support that I have received. I thank you all and apologise to anyone who has been omitted because of my 'senior moments', or any owners of copyright material who feel they may have been overlooked despite best efforts to ensure that appropriate permissions have been secured.

Keith Adam, Sharon Allison, Pat Andriou, Laura Blair, Linda Bryce, Keith Bryers, Claire Burnet, Alison Campbell, Dr Anne Cameron, Carol Curran, Mary Dharmachandran, Isobel Duguid, Lothian Health Services Archivists, Elsevier, Mary Findlay, John Getley, Donna Gilchrist, Glasgow City Archivists, Beatrice Grant, Jenny Hall, Veronica Hansmann, Ann Holmes, Diane Howie, Sharron McCall, Susan McGann, Dr Margaret McGuire, Carrie McIntosh, Dr Jenny MacLeod, Catherine MacMillan, (Robertson), Angela MacMorran, Professor Rosemary Mander, Anne Matthew, Catherine Murray John, Dr Alison Nuttall, Jenny Patterson, Elizabeth Radley, Margaret Ritchie (Nicol), Viv Riddoch, Susan Sanders, Shetland Museum and Archives, Natalie Smart, Brian Smith, Eleanor Stenhouse, Renée Stewart, Susan Stewart, Katie Strang, Kathleen Tait, Agnes Young, Norman Young, Edna Walker, Lorna Wallace, Mary Wallace, Laura Yeates.

I am indebted to all who generously talked to me at length about midwives and midwifery in the past. Oral history interviews between 1997 and 2003 have been a wonderful source of inspiration over the years since they were recorded and I have used many quotes from testimonies here. Apart from two midwives who would rather remain anonymous, they are: Dr Margaret Auld, Ella Banks, Anne Bayne, Anne Chapman, Ella Clelland, Wilma Coleman, Margaret Crombie, Alison Dale, Doddie Davidson, Margaret Dearnley, Jan Fenton, Margaret Foggie, Mary Gilhooly, Peggy Grieve, Maureen Hamilton, Annie Kerr, Margaret Kitson, Ann Lamb, Mary McCaskill, Margaret MacDonald, Anne McFadden, Margaret McInally, Fay MacLeod, Moira Michie, Agnes Morrison (Tillotson), Mollie Muir, May Norrie, Alice Porter, Gelda Pryde, Chrissie Sandison, Joan Savage, Betty Smith, Joan Spence, Linda Stamp, Mima Sutherland, James W Tweedie, Jean Woods.

Thank you also very much to the five contemporary midwives, Sarah Green, Jayne Forrest, Elizabeth Mansion, Sandra Smith and Phyllis Winters for allowing me to speak with them and record and quote from their conversations. Their words, thoughts, opinions and ideas have informed and stretched the original basic ideas for chapters 9 and 10 of this book.

To Professor Marguerite Dupree, Professor Edith Hillan and Dr Malcolm Nicolson, I would like to accord my thanks once again for their help.

I promised Dr Helen Bryers that she would have at least a line in the acknowledgements. The help that she gave is worth much more than that. I would like to thank Helen very much for her constant support, her reading and commenting on Chapters 9 and 10, her in-depth input into the text of those chapters, and her generosity in being able to share so willingly her knowledge of her subject.

Gillian Smith, Director of the RCM UK Board for Scotland, and I have known each other for a long time. I particularly remember Gillian's kindness to me when I was working at the RCM. They say, 'If you want something done, ask a busy person.' It was to Gillian, a very busy person, I turned when looking for someone to write the Foreword for *Midwifery in Scotland: A History*. I knew that she would get it done in the time available. More importantly, I also knew that she was the person I wanted to write my Foreword because of her longstanding care for midwives and midwifery in Scotland. This comes over clearly in what she has written. Thank you, Gillian.

Thank you also to Dr Iain Hutchison of The Scottish History Press, for taking the brave step of embarking on *Midwifery in Scotland: A History* and for keeping going.

I am indebted also to all others involved in the painstaking work of publication and printing.

Thanks to my family and their patience – again.

And David. He puts up with a lot. Thank you.

Lindsay Reid

Foreword

When Lindsay asked me to write the foreword for her book I was honoured and delighted, especially since I have enjoyed reading her others so much. However, this one was different. I recognised that a large part of it was taking me through my journey as a midwife in Scotland. This is when it dawned on me that I had lived through and was continuing to live through history and for those midwives starting out now, today's challenges and the ambitions of the profession are tomorrow's history.

It is fundamentally important to understand where we, as midwives, have come from and to know some of the difficulties we have encountered on our journey to getting midwifery recognised. Lindsay says it beautifully when she talks about autonomy and, as she put it, this book really does 'explore the paradox within midwifery: a legally autonomous profession yet subject to the over-riding authority of another profession.'

This is still obvious at the beginning of the twenty-first century with contemporary maternity services. The *Keeping Childbirth Natural and Dynamic (KCND) Pathway for Maternity Care*[1] recommends that midwives should be the first point of contact for pregnant women. This has met with opposition from some General Practitioners (GP) who believe that this will exclude them from the care of the women in their practice during pregnancy. At a Scottish GP conference in 2010 there was one GP who accused midwives and the Royal College of Midwives (RCM) of empire-building around this issue. I believe that this demonstrates a fear of lack of control by GPs in giving up authority to the midwife. Although the number I believe is small, some GPs do not appear to recognise the autonomy of the midwife's role. Every woman needs a midwife, not just for checking her blood pressure and urine, and for all the physical care that she can give, but for the social, emotional, educational and the wider public health needs of the whole family. However, some will also need the care of their GP or an obstetrician. There is enough work for all.

The *KCND* programme was launched with a highly visible advertising campaign run by Health Scotland. The highlight was a poster containing a picture of a young midwife from Fife on display the length and breadth of the country, on bus shelters, in pharmacy windows and anywhere else that pregnant women would go. The purpose of this was to get women to go to their midwife as early as possible upon knowing they were pregnant. This has certainly raised awareness within the Scottish community of the midwife's importance in providing maternity care and, according to the midwife from Fife, has made her a bit of a mini-celebrity.

September 2010 saw the launch of the *Midwifery 2020* programme of work which should provide a road map for the future of midwifery as a profession. This has been a piece of work led by Scotland, but with all four countries of the UK involved, from midwifery educationalists to Government lead midwives and organisations such as the

1   KCND Pathways for Maternity care, Edinburgh: NHS Quality Improvement Scotland, 2009.

RCM and the Royal College of Obstetricians and Gynaecologists (RCOG) as well as participation from women's groups who have walked hand in hand with midwives on their journey of change.

Women have been fundamental in supporting change with midwives through the years and I believe that the changes which have been brought about by midwives would not have happened if there had not been a shared vision with women. The only constant within the ever-changing Health Service is the notion of change in whatever form it takes. It is clear in this book how midwives work through that change and indeed embrace it.

It is the business of the midwife to support and deliver woman-centred care. I am always proud when I am out and about to say to colleagues from other countries 'this is what we are doing in Scotland.' Midwives in Scotland are trailblazers. Long may that continue.

As I write, I already know that a large number of abstracts for presentations have been submitted from our small nation for the 2011 Congress of the International Confederation of Midwives to be held in Durban, South Africa. All are strong candidates for acceptance. Within many of the papers, the demonstration of the midwives' growing strength and confidence in themselves as an autonomous profession is very obvious.

In 2015, all being well, I would like to assure Lindsay and the readers of this wonderful book that I will be making it the business of the RCM in Scotland to mark the centenary of the 1915 Midwives (Scotland) Act.

Thank you Lindsay, for reminding us how we as a profession got to where we are today and also about the more contemporary challenges we are facing now and indeed, those we will inevitably face in the future.

Gillian Smith
Director RCM UK Board for Scotland
July 2010

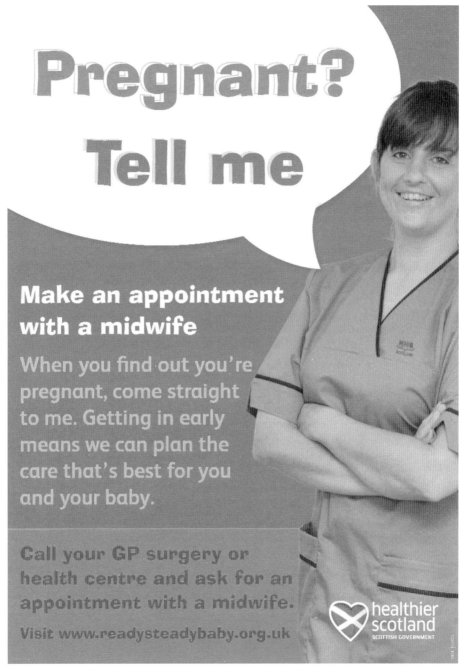

KCND Poster with Donna Gilchrist, midwife, Dunfermline Maternity Hospital. (Courtesy of NHS Health Scotland 2010.)

Introduction

The development of the profession of midwifery in Scotland from the uncertified aid-woman or 'howdie' to professional midwife has occurred alongside many changes in childbirth practice. The concurrent narratives of practical midwifery told by midwives and that of legislation and regulation of midwifery come together in *Midwifery in Scotland: A History* to present a history of midwifery in Scotland and demonstrate how issues surrounding childbirth developed.

An important issue for midwives is autonomy. The words 'autonomous' and 'autonomy', in the context of this book, indicate a freedom: the freedom of midwives to determine their own actions or behaviour when practising normal midwifery; and the freedom of the profession to make its own decisions over, for instance, education and practice. This is an autonomy which enables one professional group to co-operate with others on an equal basis, allowing parity and respect for the opinions and practice of others within a framework of partnership-working to be maintained.[1]

For much of the twentieth century, the ideals of parity within the professions of midwifery, medicine and nursing, and respect for each other's opinions were not apparent. From 1916 to 1983, the statutory regulatory body for midwives in Scotland was the Central Midwives Board for Scotland (CMBS). Research into the work of the CMBS, and the oral testimonies of midwives, have brought to light fluctuations in midwifery autonomy over the years. This can be attributed to changes in legislation and practice in the care of childbearing women, the implementation of the National Health Service (NHS) in 1948, the input and opinions of practitioners in other professions, the change in the place of birth over the years, and the actions and attitudes of midwives themselves. In each of these areas, the developing profession of obstetrics, the rise of the general practitioner in antenatal care, coupled with growing technology in the field of childbirth, contributed to the medicalisation of childbirth in Scotland and the loss of midwifery autonomy. As childbirth became more medicalised, affecting all areas of maternity care, midwives found themselves in the dilemma of obeying policies and protocols rather than acting as practitioners in their own right. In addition, the influence of the medically-dominated CMBS was significant in keeping midwives firmly in a role subordinate to General Practitioners (GPs) and obstetricians. This book investigates these issues and explores the paradox within midwifery: a legally autonomous profession yet subject to the over-riding authority of another profession.

Lack of midwives' autonomy led also to a lack of confidence and, for a time, an inability to be true advocates for mothers. Many mothers felt unable to choose how or where they gave birth. It was only in the second half of the twentieth century that childbearing women gradually began to articulate what they wanted and where they wanted it. Midwives became more educated, more confident, more able to 'stand beside' their medical counterparts, and more able and willing to work in partnership with women.

With the final decades of the twentieth century the mood for change in childbirth in Scotland became increasingly evident as joint meetings and road-shows were held for professionals, women and representatives of interested groups. In the early 1990s, the Government put into action the publication of documents, specific to each country of the UK, advocating change, informed choice, partnership between professionals and with women, and, woman-centred care.[2] Change brings its own problems such as lack of agreement, stress and unwillingness to adjust. In addition, there are differing ideas of best practice and care of pregnant, labouring and postnatal women and their babies. This, in Scotland, is partly due to the demography and geography with the relatively sparsely populated Highlands and Islands and crowded Central Belt leading to an uneven distribution of midwives and services. Maternity care can therefore depend upon area: urban or rural, island or mainland, easily accessible or difficult to reach.

Differing ideas can also be down to professional and personality diversities. However, given the history of inter-professional problems, the moves towards partnership-working, evident in the maternity care professions in the decades bordering the turn of the twenty-first century, have been significant. They have brought changes and development in midwifery practice, more inter-professional working and respect, and greater information to, choice for, and working with, women in the childbearing period.

Midwifery in Scotland: A History explores the issues within the history of midwifery in Scotland in the twentieth and early twenty-first centuries through the voices of midwives, archival research, and recent Government reports and discussions.

The voices of midwives are paramount for this book and comprise two components, oral history testimonies and contemporary conversations. Oral history, as a method of qualitative research, has become increasingly valued by historians since the 1970s and has considerable potential for the history of midwives.[3] Significantly, it can be used to obtain information where little documented evidence exists, or where the documented evidence is one-sided or suspect. It also challenges accepted, usually written, views of events and in this way revises history.[4] I found this to be very true. Between 1997 and 2003, I interviewed one local historian and many midwives from across Scotland, from Shetland to the Borders. Many of them old and retired and thinking back on their practice, the information that they gave me differed remarkably in style and content from the information given in the Central Midwives Board records. Their accounts added colour, diversity and a different dimension to the black and white picture provided by Minutes, Reports and the all-important *Rules* for midwifery practice.[5]

Secondly, *Midwifery in Scotland: A History* is also concerned with modern-day midwifery. I approached five contemporary midwives at varying stages in their midwifery careers who generously agreed to speak with me about midwifery today. These conversations took place between September 2009 and February 2010. The midwives conceded that evolution of their professional practice is still in progress and there is still much to be done to improve maternity care in Scotland. Nevertheless, these midwives, through their voices, have presented a snapshot of maternity care in Scotland in the first decade of the twenty-first century which is vibrant, hopeful, energetic and dynamic.[6]

Midwifery in Scotland has come a long way since the beginning of the twentieth century. The years since the 1915 Act have revealed a remarkable professional midwifery journey and the Scottish birthing world is the better for this. I would like to congratulate midwives in Scotland for their continuing development, confidence, sense of purpose and strength, and woman-centred care.

1.   L Reid, Introduction, in L Reid, (ed) Midwifery: Freedom to practise? Edinburgh: Elsevier, 2007, p 3.
2.   Welsh Office, Maternal and Early Child Health, (Cardiff: HMSO, 1991); Northern Ireland Maternity Unit Study Group, Delivering Choice: Midwife and GP-led Maternity Units, (Belfast: HMSO,1994); DH, Changing Childbirth, Part 1: Report of the Expert Maternity Group, (London, HMSO, August 1993); SHHD, Provision of Maternity Services in Scotland – A Policy Review, (Edinburgh: HMSO, July 1993).
3.   B Hunter, 'Oral history and research, part 1: uses and implications', British Journal of Midwifery, (1999), Vol 7 (7), pp 426-429.
4.   L Reid, Scottish Midwives 1916-1983: The Central Midwives Board for Scotland and Practising Midwives, unpublished PhD thesis for the University of Glasgow, p 309; L Reid, 'Using oral history in midwifery research', British Journal of Midwifery, (2004), Vol 12 (4), pp 208-238.
5.   Most of these interviewees agreed to allow me to use their names. They are cited in the footnotes as LR 1-128.
6.   Their names are not used in the text and are cited as LR 129-134. Each of the midwives chose her own pseudonym.

Chapter 1
The Howdies

The unique art and craft of the midwife combine to form what has been an enduring profession over many centuries. As long as women have given birth, they have needed someone to tend, support, help at the birthing, and care for them and their babies afterwards.

There have been midwives in Scotland for centuries, using instinct, ancient learnings, customs, folklore and habits, but 'unqualified' as understood today. It was not until the twentieth century that midwives achieved statutory regulation and with this the new status of being certified. This chapter looks at the work of the uncertified midwife in Scotland or, 'howdie'. This term came into common use in the later centuries of the second millennium. These uncertified midwives learned the craft of midwifery by observing other howdies, or the local general practitioner (GP), at work. When the time came for them to practise on their own, there was no regulation or registration. Other would-be midwives obtained a form of midwifery qualification from a maternity hospital; although more formal, this was still unregulated. The majority learned midwifery practice by accompanying, and learning from, a woman known for her experience and so gradually developed reputations as midwives themselves. Howdies built up a trusting clientele by word of mouth, by stepping into the shoes of their predecessors, or on the recommendation of a GP. Registration of midwifery in Scotland was introduced in 1916 upon implementation of the 1915 Midwives (Scotland) Act. The chapter explores what happened to the howdies as registration of midwifery became a reality, and those who were uncertified found that, to remain legal, they had to rethink their practice.

Before Regulation: the uncertified midwives
In Scotland, the autonomous practice of midwives caring for women undergoing a normal childbearing episode has been approved by statute since 1916 following passage of the 1915 Midwives (Scotland) Act. Before 1916, women who practised as midwives did so without need for state regulation. The majority were untrained and took the title 'midwife' by repute rather than by any specific education they received. The provisions of the Act permitted midwives to practise independently and make their own professional decisions. Yet, even before 1916, midwives did not have unlimited autonomy. Prior to the mid-eighteenth century, midwives cared for and delivered women in childbirth; male medical practitioners were called in emergency situations, such as prolonged labour, malposition of the fetus and haemorrhage. From the mid-eighteenth century, the presence of male practitioners in the delivery room became more common, even for normal births.[1]

The 1915 Midwives (Scotland) Act established a Central Midwives Board (CMBS) to oversee the registration (known at the time as 'enrolment'), training and practice of midwives; the CMBS continued until 1983. While the Act brought the first formal recognition of midwives as a group throughout Scotland and gave them a legal identity, in practice its provisions affected their autonomy.[2] Throughout the period from 1916 to 1983 the identity and autonomy of midwives were subject to negotiation and change, both in terms of the institutional frameworks within which they trained and practised, and the nature of their practice before, during and after birth.[3]

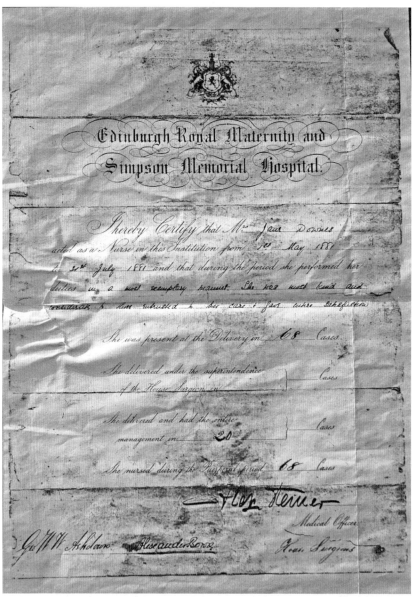

Parchment awarded to Mrs Jane Downes in 1881. (Courtesy of Edna Walker.) See Appendix 3 for transcript.

On the eve of the 1915 Act, midwives in Scotland had no unifying organisation, nor, despite some sporadic local attempts to license and educate midwives, was there any formal regulation of their practice.[4] Some had attended lectures and trained in maternity hospitals; some were trained nurses (although nursing at that time was also an unregulated profession); most relied on experience on-the-job, ranging from delivering a baby as a neighbourly act to gaining a reputation in an area through watching and learning from another uncertified midwife, known in many parts of Scotland as a 'howdie'. Chrissie Sandison from Shetland recalled:

> I had a grand-aunt [Meggie] who was the age I am now [80] when I was a teenager. She had had no children of her own, never was married, a peerie body who was in attendance at many a birth. I asked her how it was she had taken up to be a howdie for she had had no proper training. Apparently, her mother, Hannah, had been a howdie and when she began to get old she began taking Meggie along too... There were big families in those days – that would have been from about 1880 onwards. This Meggie had been born in 1858 and was in attendance at the birth of one of my nephews in 1926.[5]

Before the 1915 Act, an estimated ninety-five per cent of all births, by both the rich and the poor, took place at home. A few, especially in the cities, took place in maternity hospitals which evolved in Scotland from the second half of the eighteenth century.[6]

There was little or no antenatal care which meant that potential problems went unnoticed until the mother went into labour and called out the midwife. Although postnatal care was part of the midwife's duty, especially immediately post-delivery, it also was unregulated and of varying standards.[7]

The term 'midwife' is very old and is commonly understood to mean the 'with-woman'. That is, the woman who is with a woman in childbirth. However, midwives in Scotland have been known by other names, hence the favourite old word 'howdie'. This term was understood across Scotland with variations depending on the area, like 'howdie-wife', or in the northeast, 'howdie-wifie'. Doddie Davidson, an Aberdeenshire howdie in the 1930s and 1940s, said: 'There wis nae midwife. They ca'ed ye the howdie. Fan ye arrived they said, 'Are you the howdie?'[8] Elsewhere were other terms, like 'skilly', or 'skilful-woman', 'handy-woman', 'neighbour woman', 'helping woman'. Gaelic words were used where appropriate: 'bean-ghluine' or 'knee woman' on St Kilda and, elsewhere in the Highlands, 'bean chuideachaidh' meaning 'aid woman'.[9] Upon occasion, the howdie was called 'Mam'. Mima Sutherland, a Shetland midwife during the mid-twentieth century, said, 'My grannie was a howdie. She was called Mam Willa'.[10] Another Shetland howdie was known in her latter years as 'Aald Mam o Houbanster'. She was Betty Balfour and was so well known as a skilful howdie that people consulted her from far and wide. The story goes that once, Jeemie, her blacksmith fisherman husband, rowed her from Houbanster to the island of Muckle Röe to a labouring woman. Eventually Betty could see that prolonged labour was putting both the mother's and baby's lives in danger. She consulted Jeemie who used his blacksmithing expertise to fashion forceps. With these she saved both mother and baby and was apparently the first in the area to deliver by forceps. She died at Houbanster aged 86 in 1918.[11]

Yet the uncertified midwives were not all so competent. Commentators and historians have described midwives before the twentieth century across a spectrum from ignorant to able. At one extreme, they were 'too ignorant to recognise the signs of danger and so too late in seeking medical assistance.' At the other extreme they were 'too impatient and started to "work upon" their patients by stretching the vulva with their hands to stimulate pains, pushing on the fundus and pulling upon any part of the unhappy foetus that afforded a grip to their searching fingers.'[12]

Some historians give a more positive appraisal. Irvine Loudon firmly recognises midwives' ability in the late nineteenth century and, while Hilary Marland acknowledges great variation in midwives' skills, competence and background, she discounts with equal firmness the 'ignorant midwife' theory in Early Modern Europe.[13]

Regardless of different views on the quality of care that they provided, there is agreement that the status of midwives suffered in the eighteenth and nineteenth centuries because of their lack of formal training, lack of regulation and associated lack of professional solidarity. In addition, their standing suffered because of the rising ascendancy of the male medical profession, and because midwives were predominantly women who characteristically were 'listening, feeling [and] attached' as opposed to the more scientific description of the male medical practitioner as 'seeing, examining [and] detached'.[14]

There were efforts to formalise training and regulate midwives in Scotland before the early twentieth century. However, it was the legislation, first for England and Wales in 1902, and then for Scotland in 1915, which set the framework for the formal training, registration and regulation of midwives, gave them a legal basis for their professional status, and shaped their relationship with doctors, nurses and childbearing women.

Early attempts to formalise midwifery training in Scotland
The lack of formal training and regulation for women in midwifery were issues which medical practitioners and official bodies in Scotland attempted to address from the eighteenth century. Male medical practitioners, called originally to the birthing rooms to help in emergency situations, became a common presence even at some normal births from the mid-eighteenth century.[15] Concurrently came the introduction of formal training schools for midwives and an attempt to control their activities. The first training through lectures for midwives in the United Kingdom was said to have been established in Edinburgh in 1726 when the Town Council appointed Joseph Gibson as Professor of Midwifery. The Council made this appointment because it was appalled by the prevalence of what it called 'obstetrical disasters', many of which were blamed on midwives.[16] However, Professor Gibson was well known for his efforts to promote midwifery and had in 1723 advertised 'An Account of what Mr Gibson proposes to do in a Course of MIDWIFERY', adding that he 'may be spoke with [sic] at his house in Leith.'[17]

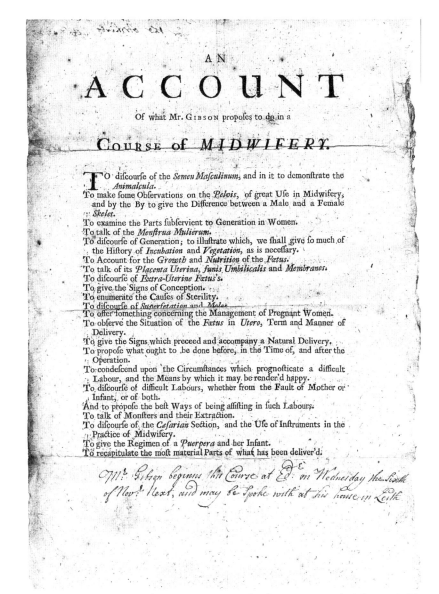

Advertisement for a Course in Midwifery, Mr Joseph Gibson, 1723.
(Courtesy of Keith Adam of Blairadam.) See Appendix 3 for transcript.

A midwifery examination and licence similar to Professor Gibson's in Edinburgh was established in Glasgow in December 1739 under the auspices of the Faculty of Physicians and Surgeons of Glasgow. The Faculty declared in their Act Anent Midwives, 'that all midwives after a certain time shall pass an examination and have a licence from the Faculty before they be admitted to practise.'[18] The Faculty's sphere of influence included Lanarkshire, Renfrewshire, Ayrshire and Dunbartonshire. Its authority for framing this Act originated in an enabling Charter granted to the Faculty by James VI (r.1567-1625). In theory, the members had the power under this Act to license midwives to practise, to try them for bad practice and to prevent them from practising further. In reality, they had difficulty maintaining the Act and the last recorded mention of a midwife being disciplined under the Act was in 1820.[19]

Other midwifery lectures and examinations followed in Scotland. In Aberdeen, although there was no similar attempt to force midwives to undertake a recommended training, the Kirk Session of St Machar's Cathedral, 'appalled by the ignorance of women practising midwifery', recommended that women wishing to practise as midwives should attend lectures given by Aberdeen practitioner, Dr David Skene.[20] The Kirk Session also had the relevant minute from their Records reproduced in the *Aberdeen Journal* of 9 January 1759 and, following the example of other Kirk Sessions, agreed to assist those 'who may not be able to afford the necessary Expence [sic] of their Education this Way' and requested Voluntary contributions from members of the public who were prepared to help.[21]

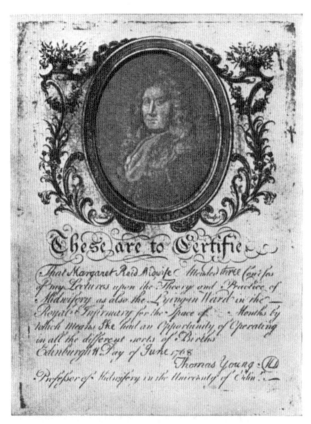

Certificate awarded to Margaret Reid, midwife, in 1768. Reprinted from M Myles, A textbook for midwives (6th ed), (E&S Livingstone, 1968), p 667 fig 448. See Appendix 3 for transcript.

Newspapers in Dundee also advertised classes in midwifery. In the *Dundee Weekly Advertiser* of Friday 16 January 1801 an advertisement stated:

MIDWIFERY

SEVERAL WOMEN having applied to Mr Grant, Surgeon in DUNDEE, for instructions in the above art, and it being inconvenient to his private practice to give the attention necessary to instruct them separately; he takes this method of acquainting them and the public, that he intends to OPEN a CLASS sometime in the month of January, 1801, for that purpose – Of the particular time and scene, information may be obtained at his house in St Andrews Street, Dundee.[22]

Throughout the UK there was no uniformity of midwifery training and nothing to regulate it. In addition, apart from the attempt at regulation in Glasgow, any woman was able to practise midwifery, and the untrained midwife was regularly in attendance at births, especially among less well-off childbearing women. Particularly in rural Scotland, trained midwives were seldom available and most babies were delivered at home by untrained midwives or howdies.[23] This old tradition is reflected fictionally in John Galt's 'The Howdie'. This howdie obtained her post through the auspices of the local minister's wife and the 'Leddy Dowager'. She succeeded her predecessor when she became ill. According to the story, she did not appear to work with doctors but found herself in competition with them:

I cannot tell how it happened that there was little to do in the way of trade all that winter, but it began to grow into a fashion that the genteeler order of ladies went into the towns to have their han'lings amang the doctors. It was soon seen, however, that they had nothing to boast of by that manoeuvre, for their gudemen thought the cost overcame the profit, and thus...whatever the ladies thought of the doctors, their husbands kept the warm side of frugality towards me and other poor women that had nothing to depend upon but the skill of their ten fingers.[24]

Uncertified midwives: a link with tetanus neonatorum

At the end of the nineteenth century, maternal and infant mortality rates remained high. This brought maternal and child health, along with a falling birth rate and fear of population decline, into the political arena.[25] One area for concern was the high incidence of *tetanus neonatorum*, described as a major disease of the Scottish islands.[26] Although it was sufficiently prevalent in many of the islands of the Inner and Outer Hebrides to warrant various entries in the *Statistical Account of Scotland* in the 1790s, it was the frequency of *tetanus neonatorum* among newborn babies on the island group of St Kilda in the nineteenth century which brought the matter to a head and played a part in the evacuation of the islands in 1930.

This small island group lies 110 miles west of the Scottish mainland.[27] In the nineteenth century, the howdie or 'bean-ghluine' delivered the babies and looked after the mothers and babies postnatally. Many of this generation of babies died of *tetanus neonatorum*. The neonatal mortality rate (NMR) is defined as the number of live-born infants who die under the age of twenty-eight days per thousand live births. The NMR for St Kilda in the decade to 1869 was 689.7.[28] This equates to twenty-nine births of which twenty babies died with *tetanus neonatorum* being the chief cause of death. This was a major contribution to the falling population and the islanders' eventual evacuation to the mainland. It took the efforts of the Rev Angus Fiddes, the local minister between 1890 and 1894, to eradicate the disease from the islands of St Kilda. This involved trips to Glasgow, firstly to recruit a nurse for St Kilda. The nurse's ten months on St Kilda was a failure, probably due to her being distrusted by the local mothers. Not to be thwarted, the minister returned to Glasgow for personal instruction after which he practised successfully on subsequent babies.[29]

There were various early theories why the babies of St Kilda were so badly affected. Speculation included: the oily fish diet of pregnant women which might inhibit lactation; improper feeding of the new babies; poor, filthy home sanitation with a smoky atmosphere; birth trauma; 'mental perturbation' of the mother prior to breast feeding; and, later, some sort of umbilical sepsis. This latter theory became the crux of the problem. To begin with, the use of communal infant clothing was blamed. However, the dressing used for the umbilical area seemed to be the key. In the Hebrides, it was the custom in the late 1800s to dress the umbilicus with a rag which had been held with tongs over the fire to burn a small hole in it.[30] This practice was not unusual elsewhere at that time. Ann Lamb, a midwife in the 1930s whose mother was a howdie around the late 1890s and 1900s in Glenlivet, Banffshire, said:

> My mother told us how she dressed the babies' cords. She washed and boiled old white linen rags, dried them and lit a candle. She cut a hole in the centre of each square of linen and held the candle over the hole until it was burning, then blew it out and rolled them up in a clean towel. That was sterilisation.[31]

Sterilisation by burning a hole in the rag seemed by itself to be a reasonable idea. However, it was what the rag was coated with that possibly introduced the infection. It is likely that the howdie on St Kilda dressed each baby's cord with a rag, possibly with a hole burned in it, but coated with fulmar-oil. Collacott uses the word 'anointing' in this context and it appears that the howdie, the *bean-ghluine*, used it as a ceremonial unguent for newborn babies. Probably either the fulmar-oil or its container, which was usually the dried stomach of a gannet, carried the tetanus virus. Possibly the fulmars themselves were the carriers. To the St Kildans, fulmars were a staple as food, and for oil for domestic uses including this lethal anointing for the babies' cord areas. On the eighth postnatal day babies became ill: 'the sickness of eight days'. By the fifteenth day many were dead. It took until 1912 to persuade mothers of St Kilda to accept new, cleaner habits.[32]

The 'burnt rag' method of cord-care was also in use on South Uist about 1914. Fulmar oil is not mentioned in this context, but it was the custom to 'put a piece of burnt rag on the cut cord, to truss the baby up tightly in clothes, and neither to wash nor change the child until the fifth day.'[33]

The theory of poor home sanitation accompanied by dirty conditions also contributed to the incidence of tetanus. The houses were so filthy that the possibility of tetanus spores being present in the muck cannot be ruled out.[34] A further theory blamed the spread of infection on midwives' use of unsterilised knives, and on the islanders' mistrust of modern medical practices. These multi-purpose knives would almost certainly have become contaminated with tetanus.[35] Stride cites accounts from a doctor who visited the island in the 19th century and found nurses were using unclean medical equipment. An analysis of the island's soil shows heavy contamination with tetanus spores. The squalid conditions in which the islanders lived, surrounded by manure from livestock, created the perfect conditions for the spores to grow.[36]

The following testimony highlights the fears of a midwife from the Outer Hebrides regarding the work of howdies:

> By the time we arrived ... the baby was born and a howdie was there. I still remember that handsome lady, she was eighty – and she was standing there and I said, 'Oh hello. Well, I'm glad you were here.' And the mother was quite happy with the baby, and the first thing I thought, 'the cord'. She had covered the baby and when I looked, the umbilical cord was intact. She hadn't touched it. That was the trouble previously. They cut the cord... But she had left it. She just said, 'I left everything for you.' She had covered the baby and the baby was fine between the mother's legs. The mother was very happy. 'Oh', she said, 'the baby's here.' And I remember that incident because I heard of the stories of howdies.[37]

In the mid-1800s, tetanus neonatorum was less prevalent in the east of Scotland than in the west and in the islands. Of live births, the number of babies who died was also lower. For instance, on the east coast of Scotland between 1863 and 1899 the neonatal mortality rate was 35.2 per 1000 live births; for the Isle of Lewis it was 44.3 per 1000. Deaths between four and fourteen days, when most tetanus neonatorum deaths occurred, were 26.5 per 1000 in Lewis compared with 13.1 in east-coast parishes under examination.[38]

There are several reasons underlying the conclusion that tetanus neonatorum was more prevalent in the west and on the islands than in the east. The number of medical practitioners, and therefore their influence, was greater in the east than in the west. Poor communication and isolation in the west Highland and island parishes inhibited development of standards of hygiene across communities, including untrained midwives. St Kilda, the farthest flung island of the group was, as far as communication was concerned, the most vulnerable and, in some areas of the Hebrides, there was the possible 'ritual' aspect of the anointing with fulmar oil.[39] A further theory linked the cause to peat-burning and subsequent soil pollution with heavy metals. This was because recent laboratory samples of fulmar oil revealed no tetanus, whereas soil from areas around the dwelling houses on St Kilda were found to be heavily infested with tetanus clostridium.[40]

Towards a Midwives Act for England and Wales
The howdie in Scotland was the same as the handywoman in England and Wales. As statutory registration in England and Wales pre-dated Scotland by some thirteen years, it is appropriate for this chapter to look briefly at how this came about.

In the second half of the nineteenth century, occupational boundaries between midwifery and medicine continued to be contested throughout Britain. In the late 1870s, members of the London Obstetrical Society proposed a Midwives Bill that would put midwives completely under obstetricians' control and seriously restrict midwives' practice.[41] Members of the women's movement opposed this legislation on the grounds that it placed restrictions on women's work.[42] In 1881, Louisa Hubbard (1836-1906), a wealthy woman working for the extension of employment opportunities for women, and three midwives including the social reformer Zepherina Veitch (1836-1894), formed the new Matrons' Aid Society, later to be known as the Midwives' Institute, the forerunner of the College of Midwives.[43] Through the Society, they 'aimed to raise the status of the midwife by the recruitment of educated women and by State registration.'[44] Realising that to achieve their aims they required approval of leading obstetricians, they announced at the outset that the Society would work 'in harmony' with the medical profession, so receiving co-operation in return.[45] However, the price for co-operation was that midwives would not be allowed to give direct care to women whose labour was not 'normal', consequently putting them into a non-competitive role.[46] It suited obstetricians to have this sort of co-operation with midwives. For them, the licensing of midwives was a way of establishing a lesser practitioner to relieve them of unproductive time-consuming work, and also a way to bypass the general practitioner (GP).[47]

GPs, therefore, opposed legislation for the registration of midwives. In particular, GP members of the General Medical Council (GMC) resisted registration for many years because to register midwives and regulate their training would increase competition for work.[48] However, the 1893-94 Report of the Midwives' Registration Select Committee argued that, with more education, midwives would recognise the abnormal and call medical aid and therefore theoretically rule out this perceived threat to medical practice.[49] This reinforced the view of the *British Medical Journal* which claimed in 1890 that the medical profession favoured registration of midwives.[50]

The different parts of the medical profession were not the only groups which had to be won over. Opposition to registration in the 1890s also came from some midwives in the Manchester Midwives' Society. They saw this development, and the projected plans of governance by a board mainly staffed by medical men, as a removal of much of their autonomy.[51]

In addition, some members of the British Nurses' Association (BNA) opposed midwives' registration. Members of the nursing profession campaigned for registration at the same time as midwives. In an attempt to strengthen the nurses' cause, Elgin-born Mrs Ethel Bedford Fenwick (1856-1947), leader of the BNA and Matron of St Bartholomew's Hospital, London, suggested a midwife-nurse alliance. However, members of the Midwives' Institute stated that their members were independent practitioners and, as such, required 'separate and prior consideration' and they declined Mrs Bedford Fenwick's invitation. From that point, Mrs Bedford Fenwick and her followers campaigned against registration of midwives. The nurses' voice, the *Nursing Record*, referred to midwives as 'obsolete', 'an anachronism', and an 'historical curiosity'.[52]

Finally, after twenty years of effort, the first Midwives Act was passed in 1902 and arrangements were made for the registration of midwives in England and Wales, but not in Scotland and Ireland. This was a major landmark in the professionalisation of midwifery and for the mothers and infants they cared for.[53] Nevertheless, this legislation restricted midwives' practice through medical dominance of the Central Midwives Board for England and Wales (CMBE&W) and by imposing *Rules* and allowing policies which promoted the idea that doctors should be the lead professionals in all areas of childbearing. In addition, by requiring an expensive education with terminology that was alien to many, it effectively barred many working-class uncertified midwives in England and Wales from achieving a formal career in midwifery.[54]

Midwifery in Scotland after 1902

Prior to 1902, the maternity hospitals of Edinburgh, Glasgow, Aberdeen and Dundee independently granted certificates to the midwives that they trained. In 1903, the medical staffs of these maternity hospitals set up a Scottish Examining Board for Obstetric Nurses which held quarterly oral and written examinations for pupil midwives. This attempt by the medical profession to regulate midwifery in Scotland and to keep midwives in Scotland as far as possible in line with those in England was reasonably successful. The newly formed CMBE&W formally recognised some Scottish maternity hospitals as training institutions, and some Scottish midwives went to England to sit its new examination even although the CMBE&W had no jurisdiction over their practice in Scotland. Despite these initiatives, most midwives in Scotland were without formal training and therefore remained uncertified during the first fifteen years of the twentieth century.[55]

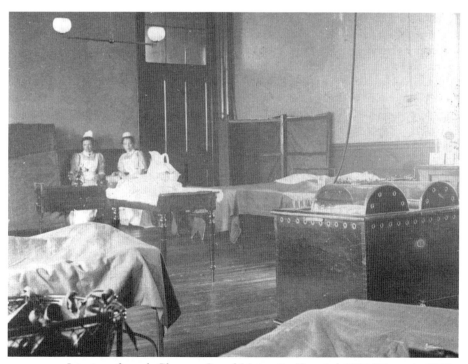

Interior of ward, Glasgow Royal Maternity Hospital (GRMH), early 1900s.
(Courtesy of Elizabeth Radley.)

It is difficult to estimate the number of midwives, trained or untrained, in Scotland before the 1915 Midwives (Scotland) Act. In the 1911 Census for Scotland, 313 females (no males) returned themselves as midwives, a decrease of seventy-two on the 385 recorded for 1901, and a further decrease on the 510 women listed as midwives in 1881. However, the 2,179 women who were recorded as sick nurses in 1881 had increased to 10,316 by 1911. While nurses were nearly five times as numerous in 1911 as in 1881, midwives were little more than half as numerous in 1911 as in 1881.[56]

It is likely that the Census underestimates the number of midwives practising in Scotland before the 1915 Midwives (Scotland) Act. When midwives enrolled following the Act, over 2,000 signed up within the first year.[57] Firstly, it is possible that women who practised midwifery without a formal certificate used terms like 'howdie' or 'neighbour-woman', which were either not recorded on the census form or were categorised differently by the Registrar General's office. Secondly, in the 1911 Census, the 313 women who described themselves as 'midwife' were unmarried or widowed.[58] It is likely that uncertified midwives or howdies included married women who practised midwifery on an informal basis without being recorded on the census return. The Central Midwives Board for Scotland (CMBS) Roll from 1916 did not contain information about marital status; however, the CMBS required marriage certificates from midwives seeking enrolment, suggesting that some midwives were married.[59] Thirdly, there was the problem of recording women's occupations on a census form written, organised and completed by men who did not see occupations of women as of primary importance.[60] Reporting of married women and their employment was seriously under-recorded in censuses of this period. It was only in 1911 that the number of married women working was listed separately for the first time. There was also a significant sexual division of labour in the home which influenced women's participation in paid work.[61] Also, as the 1911 Census Report suggests, the fall in the number of midwives and rise in the number of nurses might be partly accounted for by midwives describing themselves as nurses.[62]

One woman who described herself as a midwife and who appears in the 1901 census as such, was Elizabeth Sanderson, aged forty-four, of Young's Land, Thorniewood in the Ward of Uddingston, Parish of Bothwell. Elizabeth Rae was born in the Parish of Govan in 1854, married James Sanderson on 16 February 1872 and had six children (one boy and five girls) between 1873 and 1891. James, a roadsman in a coalmine, was 'killed [in August 1891] by being crushed by a fall of stone in No 2 Pit, Nackerty, in the Parish of Bothwell, [duration of illness] 14 hours.[63] Elizabeth, on poor relief with 'young children dependent', continued to live in damp, straitened circumstances in New Rows, Nackerton (or Nackerty; also called Aitkenhead) before moving to Thorniewood. In 1901, this dwelling accommodated six people in two rooms.

It is likely that, like many widows, Elizabeth Sanderson turned to midwifery as a way of earning a living. In 1901, there were still two of her own children at home along with her adult nephew, William, a coal miner, his wife Florence and their infant son Joseph. Elizabeth probably had no formal training. We do not know many details of how hard she had to work as a midwife, but her daughter Elizabeth Hutchison remembered her mother assisting at confinements and her dedication:

> From the confinements, she would bring home sheets for the laundering which she did at night. [I remember] as a child often joining [my] mother, at

her request, in the wash-house to keep her company while she worked there...
It was always cold in the wash-house... she was asthmatic and [I believe that]
it was the cold, damp conditions of this work that contributed to her death at
a relatively early age.

Elizabeth Sanderson died in Thorniewood at the age of 52 on 2 March 1907 of acute
broncho-pneumonia after five days' illness.[64]

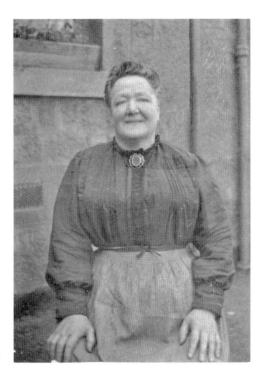

Elizabeth Sanderson (née Rae),
uncertified midwife, Uddingston.
(Courtesy of Dr Iain Hutchison.)

Whatever the nomenclature, and whether they were census-cited or not, although
there were some hospital-trained midwives in Scotland, a few of whom were certified in
England, the majority of women practising midwifery, especially in rural areas, were
untrained midwives or howdies delivering babies in the homes of the mothers.[65] In their
practice, they could call for medical aid if they had problems. Of Unst, Shetland, in
1917, MacKenzie wrote:

There are no trained midwives in the district, but there are four very capable
women who attend most of the confinements, the doctor being called in
when labour seems for some reason unknown to the midwife to be unduly
prolonged.[66]

The procedure of calling for medical aid when a mother's labour went beyond the
bounds of 'normal' also became an important rule for certified midwives and was based
on the terms of the 1915 Act.[67]

Sometimes GPs appeared to prefer working with howdies than with certified midwives, as Chrissie Sandison of Shetland illustrated:

> The doctor that I remember [in the 1920s]... [he] was a good doctor and the women liked him but he would never fetch the midwife [certified midwife] until she was required. This was my aunt's second baby. She said he sat down the stairs reading a book and he never went upstairs until he knew that the midwife had gone to the lavatory. This was a good bit from the house. It was a wee house across a burn, there was no bucket just a seat across a burn and I don't know about a toilet roll – likely it was a bit of newspaper and no buckets to empty. Well, anyway, when she had to go, he went up to inspect [how the mother was progressing] and then when she came back he would go downstairs again. When she had her next baby... that would be in 1929, she employed another woman, one who had had a big family but who wasn't a certified midwife. Then the doctor was quite happy. He didn't like working with the trained midwife... he maybe thought she knew as much as he did. I think he had a bit of a psychological blockage.[68]

Chrissie Sandison also noted the difference between a howdie and a neighbour. 'I knew another woman who was not happy with the midwife she had for her first, and ever after that she had – not a howdie – just a neighbour. You see they didn't do much – nature did it. A lot of midwifery is just waiting.'[69]

Howdies worked in some parts of rural Scotland until the 1940s and 1950s, but in the early 1900s were an accepted part of the country scene. Ann Lamb, herself a midwife, was born in Banffshire and delivered by the howdie, Meg Gordon: 'She would have been called the Howdy [sic], the midwife for the district, and she liked a dram...I was brought into the world on 25 February 1902.'[70] Ann Lamb also made clear the perceived importance of the GP in midwifery at the time: '...and there was six feet of snow and the doctor never saw me for six weeks because the roads were all blocked.'[71]

Local GPs, especially in rural areas, could be influential in obtaining positions for howdies. One in particular, Doddie Davidson, had never seen a baby born before she faced her first delivery in Aberdeenshire in the early 1940s. She was eighteen years old, the woman was in labour and her husband had gone away to fetch the doctor in the snow, with the added complication of blocked roads. She recalled:

> Meantime Babby wis gettin on wi't an I thocht, 'Oh I better get tools an things ready'. I kent foo tae dae at. So I got the tools an bilin watter an a thing for the doctor comin. But it went on fur a couple o oors, maybe langer than at – and then I could see the baby's heid comin and so here's the baby, 'Oh there's naebiddy here bit me.' Naebiddy ti help, there wisna neighbours ye see. So I thocht, 'Fit'll I dae?' So I said, 'Oh it winna be lang noo, Babby'. But the heid jist didna come ony further. I thocht, 'Oh at bairn disna look richt ti me. I na ken fit ti dae.' An I could see there wis twa cords on its neck. The heid wis oot, an the baby jist didna look richt. It wis growin bluer... So I pushed the heidie back a wee bittie and I got one finger in below the cord and I got it ower. The second bit o the cord wis easy. It wis the first ye see. An eventually, the baby wis born, nae doctor, nae hubby, naebiddy. I had ti

wrap it. Bit at the same time the baby wis motionless an blue. An I thocht, 'Oh well, the baby's deid'. But I wrappit it up wi a tool an it gaed a kin a half cough and then anither een and then sort of spluttered a bittie and I thocht, 'Well it's still here.' An then aa at aince it gaed a yell and I thocht, 'Oh God, I wis nivver so pleased to hear a bairn.'[72]

When the doctor finally appeared, Doddie was scared that what she had done might have been wrong:

But hooivver, it wis a while efter at, the doctor an her hubby came back an he looked at the baby an, he said, 'Fit, is this been corded, is it?' Ye ken, the marks wis still on the neck. An I said, 'Aye,' an I telt him. I wis fair shakkin ye ken wi fit I did. Ye ken, pushed the baby back a bit and put ma finger in. So he commended me. He said, 'Oh, at wis jist great.' He says, 'Oh I could dae wi you on the [district]'. I wis really worried aboot it, really worried, but no that wis jist it. An I wis wi him a few times efter at.[73]

This gives some indication of the deference 'ordinary' people accorded medical practitioners. It also demonstrates the GP's ability to obtain work for howdies and how they worked together.

Annie Kerr, another howdie, made a similar comment: 'Dr Welsh knew I likit these kind of jobs away oot of the road of everybody and no other body would go near them... I can min Dr Welsh gied me great jobs.'[74] However, GPs not only obtained work for the howdies and recommended them to women, they needed them to be there. Ann Lamb indicated this when describing her mother in rural Banffshire. She said:

She was a bit of a midwife as well and the Doctor always told them, 'Fetch Mrs. Lamb until I come.' He had to come all the way from Tomintoul or Achbreck and when Willie was born she didn't see him there for weeks as there was a storm.[75]

Howdies were evident in Scotland until at least the 1950s. Some appeared to be very organised and worked closely with the local GP as Johnann Roberton did in 1930s Aberdeen. Her grand-daughter wrote:

I was delivered [in 1934] by my grandmother – by Johnann Roberton who was the uncertificated midwife for the King Street and surrounding streets. She was employed by a Dr Coutts who I believe was specialising in confinements and child care. He ran the main surgery in King Street and she was called out at all hours to confinements in houses. She had her own special bag... When a birth happened unexpectedly, Dr Coutts would collect her in his little car, but otherwise she had to walk to all the other call-outs. She liked to be summoned in the first stages of labour to avoid complications where possible, and lived and worked by the idea that 'To be forewarned was to be forearmed.'[76]

However, Anne McFadden was more doubtful about the practices of howdies. In 1951, she moved from the Simpson Memorial Maternity Pavilion (SMMP), Edinburgh, to a post as district nurse-midwife in Lochgelly, Fife, where she came across howdies for the first time. She explained the situation:

> At that time there were at least five or six 'domiciliary midwives', but they really...were only...howdies... Coming straight from Simpson where everything was, you know...ahead of its time...I found it extremely difficult because I didn't get a lot of midwifery because these other people were depending on it for a livelihood... Of course the people in Lochgelly knew them. They were Lochgelly bodies, so [the mothers booked these howdies]... and the doctor might or might not be involved...they...were known to the doctor. Now...they would only be assisting the doctor, you know, fetching and carrying... So therefore the doctor would be very aware of the capabilities of certain women. Also, their integrity would be important... She was really a handywoman...with little or no training.[77]

Another midwife described a similar situation where the howdie made a habit of getting the delivery instead of the midwife:

> In that area I was in, in Central Scotland [in the 1940s], there was [a howdie]. ...she was very loath to give up. You see she was in an area of town, you know a country area, and she was kind and she was the one who would deliver the babies and I think some of [the certified midwives] had battles with her. I think she would say [to the mother], 'Oh you've time enough to send for the midwife,' and then she would be able to get the baby.[78]

Anne McFadden also indicated that the howdie learned skills from the doctor with whom she worked. 'The doctor might...take her with him, if he needed somebody. Therefore she would get a bit of experience.' But then mothers sometimes just had the howdie. 'They [the mothers] might be lucky if they had the doctor and you just had to hope that the midwife [howdie]...knew enough to know when to get the doctor.'[79] She also voiced concern that the howdies took on mothers whom she felt should have gone to hospital to have their babies:

> I had been brought up in the Simpson where...everything was done, you know, according to the book. And we were taught that...if somebody had [previously] had a prolonged labour or had to be taken in to have their placenta removed, if she'd had a whole lot of children, you know we were taught you should never accept them on the district... They should be hospitalised. Well, you see many of them were like that...to have eight and nine children wasn't unusual at one time and if you had that nurse [sic] for your first baby and everything was all right, you would go on and have another and so...[this howdie] would have delivered eight and nine of the same family...not always with the doctor. Only if...she was clever enough to spot that there was a problem. I wouldn't have wanted the responsibility of having them... I would just [have] said, 'No, no, no, I think you'd be safer to go into the hospital.' And furthermore...home conditions were sometimes certainly not suitable for home confinement.[80]

However, despite her doubts, she acknowledged that in the early 1950s when there were not enough hospital maternity beds to meet the growing demand, the howdies came in useful. 'So [if] you were forced to be at home, [as] you might if there was a lot of people due, then there wouldn't be enough [hospital beds] so they would need all these "domiciliary midwives".'[81] Anne MacFadden used the term 'domiciliary midwives' interchangeably with 'howdies'.

The situation in Lochgelly was rectified in the mid-1950s with the intervention of the depute Medical Officer of Health:

> Now, Dr Grant was a real pioneer of change when she came...She was depute Medical Officer of Health but with responsibility for maternity and child health in the area and she got...the only ones [howdies] that were left by that time to go to Forth Park [Kirkcaldy] and that was when they took their training. They'd been doing the work, but they got the theory then... I suppose they were still young enough... They'd done sterling work and it would have been a shame just to discard them. She gave them the opportunity of going.[82]

However the presence of howdies at many births seemed to be accepted at least until the 1950s. Anne McFadden said, 'I came here in '51 and they were beginning to fade out then. In the country areas...they would use them much more...where maternity facilities would be at a distance.'[83] This was despite previous legislation and the activities of the GMC to stop GPs 'covering' howdies. Some possible reasons emerge for this. Firstly Anne McFadden's comment on 'needing all these "domiciliary midwives"' [howdies] raises a question about the staffing levels of midwives in Scotland. During and after World War Two there was a rising birth rate and a shortage of certified midwives, which could have led local authorities (LA) to turn a blind eye to the activities of the howdie.[84] Secondly, Chrissie Sandison commented that doctors preferred to work with howdies rather than certified midwives. It is possible that this liaison went on far later than has been officially acknowledged. In addition, as Chrissie Sandison indicated above, mothers possibly felt more comfortable with someone they knew well.

In addition, oral evidence shows that some howdies were prepared to attend mothers in remote rural areas where sometimes there were no certified midwives. This not only emphasises the point about poor staffing levels, it also highlights the perennial problem of staffing in remote areas.

The members of the new CMBS, from its outset in 1916, were anxious about some midwives' lack of knowledge of basic care and listed what they must be capable of in detail. Their anxiety was probably justified in some cases. A K Chalmers, the Medical Officer of Health (MOH) for Glasgow, and one of the key advocates of the registration of midwives in Scotland, reflected this anxiety. He observed:

> Many of those [midwives and handywomen] who were interviewed, [in Cowcaddens in 1906] carried whatever equipment they might require, such as syringes and catheters and such disinfectants as they deemed necessary, in the pocket of their dress, and many who had a bag, misused some of the material they carried in them... Fifty-nine carried a Higginson's syringe, but twenty-two admitted using it impartially for douching or for administering

enemeta, frequently for the same patient and always without any effort to disinfect the nozzle save by external rubbing. Twenty-two also carried no thermometer ... one had a thermometer with whose use she was unacquainted, and some did not recognise a thermometer when shown it.[85]

While we cannot say that all howdies practised with such lack of knowledge and insight (see, for instance, Doddie Davidson's story above), one midwife practising in Glasgow had doubts on the ability of one uncertified midwife to write her name. She said:

> There were still a few of them on the go [in 1946-1947]. And I can tell you what I thought was a bit of a funny story about that. [Some years after that date], I went back in to the Health Department in Glasgow to do a wee bit of research, but during that I had to check over midwives' records of confinements. This particular person was still working [for the Glasgow Corporation] then, and when I read over the... postnatal reports and the midwife had to sign at the bottom the signature was always 'me'. She never signed her name. She just put 'me'.[86]

'Covering' of howdies by medical practitioners

The CMBS did its best to stop the practice of howdies. Its statutory role in the regulation of midwifery in Scotland was to a certain extent undermined by the howdies, and sometimes by working with them, members of the medical profession. An uncertified midwife was allowed to work in maternity care provided she did so under direct supervision of a qualified medical practitioner.

For many years after the 1902 Midwives Act for England and Wales came into effect, there was a problem in England with uncertified women practising midwifery by themselves, but with the co-operation of qualified medical practitioners who professed to give them medical supervision. This was known as 'covering' of howdies or uncertified midwives by medical practitioners. It was illegal and could result in a medical practitioner's name being removed from the Register of the GMC.[87]

After the 1915 Midwives (Scotland) Act was passed, the GMC, indicating how seriously it took this activity and emphasising that it was unacceptable, asked the CMBS to issue warnings about 'covering' to medical practitioners.[88] In addition to being illegal, the certified midwife's livelihood was threatened by such a practice, while those in competition with her, the medical practitioner and the howdie, could prosper.[89] According to the Act, howdies in Scotland were given one year, followed by another five years' grace, following the implementation of the Act on 1 January 1916, to become certified as midwives. Therefore, during these first years, midwifery practice by the uncertified midwife in Scotland was not illegal as long as she did not call herself a midwife or imply that she was certified.[90] It only became illegal after 1 January 1922 if she had not become certified as a midwife and continued to practise 'habitually and for gain'.[91] Similarly, in Scotland no doctor could have been disciplined for 'covering' a howdie before that date. However, the GMC's warnings drew the potential problem to the attention of the CMBS, the Local Supervising Authorities (LSA) and, through MOHs, to many GPs. In December 1921, the Board reminded LSAs of the law and requested MOHs to notify Procurators Fiscal of any cases which arose in their areas with a view to summary action being taken against women practising without certification.[92] Therefore, as well as issuing a further warning to medical practitioners about covering howdies, the Board also asked doctors to inform against them and this began to happen in 1922.[93] Howdies could disobey the law with the help of qualified medical practitioners, by the practitioner paying perfunctory visits to confinement cases, signing certificates or other documents under the National Health Insurance or Notification of Births Acts, and claiming that the howdie was acting under medical supervision. The first case noted in the CMBS Minutes of someone using the 'cover' of a doctor was in 1923. Here a 'handywoman' was prosecuted in Kilmarnock by the Procurator Fiscal for practising without enrolment, 'covered' by medical practitioners certifying for maternity benefit under the Insurance Act.[94] She was fined £5 or twenty-one days imprisonment.[95] In this instance, it was only the midwife who was punished. However, as we have seen, even with threats of prosecution, the practice of the uncertified midwife, or howdie, continued in Scotland until the 1950s.

Conclusion
This chapter has surveyed midwifery in Scotland during the era when there were no enforceable rules, but where the argument was gaining ground that there should be some sort of legal watch over the practice of midwifery. The debates lasted for many years. Midwifery courses evolved, but there was no statutory Scottish midwifery regulation until 1915. At that time, most mothers were cared for in labour by uncertified midwives or howdies whom history has praised and condemned in equal measure.

Howdies, neighbour women, skilly women, uncertified midwives, bean ghluine – call them what you like – were an important part of the birthing scene in Scotland for much of the first half of the twentieth century. However, they were still uncertified midwives, and as such, on many occasions after the passing and implementation of the 1915 Midwives (Scotland) Act, they practised outside the law. Nevertheless, they are remembered with affection and for the caring they brought to the work they did.

1   J Donnison, *Midwives and Medical Men*, (New Barnet: Historical Publications, 1988), p 34.
2   V Fleming, 'Autonomous or Automatons? An exploration through history of the concept of autonomy in midwifery in Scotland and New Zealand' in *Nursing Ethics*, (1998),Vol 5 (1), p 46.
3.   In this case 'autonomous' and 'autonomy' indicate the freedom of midwives to determine their own actions or behaviour when practising normal midwifery; and the freedom of the profession to make its own decisions over, for instance, education and practice. This is an autonomy which enables one professional group to co-operate with others on an equal basis. Thus parity and respect for the opinions and practice of others within the framework can be maintained.
4   A Cameron, "Licensed to Practise within their Bounds': The Faculty of Physicians and Surgeons and the Regulation of Midwives in Eighteenth Century Glasgow', presented at *History of Nursing Research Colloquium*, Oxford Brookes University, 18 March, 2000; D Dow, *The Rottenrow: The History of the*

Glasgow Royal Maternity Hospital 1834-1984, (Carnforth: The Parthenon Press, 1984), p 143.

5.   LR 61. Oral testimonies collected between 1997 and 2002 cited as LR 1-128; see also L Reid, 'Uncertified midwives in Scotland: the howdies', *The Practising Midwife,* (2009),Vol 12,(5), pp 40-43.

6   J M Munro Kerr, 'The Maternity Services', in J M Munro Kerr, R W Johnstone, M H Phillips, *Historical Review of British Obstetrics and Gynaecology 1800-1950*, (Edinburgh: E&S Livingstone, 1954), p 3; Dow, *The Rottenrow*, p14.

7   J Watson, *'A Complete Handbook of Midwifery for Midwives and Nurses'*, (3rd ed) (London: The Scientific Press, 1914), p 287.

8   LR 101.

9   L Reid, *Scottish Midwives: twentieth century voices*, (*2nd ed)* Dunfermline: Black Devon Books, 2008), p 2.

10   LR 56.

11   L Reid, 'Balfour, Elizabeth, (Betty), in E Ewan, S Innes, S Reynolds, R Pipes, *Scottish Biographical Dictionary of Women*, (Edinburgh University Press: Edinburgh, 2006), p 24.

12   R W Johnstone, 'Scotland's Contribution to the Progress of Midwifery in the Early Eighteenth and Nineteenth Centuries', *The Journal of Obstetrics and Gynaecology of the British Empire*, (1950), Vol 50, p 583.

13   H Marland, (ed), *The Art of Midwifery*, (London: Routledge, 1993), p 2; I Loudon, 'Midwives and the Quality of Maternal Care', in H Marland, A M Rafferty, *Midwives, Society and Childbirth*, (London: Routledge, 1997), p 186.

14   S Pitt, 'Midwifery and Medicine', in Marland, Rafferty, *Midwives, Society and Childbirth*, p 220.

15   Donnison, *Midwives and Medical Men*, p 34.

16   Munro Kerr, Johnstone, Phillips, *Historical Review*, p 348.

17   Blairadam Archives, *Colville Papers*, Box CC, paper 9/26, 1723.

18   D Dow, *The Rottenrow,* p 143.

19   Cameron, 'Licensed to Practise within their Bounds'; Dow, *The Rottenrow*, p 143. 20 G P Milne, 'The History of Midwifery in Aberdeen', in G P Milne (ed) *Aberdeen Medico-Chirurgical Society, A Bi-centennial History 1789-1989*, (Aberdeen, 1989), p 227.

21   Milne, 'Extract from the Aberdeen Journal, 9 January, 1759', *A History of Midwifery in Aberdeen, p 239.*

22   Advertisement in *Dundee Weekly Advertiser*, (Friday 16 January 1801) Vol 1(1) p 1, reproduced in *The Courier and Advertiser*, Dundee, (Tuesday 16 January 2001), p 6.

23   T Ferguson, *Scottish Social Welfare 1864–1914*, (Edinburgh: Livingstone, 1958), p 510.

24   J Galt (1779-1839) 'The Howdie: An Autobiography', in *The Howdie and Other Tales*, (Edinburgh: T N Foulis, 1923), pp 3-28, reproduced from the original manuscript; the 'Leddy Dowager' was the mother of the Laird.

25   I Loudon, *Death in Childbirth*, (Oxford: Clarendon Press, 1992), p 206.

26   Collacott R, 'Neonatal tetanus; a major disease of the Scottish islands', in Cule J,

Turner T, (eds), *Childcare through the centuries*, (Cardiff: The British Society for the History of Medicine, 1986),136-151.

27   Steel T, *Life and Death of St Kilda*, (Bungay: Fontana, 1975), 26.

28   Collacott. 'Neonatal tetanus'.

29   Steel, *St Kilda*, 154, L Reid, 'A killer on St Kilda', *The Practising Midwife,* (2009),Vol 12 (1) 50.

30   Collacott, 'Neonatal tetanus'.

31   LR 47; Reid, 'Killer on St Kilda'.

32   Steel, *St Kilda*, 154**.**

33   W L MacKenzie, *Report on the physical welfare of mothers and children, Vol 3, Scotland,* Dunfermline: Carnegie United Kingdom Trust, 1917), p 444.

34   S MacDonald, 'Dirty knives sealed fate of St Kilda people', *The Sunday Times,* 25 Jan 2009.

35   P Stride, 'St Kilda, the neonatal tetanus tragedy of the nineteenth century and some twenty-first century answers', *Journal of the Royal College of Physicians of Edinburgh, (2008)*, Vol 38, 70-77.

36   *Ibid,* Stride, 'St Kilda'; MacDonald, 'Dirty knives'.

37   Reid, *Scottish Midwives*, p 58.

38   Collacott, 'neonatal tetanus'.

39   *Ibid.*

40   Grampian TV, *St Kilda*, (2005), Thursday 8 September); www.grampiantv.co.uk/content; I Poxton, A Heffron, 'Neonatal Tetanus on St Kilda and other tales of avian neurotoxigenic clostridia', presentation to *Society for Anaerobic Microbiology(SAM), 2004,* http://www.clostridia.net/SAM/Presentations/Presentations.html.

41   Donnison, *Midwives and Medical Men*, p 94.

42   Donnison, *Midwives and Medical Men*, p 95.

43   B Cowell and D Wainwright, *Behind the Blue Door: The history of the Royal College of Midwives, 1881-1981*, (London: BailliËre Tindall, 1981), p 18.

44   Donnison, *Midwives and Medical Men*, p 111.

45   *Ibid*, p 112.

46   R Mander, L Reid, 'Midwifery power', R Mander, V Fleming, (eds), *Failure to Progress: The contraction of the midwifery profession*, (London, New York: Routledge, 2002), p 4.

47   R Dingwall, A Rafferty, C Webster, *An Introduction to the Social History of Nursing*, (London: Routledge, 1988), p 154; Cowell, Wainwright, *Behind the Blue Door*, p 24; Donnison, *Midwives and Medical Men*, p 142.

48   Donnison, *Midwives and Medical Men*, p 138.

49   B Abel-Smith, *A History of the Nursing Profession*, (London: William Heinemann, 1960), p 77.

50   Donnison, *Midwives and Medical Men*, p 128.

51   *Ibid*, pp 140, 154; Cowell, Wainwright, *Behind the Blue Door*, p 33.

52   Dingwall, Rafferty, Webster, *Social History of Nursing*, p 156; Cowell, Wainwright, *Behind the Blue Door*, p 24; Donnison, *Midwives and Medical Men*, p 142.

53   Cowell, Wainwright, *Behind the Blue Door*, p 33; Loudon, *Death in Childbirth*, p 207.

54   Mander, Reid, 'Midwifery power', p 4.

55   Dow, *The Rottenrow*, p 151; H Tait, 'Maternity and Child Welfare', in G McLachlan, (ed) *Improving the Common Weal: Aspects of Scottish Health Services 1900-1984*, (Edinburgh: Edinburgh University Press, 1987), p 415.

56   Census of Scotland 1911, *Report on the Twelfth Decennial Census of Scotland, Vol 2, Occupations*, (London, 1913), p lxxv; Ibid, lxxiii.

57   See Chapter 3, Table 3.3.

58   *Census of Scotland*, 1911, p lxxii.

59   See Chapter 3, Table 3.1.

60   A Coombs, 'Finding herring gutters' in *Women's History Notebooks*, (2001) Vol 8 (1), pp 15-16.

61   E Gordon , 'Women's spheres' in W H Fraser, R J Morris, *People and Society in Scotland Vol II, 1830-1914*, (Edinburgh: John Donald, 1990), pp 206-235.

62   *Census of Scotland*, 1911, p lxiii.

63   Death certificate, *Record of Corrected Entries*, p 68, 20 August 1891, following *Report of Result of Precognition*, cited in I Hutchison, *Elizabeth Sanderson, née Rae, 1854-1907*. Unpublished paper, 2009.

64   *Ibid*; see chapter 2 endnote 52 regarding washing accouchement linen.

65   Ferguson, *Scottish Social Welfare*, p 510.

66   MacKenzie, *Mothers and Children*, p 484. In this report of circumstances on Unst in Shetland, the GP, Dr Saxby, used the term 'midwife' throughout; Reid , 'Uncertified midwives in Scotland.'

67   Midwives (Scotland) Act, [5 & 6 Geo 5 Ch 91] 1915, 22, 1.

68   LR 61; Reid, 'Uncertified midwives in Scotland'.

69   LR 61; Reid, 'Uncertified midwives in Scotland'.

70   A Lamb, *Memories, handwritten and tape-recorded*, (Northern College, Aberdeen, 1994-1995, Unpublished), p 17. Now published as: A Lamb, 'Life at Larryvarry', in, A Roberts, *Tales of the Braes of Glenlivet*, (Edinburgh: Birlinn, 1999), pp 118-129.

71   Lamb, *Memories*, p 17; Reid, Uncertified midwives in Scotland.

72   *Ibid*; LR 101.

73   LR 101; Reid, 'Uncertified midwives in Scotland'.

74   *Ibid*; LR 110.

75   Lamb, *Memories*, p 9; Reid, 'Uncertified midwives in Scotland'.

76   Written communication, LR 3.

77   Reid, 'Uncertified midwives in Scotland'; LR 108; the use of the term 'domiciliary midwife' here means uncertificated midwife.

78   Reid, Scottish Midwives, p 59; Reid, 'Uncertified midwives in Scotland'.

79   LR 108.

80   *Ibid;* Reid, 'Uncertified midwives in Scotland'.

81   LR 108; Reid, 'Uncertified midwives in Scotland'.

82   LR 108;

83   *Ibid;* Reid, 'Uncertified midwives in Scotland'.

84   There is further oral evidence, LR 27, that Glasgow Corporation used howdies (again called 'domiciliary midwives'), for postnatal visiting in Glasgow: 'There were still a few of them on the go.'

85   A K Chalmers, *The Health of Glasgow 1818-1925*, (Glasgow: Corporation of Glasgow, 1930), p 262.

86   LR 27.

87   National Archives of Scotland (NAS), CMB 1/2, *CMBS Minutes*, 28 September, 1916, Vol 1, p 28.

88   *Ibid*, 8 February, 1917, p 46; NAS, CMB 1/2, *CMBS Minutes*, 19 July, 1917, Vol 2, p 23.

89   Donnison, *Midwives and Medical Men*, p 181.

90   *Midwives (Scotland) Act*, 1, (1), (2).

91   *Midwives (Scotland) Act*, 1, (2).

92   NAS, CMB 1/2, *CMBS Minutes*, 19 January, 1922, Vol 6, p 60.

93   NAS, CMB, 1/2, *CMBS Report*, 11 May, 1922, p 5.

94   NAS, CMB 1/2, *CMBS Minutes*, 28 September, 1916, Vol 1, p 28.

95   NAS, CMB 1/3, *CMBS Minutes*, 21 June, 1923, Vol 7, p 24.

Chapter 2

The need for midwifery regulation

For midwifery in Scotland to move forward statutory, legislation was necessary. This was provided in England and Wales by the 1902 Midwives Act which epitomised a major legislative milestone in the professionalisation of midwifery. It included neither Scotland nor Ireland. It was to be another thirteen years before the Midwives (Scotland) Act was passed in 1915. This chapter discusses the reasons for this thirteen-year gap, what was occurring in Scotland regarding maternity care in the years between the two Acts, and the key issues and the advocates behind the eventual passing of a Midwives Act in Scotland.

The Background

Legislation for midwives was debated in Parliament from the mid-1890s. The debates culminated in the 1902 Midwives Act which governed midwives in England and Wales. Although Scottish legislation was omitted at this time, the Scottish Act of 1915 had parallels with that of the 1902 Act for England and Wales in that both were debated in Westminster and included all members of Parliament. Despite this, the proposals for Midwives' Registration Bills under discussion in the mid-1890s were not intended to apply to Scotland.[1] One reason given for this in the House of Commons in 1902 was the different administrative structure in Scotland. Heywood Johnstone, MP for Horsham, Surrey, and a former medical practitioner, said that '...with regard to Scotland there did not exist at present any machinery which they could invoke to put the Bill into operation, and a large number of provisions and Amendments would require to be introduced to make the Bill apply to Scotland.'[2] The Rt Hon Eugene Wason, MP for Clackmannan and Kinross also explained to the House that 'a joint Bill would have been difficult because of differences in the legal systems.'[3] In addition, Wason suggested that the situation at the time in Scotland was satisfactory as 'these things are managed better in Scotland'.[4] In other words, Scottish midwifery legislation was not necessary.

Wason's argument reflected the view of both the GPs and consultants in the Scottish medical profession. While parliamentary debates were going on in the 1890s, members of the Edinburgh Obstetrical Society (EOS), made up of GPs and consultants, took up the discussion in Edinburgh. A majority of the members present demonstrated their opposition to registration of midwives in Scotland.[5] Some thought that it would be a long time before the establishment of adequate midwifery training, creating a danger of 'launching a large number of unqualified women on the public.'[6] There was also the continuing fear that registered midwives would encroach on their livelihoods. Dr Berry Hart opposed registration of midwives because 'it is doubtful if we can persuade the Legislature to interfere with the right of any woman to call herself midwife.'[7] Instead, he suggested midwifery nurses should be trained and registered. The advantage of midwifery nurses over midwives was that 'the public would more readily understand the position of such, and that the women [midwives] themselves would not be put in the false position of being considered duly competent to attend labour cases on their own responsibility.'[8] Midwifery nurses would not work on their own responsibility but under the direction of a medical practitioner. In short, while the uncertified midwife or howdie would be there for a time, 'he would leave midwives to die a natural death.'[9] Sir William Turner agreed that 'it seemed as if the midwife in Scotland was rather an accident. She did not seem to be required, but undoubtedly she was required in England.'[10] There was a dissenting voice when Dr Thatcher, arguing the case for examined, registered midwives, was quoted as saying that

> ...he considered that he was supported in his opinion by a great number of country practitioners, that midwives were absolutely essential in Scotland. In large colliery districts and large manufacturing districts the practitioner had not time to do the work, and it was very important that women expecting to have children should be properly attended to.[11]

In summing up, the President, Dr A H Freeland Barbour, commented that in Scotland there was no great need for the registration of midwives. However, he advised his colleagues to watch the progress of the Midwives Bill for England and Wales very closely as 'if anything was passed for England it would sooner or later cross the border.'[12]

The first major reason for the implementation of midwifery legislation in Scotland was the increasingly influential views of another section of the Scottish medical profession, the Medical Officers of Health (MOH), who argued that these things were not 'done better in Scotland'. Members of the Society of MOHs for Scotland opposed the EOS and campaigned vigorously in the early twentieth century for legislation for the training, registration and regulation of midwives in Scotland.[13] The heart of their case was that infant and maternal mortality rates in Scotland in general, but more specifically in Glasgow, were very high. Key figures in this campaign were two MOHs, Dr A K Chalmers of Glasgow and Dr Campbell Munro of Renfrewshire, whose work with other members of the Society of MOHs for Scotland formed the basis of the first Scottish Midwives Bill.[14] In 1906, Chalmers, stimulated by work on infection surrounding childbirth and an investigation into the causes of infant deaths, began the practice of keeping records of who attended births in Glasgow.[15] The 1907 Notification of Births Act, which required notification of births to the MOH within thirty-six hours of birth, reinforced this practice. Although not compulsory initially, the Local Authorities (LA) in Edinburgh, Glasgow, Stirling, Paisley and Renfrew adopted the Act from the outset.[16] The implementation of the Act highlighted the absence of a systematic record of the qualifications of midwives and further investigation revealed that 'a considerable proportion of them held no certificate of proficiency of any sort'.[17]

The growing acknowledgement of the poor physical stature of children in Britain, highlighted by the rejection of army recruits for the Boer War, further stimulated interest in the importance of maternal and infant welfare at the beginning of the twentieth century. In 1905, a delegation from Glasgow and Edinburgh attended the Congrès Internationale des Gouttes de Lait in Paris which resulted in the First National Conference on Infant Mortality in Britain, held in London 1906.[18] Attended by influential representatives from across Britain, including Chalmers, this conference was the forerunner of a permanent national body that worked for the Infant Welfare Movement. One of the major achievements of this pressure group was the passing of the first Notification of Births Act in 1907.

However, the group did not stop there. In 1908 a deputation of three representatives from the Infant Welfare Movement met with the Prime Minister, Herbert Asquith. One of these was Chalmers who pressed for a Scottish Midwives Act on the grounds that women who were attended by untrained midwives in Glasgow had a very high rate of puerperal fever. These women accounted for over half the annual births in Glasgow.[19] On further investigation in Glasgow in 1913, Chalmers again found that there were many more cases of mothers with puerperal fever where they had been attended by a midwife rather than a doctor: the rates were 3.4 per 1000 births for women attended by a doctor and 6.6 per 1000 for women attended by a midwife. Chalmers reasoned that the higher rate was beyond the midwife's control and not necessarily that the midwives were somehow deficient in knowledge or practice. As midwives charged less than doctors for their services, the women the midwives attended were usually poorer, poorly nourished and less able to withstand infection than the clients of the doctors. Nevertheless, Chalmers said that there was a definite correlation between the number of untrained midwives and the number of mothers experiencing puerperal fever.[20] While Chalmers removed some of the blame for maternal mortality from the shoulders of midwives, he implied that because of the high MMR, midwives' practice required regulation. Although he refused to blame midwives, Chalmers still reflected the claims of doctors to the House of Commons Select Committee on Midwifery Registration 1891-1893 who asserted that 'the untrained midwife was the cause of much unnecessary maternal and infant mortality.'[21]

Although persuasive at the time, Chalmers' data and views are contrary to other contemporary and recent studies. They show that maternal mortality figures in Britain for the late nineteenth and early twentieth centuries were, on average, better for those mothers who were delivered by midwives than by doctors.[22] According to Dr W C Grigg, physician to Queen Charlotte's Lying-in Hospital, London, 'more cases of "injury and physical disaster" resulted from the imprudent use of forceps and turning [version] by medical men than from the negligence and ignorance of midwives.'[23] In addition, Dr W S Playfair, consultant to the General Lying-in Hospital, London, criticised doctors' incompetent use of antiseptics and accused them of being the 'principal vectors of the devastatingly infectious puerperal sepsis.'[24] Fourteen years after the Midwives (Scotland) Act, the MMR figures in both England and Scotland were better for mothers who were delivered by midwives than by doctors.[25] Although Loudon emphasises that midwives should be formally trained, he has no doubt that midwives were able to provide a maternity service with very low MMR.[26]

A second major reason why legislation was enacted for midwives in Scotland was because of the new welfare legislation of the early twentieth century. This provided the administrative basis said to be lacking in Scotland during the debate leading up to the 1902 Midwives Act. The Midwives (Scotland) Act was part of the Schemes of Maternity and Child Welfare. The Schemes emerged in Scotland in the early twentieth century and resulted in other related Acts (see table 2.1) which laid an administrative basis for the Midwives Act.[27]

Table 2.1 Acts resulting from the Schemes of Maternity and Child Welfare.

Act	Purpose
1907 Notification of Births Act	Early notification of births and subsequent care and supervision of infants by emerging system of health visiting.[28]
1908 Children Act	To protect disadvantaged children through thorough investigation of infant deaths. Preceded significant reduction in IMR.[29]
1908 Education (Scotland) Act	To provide medical inspection and treatment where needed for schoolchildren.[30]
1915 Notification of Births (Extension) Act	To make the provisions of the 1907 Notification of Births Act compulsory.

The Notification of Births Acts and the Children Act meant that health visitors could use their knowledge that births had taken place to visit homes with infants and encourage good feeding and attendance at infant clinics. There were significant reductions in infant mortality rates.

The Notification of Births (Extension) Act and its particular timing added considerable strength to a concerted appeal from a cross-professional group, who became known as Memorialists, for a Midwives (Scotland) Act and who stated that they were:

> In favour of taking immediate action, [and] we would...urge the recent precedent by which the Notification of Births Act was by special legislation made applicable to the whole country in order to meet a national emergency arising out of the war conditions. This measure will fail of its full beneficial effect in Scotland unless it is supplemented by the Midwives Act for which we desire to plead.[31]

In addition, the Notification of Births (Extension) Act gave wide powers to Local Authorities (LA) in Scotland through the Local Government Board for Scotland (LGBS), stating that:

> Any Local Authority within the meaning of the principal Act may make such arrangements as they think fit, and as may be sanctioned by the Local Government Board for Scotland, for attending to the health of expectant mothers and nursing mothers, and of children under five years of age.[32]

Although 'enabling' rather than compulsory, the extended powers of Scottish LAs were put to even greater use with the passing of the Midwives (Scotland) Act in 1915. Scotland was excluded from the 1902 Midwives Act because of a possible lack of administrative structure and a differing legal system. Now, with LA powers in place, any objection to a Midwives Act for Scotland was invalid. Therefore, in the long term in Scotland, the increasing influence of the MOHs, and the welfare legislation of the first decade of the twentieth century, overcame the initial opposition of GPs and consultants.

Moving towards legislation for midwives in Scotland.

The first Midwives (Scotland) Bills were proposed before the outbreak of World War One. Although the War initially intervened, it put the Act's passage beyond doubt when its provisions were portrayed as part of the war effort. The first reading of a Midwives (Scotland) Bill took place in the House of Commons on 23 April 1912. Its purpose was 'to secure the better training of Midwives in Scotland, and to regulate their practice.'[33] It was drafted as a consequence of the efforts of the 'infant mortality movement' by the Society of MOHs, and in particular Dr Campbell Munro, MOH for Renfrewshire, but it failed to pass into law.[34]

The next Bill was put forward in April 1914. The Scottish Examining Board for Midwives, set up in 1903 by the hospitals in the four Scottish cities, eventually ceased to function in 1914 because of lack of Government support. Certificates given to midwives' training through the hospitals were the only protection against the work of the untrained midwives or howdies, many of whom were employed by families obtaining maternity benefit under the National Insurance Act of 1911.[35] In February 1914, recognising the need for action, representatives from the hospitals of the four cities prepared for a privately sponsored bill promoting legislation for midwifery in Scotland. The result was the presentation of an amended Midwives (Scotland) Bill to the House of Lords on 1 April, 1914. Lord Balfour of Burleigh, who had been 'in charge' of the 1902 Midwives Bill for England, hinted why the Act was not passed in Scotland at the same time:

> I became aware that opinion was not sufficiently ripe in Scotland to make it expedient at that time to extend similar proposals to the country north of the Tweed. I need not go into the reasons for it. There are certain differences of practice, and opinion was not in favour of the change at that time. [36]

However, opinions had now changed. Lord Balfour went on to emphasise the changes in attitudes in Scotland towards midwifery legislation and how, in 1914, opinion in favour of a Bill was 'practically unanimous'.[37] This included opinions from the Committee of the British Medical Association (BMA) for Scotland, the LGBS, the Medical Service Committee for the Highlands and Islands of Scotland, the MOHs of many large towns, the medical staff of the 'four great centres of medical education – Edinburgh, Glasgow, Aberdeen and Dundee' and nurses at an 'important nursing conference in Glasgow' held the previous month.[38] There is no mention of any opinion from midwives. However, because of the frequent use of the term 'nurse' for 'midwife' it is possible that some of these nurses were midwives.

This Bill was held up for a long time. It might have become law in 1914 if war had not broken out, diverting Parliamentary attention. It was therefore 'dropped in the House of Commons mainly for want of time at the end of a busy session'.[39] There were also Parliamentary rules about measures Parliament could address during wartime. There was a skirmish in the Commons over a Scottish Bill taking precedence over English measures especially during wartime with the argument that the Midwives (Scotland) Bill was not directly to do with the war. However, some MPs saw it as an emergency measure and it also had the approval of the Minister of Munitions.[40] The Lord President of the Council, the Marquess of Crewe, defended the Bill's passage during wartime:

The Bill was urgent and a war measure due to the mortality of war; there was a current awareness to preserve new life; and, war was instrumental in many doctors being called up for military service. Their absence created a void in maternity care which was rapidly being filled by midwives, many of whom were unqualified and uncertificated.[41]

According to the obstetrician Sir John Halliday Croom, the action of influential medical personnel was the origin of the 1915 Midwives (Scotland) Act.[42] The Memorial anent a Midwives Bill for Scotland, sent to the Secretary for Scotland and the Lord President of the Privy Council on 19 August 1915, carried thirty influential signatures.[43] These included medical practitioners, obstetricians, MOHs, lecturers and examiners from Scottish universities and other university professors and deans. The urgency of the need for a Midwives Bill for Scotland was made clear at its second reading in the Commons on 25 November 1915, by McKinnon Wood, Secretary for Scotland. He had been inundated by approaches from those making a case for a Midwives Act for Scotland, particularly at this time of war:

> As the House is aware, the medical profession has been sadly depleted. A great many doctors have gone to the front, leaving rural districts inadequately provided with medical practitioners; so that competent midwives are absolutely necessary throughout Scotland ....The Scottish midwife is not able to obtain a formal qualification except in England. When she returns to Scotland she is *not* [author's italics] under the same control as the English midwife is. Altogether, I think, the case for treating this as a matter of urgency is virtually made out on very high authority indeed.[44]

The Midwives (Scotland) Bill received the Royal Assent on 23 December 1915 and came into operation on 1 January 1916.[45] However, the speedy enactment of the Bill was due primarily to the war-time shortage of doctors in Scotland and not because of the need to recognise the importance of the profession of midwifery and its place in the health care of the people of Scotland.[46] The Bill's passage through the Houses of Parliament was helped by many of its clauses being similar to those in the Midwives Act pertaining to England and Wales, and as Wason, who had previously argued against midwifery legislation in Scotland, said, 'that measure has, I believe worked exceedingly well.'[47]

Provisions of the Midwives (Scotland) Act 1915[48]

The Provisions of the Midwives (Scotland) Act were very similar to those of the Midwives Act 1902, but with a few specific differences. Its twenty-nine sections lay down rules regarding:

> Certification of midwives and provision for existing midwives; the Constitution of the Central Midwives Board for Scotland, its future revision, and duties and powers of the Board; Rules pertaining to suspension of midwives, offences, expenses, return of the certificate after suspension and removal of names from the Roll; Rules about local supervision of midwives; annual reports and definitions.

As in England and Wales, a Central Midwives Board (CMBS) was set up in Scotland as an examining and supervisory body and to establish a Roll of midwives. Its duties included the regulation of the issue of certificates, conditions of admission to the Roll of midwives, the course of training in midwifery, and conduct of examinations and remuneration of examiners. Also, as with the CMBE&W, the CMBS initially recognised three categories of midwife:

- those who were enrolled 'by virtue of *bona fide* practice' who were nicknamed the '*bona fides*';
- the 'certificated midwives' who had obtained a certificate from one of a variety of institutions ... and were enrolled 'by virtue of prior certification';
- and ... those who had taken and passed the CMBS examination.[49]

The '*bona fides*' had to have been in practice (as uncertified midwives or howdies) for a minimum of a year before the passing of the Act and had to be of 'good character'. Although the '*bona fides*' could be registered without examination, one third of the candidates presenting themselves for the first CMBS examination were already on the new CMBS roll of midwives in Scotland as *bona fide* midwives and had voluntarily come forward for examination.[50]

One of the first *bona fides* to register was Mary Bryce Smellie Henderson. She was one of the first midwives in Scotland to be certified as a midwife after the implementation of the 1915 Midwives (Scotland) Act. She lived and worked as a midwife in Larkhall, Lanarkshire, about twenty miles from Glasgow city centre. Her grand-daughter, Agnes Young, wrote:

> She worked ... on many cases, living with her patient for some three weeks at a time and bringing home the accouchement linen to be washed. She had six children of her own, five surviving to adulthood. Born in 1854, she married on 29 July 1880...and died in 1938.[51]

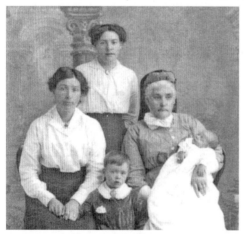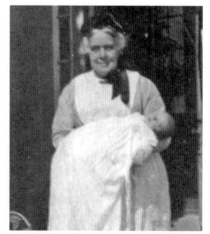

Left – Mary Henderson, midwife, Larkhall, (right) with members of her family. (Courtesy of Agnes and Norman Young.); and right – Annie Lindsay (née Robertson), uncertified midwife, late 19th and early 20th centuries. (Courtesy of Diane Howie.)

Although bringing home the accouchement linen to be washed seems over and above the call of duty,[52] the practice of staying with the mothers for a few weeks was common among howdies, and later among some certified midwives acting as a 'maternity nurse' while some, because of geographical difficulties, had to stay. Two of the howdies cited in Chapter 1 made a practice of booking mothers for a certain number of weeks. Annie Kerr, a howdie in the Borders in the 1940s, said:

> I went a wee while before the baby wis born. Not as much as a couple o weeks. I was there before, I know that. I wis wi them and did everything that wis to be done, ye know, to give her a rest. That workit in fine...I took care of the baby afterwards until she wis fit. I wid mebbe be there a fortnight.[53]

Doddie Davidson, howdie, Aberdeenshire, 1930s and 1940s, said:

> I went an lived in the hoose afore the bairns were born. The babies delivered themselves. There wis naebiddy there bit me. Sometimes, if there wis a neighbour handy she wid have come in, bit often ye see, in a fairm it's usually on its own an it wis maistly cotter hooses or fairms... There wis nae midwife...I aye kent in time afore...Usually they were needin some help especially fan there wis some little anes. An then ye stayed, sometimes a week, sometimes mair, sometimes ye didna hae time ti spare but ye aye hid aboot a wik wi them or ten days.[54]

Doddie also saw living-in as part of her payment. She said:

> The pey wis jist naethin then ye ken. Fan I stairted first it wis five shillins a wik. That is nowadays, twenty-five pence. Then it gid up. I think it wis aboot ten shillins fur a lot o the babies. Some o the folk couldna afford at. But ye aye hid yer food an yer bed wi them. Ye hid yer keep. But it didna seem ti be important tae me, the money. As lang as I could dae fit I wis needed tae dae.[55]

Most certified midwives did not 'live-in' the mother's home. However there were exceptions, particularly in rural areas. For instance, Mima Sutherland, on Raasay in the 1930s, gives a description of difficulties she encountered as an island midwife when she said:

> I remember being called to Fladda [from Raasay] one 21st of June. It was a terrible day for midsummer. The garage-man put me the nine miles then I had to start walking. It was all up and down hills. I ran down all the hills...and toiled up the next. It was about five miles before I came to the shore and you could see the banks on the opposite side. If the tide was in, the boatman came across for me but if the tide was out you could walk across. On that day, the baby had been born before I arrived and it was just wrapped up and I was able to do the rest. Then I had to stay three days that time – stayed in the same room as the mother. The beds had lovely fresh chaff.[56]

Midwives who chose to work privately also sometimes lived in. One midwife said 'When I started off [in 1952] it was usually for four weeks, depending [on] what the mother wanted or how many other children she had.'[57] This particular midwife had a difficult time during her midwifery training in 1951 because she was one of the few who, by then, did midwifery without first training as a nurse and she felt that she was unduly picked upon for that reason.[58] She recalled:

> I sat my final SCM [examination] in February 1952 and I decided I was going to do it privately because I couldn't bear all these nurses (sic) in the hospital... I couldn't bear working in the hospital because of these women. So he, my GP...got me my first patient. And he said, 'it's her fourth baby. She knows far more about it than you will'... So, all was well. That was my first, and from then on it became a snowball thing. [I went to someone else] and that was it started and of course she passed the word. I never advertised, ever. She passed the word on to somebody who was having a baby and so it went on.

This was a situation where the midwife was working very closely with the GP. On being asked, 'When you had a home confinement, were the doctors there?' she said, 'Sometimes they didn't get there in time. But I phoned them, yes, they should have been there.'

She also, as a midwife, had to comply with the law, notify the birth, and attend the statutory refresher courses. Here she ran up against those who did not approve of private midwifery practice. She said:

> I had to go to five-year refresher courses which I hated. Then again I met these awful women. Whenever I said I was doing private they closed down like that. They didn't approve of it at all. I think they thought I was earning far more than they were. I don't know what they were earning but whenever I said 'Private' ....they looked down their noses at me.[59]

Ann Lamb also had a problem with early twentieth century direct entry training as a midwife. She did not have the qualifications to get into nursing and used the midwifery training and qualification as an alternative route. She said:

> I met a girl and she said 'Why don't you try nursing' and I said, 'Well I've thought about it but I can't get in.' She said, 'You would get into Edinburgh Royal if you have one certificate.' I said, 'Oh what's that?' 'Midwifery.' 'Oh my', I said, 'I can't do that'. She said there was a place where I could train. It was small but where you got a good training. You get to the Canongate and the Cowgate and all the poor quarters [of Edinburgh]. So, she introduced me to this doctor and he said 'Oh, you'll get by, you're from the country' and so I went in. We stayed in the building and there were only, I think about ten of us. We were all doing the same thing to get into the Royal. It was a hard training [1927-28]. I wasn't in the big place – the Simpson – I wasn't there but I became a midwife.
>
> Then I got at last to Edinburgh Royal. I had to meet the Matron...I hated her... because she said, 'Don't forget that you are the only midwife in this hospital,' of about five hundred beds at that time.[60]

This attitude was a repeat of the pre-midwifery legislation mindset of many nurses who looked on midwifery as obsolete and anachronistic.

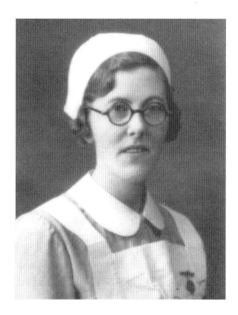

*Ann Lamb, midwife, 1920s to
1960s, mainly north-east Scotland.
(Courtesy of Ann Lamb.)*

For decades after the 1915 Midwives (Scotland) Act, there was argument and discussion about who may act as a midwife. This debate particularly surrounded the howdies. Initially, after a year's grace, no woman could call herself, or even imply that she was a midwife without being certified under the Act.[61] Also, after 1 January 1922, the culmination of another five years' period of grace, it was stated that no woman in Scotland 'shall habitually and for gain attend women in childbirth otherwise than under the direction of a registered medical practitioner unless she be certified under this Act.'[62] This breathing space was similar to that which had been allowed in England and Wales and was seen as a reasonable time to effect the change necessary for midwives to conform to the Act.[63]

The use of the term, 'habitually and for gain' which appeared in both Midwives Acts was controversial.[64] It allowed uncertified women (howdies) to practise midwifery as long as it could be seen that they were not doing it 'habitually and for gain'. This, and the phrase 'otherwise than under the direction of a registered medical practitioner', left loopholes in the law for exploitation by some uncertified midwives and some medical practitioners.[65] However, Sir John Halliday Croom, the CMBS's first Chairman, said:

> There is one point of regret, namely, that the qualifying words 'habitually
> and for gain' which was a distinct flaw in the English Act, is perpetuated in
> the Scottish one, but we have good reason to believe that had the abolition of
> these words been insisted upon the Act would not have been passed.[66]

Under the provisions of the Act, the separate CMBS comprising twelve members was set up early in 1916. The CMBS had the power to frame rules which were valid only after approval by the Privy Council who had to take into consideration comments from the GMC.[67] However there is nothing to say that the Privy Council had to act upon any recommendations which the GMC might have made.

To a certain extent, the CMBS benefited from observation of the working of the CMBE&W and the introduction of certain improvements within the Scottish Act not yet acquired by the CMBE&W. An important difference between the two CMBs was that the CMBE&W comprised just nine members; having twelve members on the CMBS made room for the statutory inclusion of two midwives. Initially, the CMBE&W had no statutory midwife members, although midwives sat on the CMBE&W as representatives of other bodies.[68] Other differences were financial. Scottish LAs had authorisation to contribute towards financial costs such as training of midwives (although for many years midwives in Scotland had to pay for their training and had no training income), midwives' expenses, for example, compensation for loss of income due to suspension; payment and supply of official forms and stamped envelopes; and payment of a doctor's fee when called out in an emergency by a midwife. This fee was recoverable from 'the husband or guardian of the patient if possible.'[69] These differences were eliminated with the implementation of the 1918 Midwives Act for England and Wales.[70] This included the Treasury's decision, in 1919, to make a grant of £20 to each pupil midwife in England and Wales who guaranteed to practise on qualification.[71]

The CMBS also had the power from its outset to suspend, or, if necessary, strike from the Roll, midwives who broke the rules; the CMBE&W could not use suspension as a punishment but it could strike midwives from the Roll.[72] Another difference (and initially a sore point) between the two Acts was to do with reciprocity of midwifery practice. The Midwives (Scotland) Act contained a clause enabling certified midwives from, for instance England, to be certified in Scotland.[73] This was not reciprocal to begin with as Scottish certified midwives could not practise as such in England. However, this was also amended with the 1918 Act after which midwives who had passed statutory examinations elsewhere in the UK could practise in any of the countries on payment of an enrolment fee.[74] In 1950, the Midwives (Amendment) Act ensured further reciprocal recognition and certification of midwives enabling them to practise freely between the four UK countries without re-enrolling.[75]

The 1915 Midwives (Scotland) Act, like the 1902 Act for England and Wales, placed much of the responsibility for supervising midwives and regularising midwifery with LAs. Under the Act, each LA became the Local Supervising Authority (LSA) over midwives.[76] The power of LAs in Scotland was strengthened in 1915 by a clause in the 1915 Notification of Births (Extension) Act, which did not apply to England and Wales, and which heralded the evolution of the Maternity Services Schemes in Scotland.[77] However, even with their wide supervisory powers, LAs were obliged to work under the rules of the CMBS. As Sir W L MacKenzie noted:

> It is therefore not merely an Act for the registration and training of midwives, itself a sufficiently important purpose; but it is also an administrative Act placing on the Local Authority an obligation to see that the work of the midwives is kept on the highest professional level.[78]

Therefore, with regard to the LAs' responsibilities for the supervision of midwives, the term 'LSA' emerged, carrying with it extensive powers and duties as shown in Table 2.2, following.

Table 2.2 Powers and duties of the LSA[79]

1	Supervision of midwives practising within their district in accordance with the Rules framed by the CMBS.
2	Investigation of charges against a midwife of malpractice, negligence or misconduct, conviction or unprofessional conduct.
3	The power to suspend a midwife to prevent the spread of infection.
4	'Power of Entry' to premises where a midwife was known to be practising and also where a woman who was not a certified midwife might be practising in contravention of the Act.[80]
5	An obligation to report these activities to the CMBS as they happened and also through the MOH, on an annual basis.
6	Receive and supply to the CMBS names of all midwives who had notified their intention to practise within the district.
7	Ensure that all midwives knew that they had to notify their intention to practise annually as well as the new rules about certification.
8	Keep a current copy of the Roll of midwives accessible for public inspection. This enabled the public if they wanted, especially to begin with, to find out which midwives were certified.

The 1915 Midwives (Scotland) Act, implemented speedily because of the war and a shortage of doctors, was also part of a move to benefit the health of mothers and babies through the provision of a practical, educational and administrative midwifery service in Scotland.

Conclusion
Before 1915, midwifery in Scotland was 'alegal' with no existing regulations or licensing requirements.[81] Early attempts to formalise midwifery training in Scotland preceded the eventual statutory regulation of midwifery in Scotland in 1915, thirteen years after a similar Act for England and Wales. Scotland's unique 'Schemes of Maternity and Child Welfare in Scotland', and the removal of doctors to the Front during World War One, acted as significant levers for the Act's passing at this time. An important objective was to prevent unqualified, unsupervised midwives attending women in childbirth.

The CMBS, as an examining and supervisory body, oversaw midwives who became legal practitioners of normal midwifery. This new professional group, still under the control of the CMBS and LSA, had two statutory midwife places on the CMBS which was in contrast at that time to the CMBE&W which had none, and this indicated a developing level of respect for the midwifery profession. Yet, real power remained with the medical profession, members of whom comprised the largest professional group in the early CMBS. In addition, traditionally Scotland's medical practitioners maintained a greater input into maternity care than their English counterparts. Their early broad medical education enabled them to function as general practitioners as the

Scottish university medical schools taught and examined in medicine, surgery *and midwifery* before it became compulsory in Britain in 1886.[82] Also, after 1915 the wide powers of the LAs acting as LSAs over midwives, and the evolution of the Maternity Services Schemes in Scotland strengthened the power of the medical profession. Thus, the medically dominated CMBS, the Maternity Services Schemes, LAs and their MOHs held power when it came to organising maternity care.

1.   J Jenkinson, *Scottish Medical Societies*, 1731-1939 (Edinburgh: Edinburgh University Press, 1993), p 83.
2.   *Hansard*, Commons, Vol 109, 6-24 June 1902, cols 58-59, quoted in Jenkinson, *Scottish Medical Societies,* p 83.
3.   Dow, *The Rottenrow*, p 151; see also: L Reid, 'The development of midwifery legislation in Scotland: a history to be proud of', (2003), *RCM Midwives Journal*, Vol 6 (4), pp 166-169; L Reid, 'Midwifery in Scotland 1: the legislative background', *British Journal of Midwifery*, (2005) Vol 13, (5), 277-283.
4.   Dow, *The Rottenrow*, p 151.
5.   Jenkinson, *Scottish Medical Societies*, p 83; 'Should midwives be registered in Scotland?' *The Transactions of the Edinburgh Obstetrical Society*, (EOS) Vol 20, Session 1894 -95, (Edinburgh: Oliver and Boyd, 1895), p 167.
6.   Jenkinson, *Scottish Medical Societies*, p 83.
7.   'Should midwives be registered in Scotland?' *Transactions*, EOS, p 167.
8.   *Ibid*, p 181.
9.   *Ibid*, p 181.
10.   *Ibid*, p 177.
11.   *Ibid*, p 180.
12.   *Ibid*, p 182; Twenty years after this discussion, he demonstrated a change of mind in keeping with the changed circumstances of a country at war. He was one of those, known as memorialists, who signed the Memorial to the Right Honourables H M Secretary for Scotland and The Lord President of H M Privy Council pleading for 'the passing without delay of a Midwives Bill for Scotland': NAS, CMB 4/2/6, Memorial of the Medical Faculties of the Universities, the Royal Medical Corporations, and the Medical Officers of the Maternity Hospitals in Scotland, to the Right Honourable H M Secretary for Scotland and the Right Honourable The Lord President of H M Privy Council anent a Midwives Bill for Scotland, 19 August 1915.
13.   *Tait*, 'Maternity and Child Welfare', in McLachlan, *Common Weal*, p 415; NAS, CMB 1-5, A K Chalmers, 'On the need for a Midwives Act in Scotland', in *The Journal Of Midwifery, A Weekly Record for Midwives and Maternity Nurses*, in *The Nursing Times*, (21 February 1914), pp 251-254.
14.   Chalmers, 'On the Need for a Midwives Act in Scotland', pp 251-254.
15.   A K Chalmers, *The Health of Glasgow, 1818-1925* (Glasgow: Corporation of Glasgow, 1930), p 259.
16.   T Ferguson, *Scottish Social Welfare*, 1864-1914 (Edinburgh: E and S Livingstone, 1958), p 546.
17.   Chalmers, *Health of Glasgow*, p 261.

18. Tait, 'Maternity and Child Welfare', in McLachlan, *Common Weal*, p 415.

19. A MacGregor, *Public Health in Glasgow 1905-1946* (Edinburgh: E and S Livingstone , 1967), p 110.

20. Ferguson, *Scottish Social Welfare*, p 509; MacGregor, *Public Health*, p 110.

21. Chalmers' view was subsequently reiterated. Sir John Halliday Croom, the CMB's first Chairman, implied that non-regulation of midwives in Scotland before the 1915 Act was a significant factor in the maternal mortality rates: NAS, CMB 4/2/17, Sir John Halliday Croom, 'The Midwives (Scotland) Act: its Object and Method', the *Maternity and Child Welfare Conference*, Glasgow, (March 1917).

22. M Tew, *Safer Childbirth? A Critical History of Maternity Care,* 2nd ed, (London: Chapman and Hall, 1995), pp 273, 281 and 283; Loudon, *Death in Childbirth*, p 241, also cites a lack of improvement in MMR figures in the years 1910-1934 associated with increased [iatrogenic] interference and the 'employment of surgical measures in normal and moderately difficult labours'.

23. BMJ, 1891, 1, p 230, quoted in Tew, *Safer Childbirth?* p 274, and Donnison, *Midwives and Medical Men*, p 137.

24. Donnison, *Midwives and Medical Men*, p 138, refers to, *Obstet. Soc. London, Transactions*, 1885, Vol xxvii, p 218; Tew, *Safer Childbirth?* p 274.

25. I Loudon, *Death in Childbirth*, (Oxford: Clarendon Press, 1992) p 244.

26. Loudon, I, 'Midwives and the quality of maternal care', in H Marland, A M Rafferty, *Midwives, Society and Childbirth*, (London: Routledge, 1997), pp 180-200.

27. W L MacKenzie, *Report on the Physical Welfare of Mothers and Children, Vol 3, Scotland*, (Dunfermline: The Carnegie United Kingdom Trust, 1917), chapter 49, pp 535-561.

28. MacGregor, *Public Health*, p 111.

29. Chalmers, *Health of Glasgow*, pp 195-204; Ferguson, *Scottish Social Welfare*, pp 551-553.

30. MacKenzie, *Mothers and Children*, p 535.

31. NAS, CMB 4/2/6, *Memorial anent a Midwives Bill for Scotland*, 19 August, 1915.

32. 'Notification of Births (Extension Act) 1915', quoted in *MacKenzie, Physical Welfare of Mothers and Children, Vol 3*, p 535; this clause was not included in the corresponding Act for England and Wales.

33. *Hansard*, Commons, Vol 37, 15 April-3 May 1912, col 942.

34. Chalmers, 'On the Need for a Midwives Act in Scotland', *The Journal of Midwifery, Nursing Times*, (21 February 1914), pp 252; J H Croom, 'Midwives (Scotland) Act, Its Object and Method', *Maternity and Child Welfare Conference*, Glasgow, March 1917, p 1.

35. Dow, *The Rottenrow*, p 152.

36. *Hansard*, Lords, Vol 15, 1 April 1914, col 877; *ibid*.

37. *Ibid*.

38. *Ibid*, col 879.

39. Dow, *Rottenrow*, p 152; NAS, CMB 4/2/6, *Memorial anent a Midwives Bill for*

Scotland.

40. *Hansard*, Commons, Vol 25 10 November 1915, col 1167; *Hansard*, Commons, Vol 26, 1 December 1915, col 814.
41. *Hansard*, Lords, Vol 20, 8 December 1915, col 569-570.
42. Croom, 'Midwives (Scotland) Act: its object and method', p 1.
43. NAS, CMB 4/2/6, *Memorial anent a Midwives Bill for Scotland.*
44. *Hansard*, Commons, Vol 26, Nov 22-Dec 17 1915, col 480-481.
45. *Hansard*, Commons, Vol 27, Dec 23 1915, col 806.
46. Jenkinson, *Scottish Medical Societies*, p 84.
47. *Hansard*, Commons, Vol 26, Nov 22-Dec 17 1915, col.482.
48. Acts of Parliament, *1915 Midwives (Scotland) Act*, [5 & 6 Geo.5 Ch 91].
49. Loudon, *Death in Childbirth*, p 208.
50. J H Croom, 'Midwives (Scotland) Act: its object and method', p 3.
51. LR 36.
52. But see also Elizabeth Sanderson Chapter 1, endnote 64.
53. LR 110.
54. LR 101.
55. LR 101.
56. LR 56; L Reid, Shanks's pony to Council 'caur', The Practising Midwife 2008, Vol 11 (5), p74; For a flavour of life on Raasay and Fladda during this period, see R Hutchinson, *Calum's Road* (Edinburgh: Birlinn, 2006).
57. LR 89.
58. LR 89.
59. LR 89.
60. LR 47.
61. This rule was similar to Section 3 of the 1878 Dentists Act: R M Ross, *The Development of Dentistry: A Scottish Perspective Circa 1800-1921*, unpublished Ph D Thesis, University of Glasgow, (1994).
62. *Midwives (Scotland) Act*, 1915, 1,(2).
63. Cowell, Wainwright, *Behind the Blue Door*, p 43.
64. *Hansard*, Commons, Vol 26, Nov 22-Dec 17 1915, col 482.
65. *Midwives (Scotland) Act*, 1915, Section 1, (2).
66. J H Croom, 'Midwives (Scotland) Act: its object and method', Croom did not explain why he felt the Act would have not been passed if the words 'habitually and for gain' had been omitted. MPs may have felt that to do so would have made too much of a difference between the Acts for Scotland and England and Wales.
67. NAS, CMB 4/1-5, A Fitzroy, Preliminary Statement to the Schedule of Rules Framed by the Central Midwives Board for Scotland (London: His Majesty's Stationery Office, 1916).
68. Donnison, Midwives and Medical Men, p 177; Dingwall, Rafferty, Webster, Social History of Nursing, p 158; Cowell, Wainwright, Behind the Blue Door, p 36; The Privy Council, the Queen's Nursing Institute and the Royal British Nursing Association each nominated a member of the Midwives' Institute to the CMBE&W as its representative. The 1918 Midwives Act for England and Wales

made statutory provision for two midwives to sit on the CMBE&W.

69.   *Midwives (Scotland) Act*, 6 (2); *ibid*, 22 and 7.

70.   J Towler, J Bramall, *Midwives in History and Society*, (London: Croom Helm, 1986), pp 185, 203.

71.   Towler, Bramall, *Midwives in History and Society*, p 205.

72.   *Midwives (Scotland) Act*, 1915, 6; Cowell, Wainwright, *Behind the Blue Door*, p 49.

73.   *Midwives (Scotland) Act*, 11, (1).

74.   Cowell, Wainwright, *Behind the Blue Door*, p 50; NAS 1 /2, *CMBS Report*, 31 March 1919, in *CMBS Minutes*, 24 July 1919, Appendix III, p 6.

75.   NBS, *Supervision of Midwives in Scotland*, (Edinburgh: NBS, February 1998); This was consolidated the following year with the *Midwives (Scotland) Act*, 1951, 14 and 15 Geo 6 Ch 54.

76.   *Midwives (Scotland) Act*, 1915, 16.

77.   MacKenzie, *Mothers and Children*, p 535.

78.   MacKenzie, *Mothers and Children*, p 540.

79.   NAS, CMB 1/2, *CMBS Minutes*, 11 August 1916, Vol 1, p 23; see also, L Reid, *Scottish Midwives 1916-1983: The Central Midwives Board for Scotland and Practising Midwives*, unpublished thesis for the University of Glasgow, 2003, Chapter 1, p 46, Chapter 2, p 64.

80.   Donnison, *Midwives and Medical Men*, p 180; the CMBE&W could also suspend a midwife to prevent the spread of infection; *Midwives (Scotland) Act*, 7.

81.   A term used to describe midwifery in New Brunswick before 1985. See: J Relyea, 'The rebirth of midwifery in Canada: an historical perspective', in *Midwifery*, (1992), (8), pp 139-169.

82.   J Hogarth, 'General Practice' Part II Chapter 1, in G McLachlan, *Improving the Common Weal* (Edinburgh: Edinburgh University Press, 1987), p 166; M Dupree, A Crowther, 'A profile of the medical profession in the early twentieth century: the Medical Directory as a historical source', in the *Bulletin of the History of Medicine*, (1991),(65), p 220, suggest that approximately 85% of practitioners in Scotland in 1911 were graduates of Scottish universities.

Chapter 3

New status

The 1915 Midwives (Scotland) Act and statutory regulation brought new status for the profession of midwifery in Scotland. With status came the provision for the constitution of a statutory body, the Central Midwives Board for Scotland (CMBS).[1] The CMBS was set up as an examining and supervisory body and to establish a Roll of midwives in Scotland. Its constitution, duties and powers required it to comply with statutory rules within the Act. A major task was to frame *Rules* involving midwifery practice and education with which certified midwives had to comply.[2]

It was the Board's responsibility to implement measures to fulfil the aim of the Act 'to secure the better training of Midwives in Scotland, and to regulate their practice.'[3] The 1915 Act, and similar subsequent Acts, provided the statutory framework pertaining to midwives and maternity care in Scotland until 1983 when the 1979 Nurses, Midwives, and Health Visitors Act took effect, superseding all previous Acts and effectively ending the life of the CMBS. On 1 July 1983, many of the functions of the CMBS and the General Nursing Council for Scotland were taken over by the new National Board for Nursing, Midwifery and Health Visiting for Scotland (NBS).[4]

There was also an ongoing long-term problem of maternal mortality in the UK with maternity care cited as one of the contributory factors to the high Maternal Mortality Rate (MMR). From 1922 to 1938 the MMR remained a cause for national concern and only began to fall in the late 1930s.[5] The CMBS responded to the expression of this concern in Government Reports and legislation by endeavouring to raise midwifery standards, to improve the education of midwives and to recruit and retain midwives of optimum quality.

The CMBS's membership comprised a majority of the medical profession for many years. This did not auger well for the midwifery profession. For a long period the CMBS's influence played a part in preventing midwives from achieving parity with those with whom they worked. It kept midwives firmly in a role subordinate to general practitioners and obstetricians.

This chapter explores issues and conflicts posed upon the midwifery profession during World War One and the inter-war years. On the one hand midwifery was dominated by a Board that was top-heavy with the medical profession; on the other, it was urged to raise midwifery standards but governed by *Rules* so inflexible that they imposed a serious handicap.

Setting up the Board

The first CMBS meeting was held on 18 February 1916 in the offices of the Local Government Board for Scotland (LGBS), 125 George Street, Edinburgh. These were one of several locations that the CMBS rented in Edinburgh until 1963 when it bought premises at 24 Duke Street, for £5,000.[6] The Board's last home was at 24 Dublin Street, sold just before the Board handed over to the NBS.[7]

The initial twelve CMBS members comprised 'two...certified midwives practising in Scotland', others drawn from the medical profession, and lay personnel.[8] At the first meeting, ten members were present, leaving two midwives to be appointed when enough midwives were certified.[9] A five-yearly re-appointment rule was in place, election of chair and office bearers was internal, and the Board could also replace any member who resigned or died before the five years were up.[10]

Between 1916 and 1983, a significant feature was the increase in the number of midwives appointed to the Board, and, particularly latterly, largely without a statutory change (see Appendix 1). By July 1916, the Board included: two midwives; six members of the medical profession comprising three obstetricians, one MOH and two medical practitioners appointed by the Scottish Committee of the BMA; and four 'lay' members, two of whom were 'ladies' 'acknowledged to be well informed on the conditions under which midwives and nurses worked.'[11] After the first five years, although the statutory Constitution remained the same, another midwife was appointed by the Scottish Board of Health (SBH) and the number of medical practitioners on the Board rose to seven, reducing the number of lay members to two.[12] The *statutory* minimum number of midwives remained the same until 1936.

In 1936, the CMBS raised its total membership to sixteen and included four certified midwives practising in Scotland.[13] Officially, midwives remained a minority even after 1951 when the Board discussed increasing the number of midwife members to eight out of the sixteen.[14] Chairman, Professor R W Johnstone (1879-1969), disagreed with this proposal, stating: 'It seemed unnecessary, and indeed, inadvisable, to give them fifty per cent of the total seats.'[15] Finally, the members agreed to have seven midwives on the Board from 1953, four of whom would be directly elected by practising midwives in Scotland.[16] This new Constitution remained until 1983. In time, and especially in the 1970s, more bodies chose a midwife than chose a lay person as their Board representative. By 1983, even though the statutory number of midwives remained at seven, there were ten midwife and six medical members.

The 1970s saw further evidence of the growing stature of midwives on the Board. For many years male obstetricians held the positions of chairman and deputy chairman. Finally, in 1973 Sheelagh Bramley (1922-2004) became the first midwife to hold the office of deputy chairman, and in 1977 she made the final breakthrough when she was elected chairman with another midwife, Mary M Turner, as her deputy.[17] Mary Turner succeeded Sheelagh Bramley as chairman in 1978 and was the last chairman of the CMBS.

Initial proceedings of the CMBS

The LGBS summoned the first CMBS meeting on 18 February 1916 initially with Dr Leslie MacKenzie, medical member of the LGBS, in the chair. The tasks were to elect a chairman, appoint a secretary and set up committees. The Board agreed that the chairman should be one of the medical members. In a tight ballot, Sir John Halliday Croom (1847-1923) won the day over Dr James Haig Ferguson (1862-1934).[18] Both were eminently suitable, but perhaps glamour won. John Halliday Croom had been Professor of Midwifery at Edinburgh University since 1905 and was renowned for his lecturing abilities: 'no student's course was considered complete if he had not attended Croom.'[19] Halliday Sutherland (1882-1960), an ex-student, described him as follows:

Sir John Halliday Croom...tall, slender, debonair, with a short well-trimmed beard, he lectured in a swallow-tailed, silk-faced evening coat, worn over a fancy waistcoat, and well-creased cashmere trousers. This combination of garments looked unusual, especially when he raised his hand and exclaimed, 'Mark me, gentlemen, and mark me well. Orange paste for your nails, a clean shirt every day, a flower in your buttonhole, and your fortune's made.'[20]

James Haig Ferguson, also of Edinburgh, who became deputy chair, was an obstetrician, lecturer at the University of Edinburgh and examiner in Midwifery and Gynaecology.[21] His forte was the importance of the mother's life and health, arguing that their preservation was a 'prime duty for obstetricians.'[22] He also devised the eponymous mid-cavity forceps still used in obstetrics today.

Other important appointments were: secretary to keep Minutes and the Roll of Midwives; and two main committees, Finance and Penal Cases, to undertake appropriate duties and report to full Board meetings. A place was reserved in each for a midwife member when available.[23]

Election of the two midwife members proved to be a lengthier process than first envisaged. The Act stated that they should 'be first appointed when ...midwives so qualified are available in number sufficient to warrant such appointment.'[24] But, 'there seemed to be some doubt as to whether any such midwives within the meaning of the Act were available.'[25] In short, the midwives had to be certified by the CMBS.

The lack of midwife appointments to the Board at this time played a part in delaying the initial drawing up of CMBS Rules. Initially, the Board had to frame enough *Rules* to regulate its proceedings and get the Roll into operation. The ten members agreed to go ahead with this, but to delay the final drawing up of remaining *Rules* until the appointment of two midwife members.[26]

The next step was to encourage midwives to apply for enrolment. The Board advertised in newspapers, informed MOHs and LSAs and requested from them a provisional list of midwives practising in each area. This led to over 1,700 women who were in practice, receiving copies of Rules D (Table 3.1) and enrolment application forms.[27] The Board was then able to appoint its first two newly enrolled midwives, Alice Helen Turnbull, Matron of the Deaconess Hospital, Edinburgh, and Isabella Lewis Scrimgeour, Matron of Govan Cottage Hospital, Glasgow, who attended their first meeting on 6 July 1916.[28] The CMBS Rules were finally revised, adjusted and approved six months after the Board's first meeting.[29] They were presented as Rules A, B, C, D, E, F, G and H with a Schedule of required Forms of Applications and Certificates.

Rules C were very detailed and included specifications as meticulous as 'the use of the clinical thermometer and of the catheter, and the taking of the pulse.'[31] Other specifically mentioned topics were to do with cleanliness such as antiseptics in midwifery, disinfection 'of person, clothing and appliances', and principles of hygiene and sanitation. Rules E also instructed on cleanliness: 'the midwife must be scrupulously clean in every way... she must keep her nails short, and preserve the skin of her hands as far as possible from cracks and abrasions'; and instrumental: 'all instruments and other appliances must be disinfected, preferably by boiling, before being brought into contact with the patient's generative organs.'[32]

Table 3.1 Summary of first CMBS *Rules*[30]

Rules A	Regulating the proceedings of the Board. Monthly; other meetings if/when necessary.
Rules B	Regulating the issue of Certificates and the Conditions of Admission to the Roll of Midwives: sufficient education; proof of marriage where appropriate, proof of midwifery training; good moral character.
Rules C	Regulating the course of training, the conduct of examinations and the remuneration of examiners: training should be not less than 6 months with 2 month exemption with proof of general nurse training.
Rules D	To do with enrolling women already in practice as midwives when the Act was passed. For example the *bona fide* midwives: they had to be 'trustworthy, sober and of good moral character'.
Rules E	To do with regulating, supervising and restricting the practice of midwives: included 'directions to Midwives concerning their Person, Instruments, etc; their duties to Patient and Child; and their Obligations with regard to Disinfection, Medical Assistance and Notification'.
Rules F	Re: the duty of a LSA to suspend a midwife from practice for the purpose of preventing the spread of infection. Added later: power to suspend any midwife accused of disobeying Rules until case settled.
Rules G	Re: particulars required on a prescribed form when a midwife notified her intention to practise.
Rules H	Applied to removal and restoration of names from the Roll.

It was not uncommon for a LSA to use Rules F to suspend a midwife in order to prevent the spread of infection. For example, in the early days of the CMBS, if a mother had a temperature of over 100 degrees Fahrenheit for over twenty-four hours, the midwife had to call for medical assistance. Subsequently, until 1980, the *Rules* stated that the presence of an elevated temperature (degree not specified) for over twenty-four hours, signifying possible infection, required the midwife to call for medical assistance and notify the LA.[33] Mary McCaskill, a Glasgow Municipal Midwife or 'Green Lady' in the 1940s and 1950s, recalled:

If one of your postnatal mothers developed a [raised temperature]... [which] was maintained over... twenty-four hours... you were suspended from practice and a ... general... district nurse... who was a midwife, [but] who wasn't doing midwifery, took over the postnatal care and I would be suspended from practice. You see, there was always this big danger in these years of puerperal fever. And this is why it could not be a midwife [so that infection would not be spread to other postnatal mothers]. I had to go home and wash my hair, have a bath and change my uniform. I had to have a throat swab taken to make sure I wasn't carrying the infection and then the supervisor would arrange a day and a time when she would come to the house and inspect all my equipment and see that I had a clean lining in my bag. You changed your bag [lining] every week of course. [Antibiotics were] in their infancy. It was sulphonamides then you know... M & B, the great 693, the first one... we gave mothers sulphonamides if they thought there was a rise in temperature. I would say they weren't used as widely as antibiotics are nowadays. They were new but they were used. They were considered a great boon to controlling infection. I hadn't worked as a midwife before the days of sulphonamides.[34]

CMBS *Rules* for midwives emphasised the physical care of mother and baby. They were not always kept to the letter, especially early in the century and where howdies were practising although, as shown above, suspected infection was taken seriously from an early stage.

Under the terms of Rules H, the CMBS could ask a LSA or its solicitor to investigate and report on the legal conviction of a midwife or accusation of disobeying CMBS *Rules*.[35] The Penal Cases Committee then considered the case and reported further to the Board. The Board's penal cases procedure was complicated and carefully undertaken; there was time for evidence-gathering, for notifying the accused midwife of what was happening, the date of the hearing and of her rights and requirements. If an accused midwife did not attend her hearing, the Board could proceed and decide upon the charges in her absence. It could remove the midwife's name from the Roll and cancel her certificate, or punish her by censure, caution or suspension. A de-certified midwife could apply for reinstatement and a new certificate for 10/- (50 pence) after six months.[36]

The quinquennial review and update of the *Rules* laid down by the Act was waived many times. This was because of the work involved in changing *Rules*, difficulties ensuring reciprocity with the CMBE&W, later Acts affecting the *Rules*, and World War Two which diverted the Board's attention to other activities.

Education of midwives
Formal statutory education and training for midwives in Scotland began in 1916 as the CMBS responded to the 1915 Midwives (Scotland) Act. This included 'regulating the course of training [for pupil midwives]',[37] inspecting and approving potential and existing training schools or institutions, and monitoring examinations.

During training, the candidate had to attend twenty labours, personally delivering each mother, look after twenty mothers and their infants for ten days following labour, and attend a course of twenty theoretical lectures given by a Registered Medical Practitioner recognised by the Board as a lecturer. On fulfilment of these requirements for the CMBS examination, she had to notify the Board, enclosing the required certificates and a one guinea (£1-1/- or £1.05) fee. The examination included normal and abnormal midwifery. The normal included anatomy and physiology, pregnancy and normal labour, the care of the mother in the puerperium, and the management and feeding of infants, all in detail to comply with *Rules* C.[38] Listing these items with such detailed specification demonstrates the anxiety of members of the Board about some midwives' lack of knowledge of basic care.

Examinable subjects in abnormal midwifery included: signs of postnatal diseases, for example, puerperal fevers, obstetric emergencies and their management until medical help arrived, and the care of children born 'apparently lifeless'.

Table 3.2 Summary of changes in midwifery education since 1916[41]

Date	Midwifery training /education	Length of course	Comments
1916	With 3 years general nurse training Without nurse training	4 months 6 months	There were also the '*bona fide*' or uncertified midwives.[42]
1926	With nurse training Without nurse training	6 months 12 months	
1938	With nurse training Without nurse training: direct entry	12 months 24 months	Course now in 2 parts, each 6 months. Also 2 parts: 6 and 18 months. Women with Part 1 only could work under direct GP supervision.
1961	Enrolled nurses (hitherto treated as direct entry)	18 months	
1968	Direct entry midwifery training ceased in Scotland. One year integrated midwifery course for 3 year trained nurses.	12 months	End of 2 part midwifery.
1981	In response to European Economic Community (EEC) Midwives Directives[43] the midwifery course was lengthened. It was now for registered general nurses only.	18 months	The alternative would be a 3 year direct entry midwifery course which was planned.
1992	To comply further with EEC Midwives Directives, first cohort of 'new' single registration midwifery students started in Scotland.	3 years	The 18 month course continued in certain colleges/universities to supply dual-qualified staff for mainly rural areas. Also, for nurses who then wished to do midwifery although this is not considered to be cost effective.
1995	First cohort qualified with Higher Education Diplomas.		They were offered the option of taking a 'top-up' degree post-qualification.
2008	All student midwives in Scotland study a three year degree programme with an Honours option.	3-4 years	

As Table 3.2 shows, the initial period of midwifery training was very short, even for women who had no nursing training. Bryers argues that, at a time when countries, such as the Netherlands, already had a two-year training programme, the decision to set the training period at six months was detrimental to the development of midwifery in Scotland. It restricted the status of midwives in comparison with medical practitioners and so played a part in limiting the development of midwifery as a profession.[39] This equates with Foucault's power knowledge analysis of discipline in terms of theoretical knowledge described by Stephens.[40] Obstetricians with a lengthy training have power, rank and status, while midwives' shorter length of training gives them less status and power.

Midwifery training and education in Scotland extended gradually over the decades: in the 1920s in response to concerns regarding high mortality rates; the widening of the role of the midwife; more in-depth learning, education and research; and, as a response to events and changes in thinking as the century evolved.

The CMBS decided to divide the training into two parts in 1938. This was an effort to dissuade nurses with no desire to practise midwifery, but who used the qualification as a career move, from taking the full training. This custom represented considerable wastage of resources and depleted the anticipated numbers of practising midwives. In addition, it was not helpful in the campaign which later developed to establish midwifery as a profession in its own right.

Central Midwives Board for Scotland

We hereby certify that

MARGARET BOLTON NICOL

a Candidate entitled to admission to examination on completion of six consecutive calendar months' training, has passed the First Examination of the Board on ____4th DECEMBER, 1958

Chairman of the Board

Janet L. Renton
Acting Secretary

Note.—This Certificate does not entitle the pupil whose name is enscribed hereon to admission to the Roll of Midwives, or authorise her to hold herself out as certified under the Midwives Act.

CMBS Certificate Part 1,
Margaret Nicol (now Ritchie).
(Courtesy of
Margaret Ritchie.)

Central Midwives Board for Scotland

No. 2408? ____   Date 9th April 1959

We hereby Certify

That ____*Margaret Bolton Nicol*____
having passed the Examination of the Central Midwives Board for Scotland, and having otherwise complied with the rules and regulations laid down in pursuance of the Midwives (Scotland) Act, 1951 is entitled by law to practise as a Midwife in accordance with the provisions of the said Act and subject to the said rules and regulations.

Chairman of the Board

Janet L. Renton
Acting Secretary

CMBS Certificate Part 2,
Margaret Nicol (now Ritchie).
(Courtesy of
Margaret Ritchie.)

Teachers of midwifery

Following the 1915 Act, the CMBS approved certain institutions in Scotland as teaching institutions for running midwifery courses.[44] Those who taught pupil midwives were lecturers and teachers: lecturers were medical practitioners with sufficient experience and expertise; teachers were experienced midwives. All had to be approved by the Board.

To begin with, there was no formal teacher training course available for midwives. A qualification in teaching, the Midwife Teachers' Diploma (MTD), developed during the late 1930s. Up until then, would-be teachers of midwives in Scotland had to belong to an approved training institution and apply to the Board with references of good practice and ability. The Board upgraded this after the 1937 Maternity Services (Scotland) Act to a basic requirement of at least three years' midwifery practice and satisfactory evidence of teaching competence. The midwife also had to be on the staff of, or associated with, an approved training institution, must have attended at least sixty cases in the previous year, and had to provide adequate accommodation and facilities for her pupils. These stipulations became particularly relevant as district midwifery changed.[45] The number of hospital births increased with a corresponding drop in available district 'cases' for pupil midwives within a training catchment area. In the late 1940s, the CMBS also invited other midwives to apply to teach pupils.[46]

Further changes followed. The CMBS excluded from teaching any midwife, whether MTD or not, who was not also a registered nurse.[47] In 1951, the RCM asked the CMBS to reconsider this decision for non-nurse midwife MTDs.[48] This stipulation remained until 1968 when the CMBS once again approved non-nurse midwives (without the MTD) as teachers. Ironically, 1968 was also the year when the CMBS stopped midwifery training in Scotland for non-nurses.[49]

The CMBS was slow to establish the MTD course in Scotland. In England, in 1926, the Midwives' Institute inaugurated a Midwife Teacher's Certificate which evolved until 1936 when the Midwives Act for England and Wales made statutory provision for the MTD.[50] The Scottish Board of the College of Nursing initiated similar course plans with the CMBS in 1936. After an enthusiastic start, the CMBS admitted to the Scottish Board of the College of Nursing in 1937 that it was not ready to put its plans into operation.[51]

Two circumstances appear to have galvanised the Board into action. Miss Jean P Ferlie (c1898-1974), Matron of the Edinburgh Royal Maternity and Simpson Memorial Hospital, the 'old Simpson', wrote to the CMBS in December 1937 with a suggested MTD syllabus.[52] Miss Ferlie was recognized for her leadership qualities and her work in midwifery, and she was backed by Mrs Margaret Myles (1892-1988), midwifery tutor at the Simpson, and eventual well-known author of midwifery text-books.[53] It is likely that Miss Ferlie's letter was designed to persuade Board members to expedite matters. As further incentive, the 1937 Maternity Services (Scotland) Act gave the CMBS the power to grant the MTD.[54] Scotland's first MTD course got underway in 1938, and the next in 1942-1943.[55] However, although by 1953 forty-six midwives in Scotland had achieved the MTD, the courses were sporadic and represented a slow start for the MTD in Scotland compared to the regularity of English courses in Kingston-upon-Thames.[56]

The MTD course in Scotland remained in operation while the Board existed. It developed from a part-time day-release course into a full-time nine-month course run by the RCM Scottish Council, with plans for a Clinical Teachers' Instruction Course.[57] When financial constraints prevented the RCM from continuing, the Board negotiated places for midwives at Jordanhill College of Education on a Nurse Tutors' course beginning in October 1971.[58] This course, with specific midwifery support and supervision, emphasising teaching methods and educational subjects, was a successful and welcome innovation from the more traditional MTD. It remained as the accepted course for the MTD until well into the 1980s when more midwife teachers were educated to degree level.

The establishment of a MTD in Scotland, however slowly it happened, was part of a bid to improve midwifery practice and education, and make midwifery an attractive profession to which intelligent women would aspire. This was particularly important during World War Two and afterwards when the shortage of midwives reached unprecedented levels.

The Local Supervising Authority (LSA)
The Central Midwives Board for Scotland also had to deal with Local Supervising Authorities (LSA). After 1915, Local Authorities (LA) in their role as LSAs had to cope with new statutory duties and responsibilities which the CMBS circulated to all LAs and their MOs.[59] An important point was the association between the administration of the Act and that of the Maternal and Child Welfare Schemes under the 1915 Notification of Births (Extension) Act.[60] This highlighted LAs' financial responsibilities with consequent anticipated improvements in maternity care. The Act authorised LAs to contribute towards the training of midwives and there is no doubting the CMBS's hope that LAs would fulfil their obligations towards the training of midwives and help more midwives to train thereby ensuring better maternal and infant care. This was particularly important in 1916 when the Board expected a decline in the number of midwives as the 1915 Act took effect. At the same time there was a dearth of medical practitioners due to World War One. The Board also encouraged LAs to help where there was family financial hardship so that mothers would have skilled and prompt attention without worrying about their ability to pay and it would help midwives secure a reasonable salary.[61]

LSAs were also involved in the Board's finances. According to the Act, midwives' examination and enrolment fees should go via the LSA to the Board. If there was a negative balance at the end of the year, each LSA paid the Board its share of the balance in proportion to the population in its area.[62]

The Board frequently had to remind LSAs and their MOHs to report changes at the local level.[63] It finally resorted, in December 1920, to sending out an annual circular to LSAs.[64] This document asked for information regarding midwives' notifications of intention to practise, the percentage of births attended by midwives, the number of emergency cases to which medical practitioners were called, the number of cases of ophthalmia neonatorum, puerperal septicaemia and stillbirths notified by midwives, and the relation of these numbers to the total number of births attended by midwives. Eventually, after five years, the Board appeared to be satisfied that the LSAs recognised their joint 'grave responsibility for the supervision of midwives.'[65]

Midwives and the CMBS

One of the CMBS's main duties was to establish and maintain the Roll of midwives in Scotland. The Board decided that every woman practising midwifery should apply to be enrolled and by 6 July 1916 it had received five hundred applications. By 7 December 1916, the Roll of midwives stood at 1,225.[66] This included midwives who had been practising before the Act, and sixty-nine midwives who had passed the first CMBS examination held on 30 October 1916. So, to begin with, many more midwives who had been *bona fides* were enrolled than those with certificates. This pattern changed dramatically over the first five years of the Board's existence as it became the norm for midwives in Scotland to sit the CMBS examination (See Table 3.3).

Table 3.3 Numbers of midwives enrolling with the CMBS for Scotland in 1916-1921.

Year.	By Certificate of an approved body	*Bona fide*	CMBS Exam	Total
1916-17	728	1229	69	2026
1917-18	624	465	195	1284
1918-19	45	20	216	281
1919-20	36	75	328	439
1920-21	15	6	470	518

(Source: Annual Reports of the CMBS for Scotland.)

The total number of midwives who enrolled in the first five years was 4,548. The number of practising midwives, elicited by the numbers of notifications of intention to practise received by the Board, was approximately 2,165.[67] Therefore, according to these figures, only forty-eight per cent of enrolled midwives were practising in 1921. Possible reasons for the discrepancy include:

- LSAs were initially slow to send details of midwives notifying their intention to practise.
- Possibly midwives did not fully understand that they had an annual statutory duty to notify their intention to practise.
- If a midwife resigned voluntarily, her name remained on the Roll to ensure continuing LSA supervision. This complied with GMC recommendations re 'covering'.[68]
- Some midwives enrolled but did not practise.
- Some midwives had no intention of practising, but to be a certified midwife was a requirement for various senior nursing appointments.[69]
- The possession of the CMBS certificate came to be seen as necessary for nursing career advancement.[70]
- Inspectors of Midwives (see below) had to hold the CMBS certificate, but did not have to practise.[71]

According to the Act, any woman who wanted to call herself a midwife had to be certified by 1 January 1917.[72] A woman with a certificate previously granted by an approved body, or who had been in *bona fide* practice for a year before the Act, was given two years to enrol with the CMBS. After the deadline of 31 December 1917, enrolment necessitated passing the CMBS examination, although the Board could and did accept some late applications and for many years allowed late enrolment reasonably freely, especially if a good case such as war service, was put forward.[73]

Inspectors of Midwives (IOM)
To comply with the 1915 Act, supervision of midwives was necessary.[74] LSAs were required to appoint appropriately qualified people to supervise midwives in their area. Supervision of midwives involved a LSA making arrangements through an IOM for inspection of midwives, their register of cases, clothing, equipment, premises if appropriate, and how they practised. Midwives had to co-operate and 'give every reasonable facility for such an inspection.'[75] On the district, even though midwives worked on their own, the LSA checked that they obeyed the *Rules*. Mary McCaskill, practising in Glasgow in the late 1940s as a Green Lady, said, 'You had to have your *Rule* book and that had to be produced at all times and of course we were subject to inspection [at home] of your uniform and your equipment – your bag'. She also described midwives working together to make sure their equipment was complete when they knew an inspection was pending:

> And of course I'd be telling tales out of school – I had no disposable equipment. I had steel bowls and kidney dishes and gallipots, nail-scrubbers and... thermometer, stethoscope, but if you were short of something [and an inspection was pending], say I was supposed to have two gallipots and I only had one, I just phoned [another midwife] and said, 'I'll have a gallipot for tomorrow.' And so [that was the way] it went. [They actually came] yes, very much in the image of the hospital matron.[76]

Responsibility for the appointment of an IOM lay with the LSA. The Board initially recommended that any IOMs appointed should hold the CMBS certificate and 'their appointment should be determined from the qualifications held, tact and experience.'[77] Later, the CMBS pointed out to LSAs that IOMs should be a medical officer or a health visitor holding the certificate of the CMBS or CMBSE&W and subject to the approval of the LGBS.[78] Some health visitors were used as IOMs in England and Wales and this is possibly why the CMBS recommended that health visitors be used in Scotland. However, the decision to appoint health visitors, even with the CMBS certificate, as IOMs, caused problems. The Board started receiving complaints 'anent the interference of health visitors with the duties of the midwife' and this led the CMBS to clarify beyond all doubt the division of labour between midwives and health visitors.[79]

The strict rules in Scotland about qualifications for IOMs may well have come about as a result of the English experience. Donnison points out that:

> [In England] in many areas...the work of inspection was left to persons without suitable qualifications. These were commonly health visitors,

women generally of higher social status than midwives, but with little or no practical experience of midwifery, who in consequence were resented by midwives as ignorant and overbearing. In some areas, the duty was laid on the sanitary inspector, who came to it 'straight from rubbish tips and drains', in others, on the poorly remunerated Medical Officer of Health himself, 'who had forgotten most of the midwifery he had ever learnt'.[80]

Nevertheless, for the CMBS to state that an IOM should be a medical officer or a health visitor albeit with a CMBS certificate indicates a hierarchy that implied seniority of health visitors over midwives that lasted for many years.

Medical Aid
According to the Act, a midwife had to summon medical aid in an emergency. The LSA was responsible for his fee.[81] The midwife also had to inform the LSA, give the reason for the emergency and the name of the medical practitioner. The medical practitioner also had to report the nature of the call-out to the LSA and tender his account for fees and mileage. The fee was fixed at £1-1/- (one guinea, £ 1.05) for consultation, to cover one subsequent visit if required, with mileage at the rate of 1/- (5 pence) per mile. The LSA could try and recover the debt from the mother or her family.[82]

It soon became apparent that some midwives had problems obtaining emergency medical aid.[83] This was an issue which, strictly speaking, was outwith the Board's control and yet had a direct bearing on the work of midwives. In England and Wales the same problem existed, exacerbated because, under the rules of the CMBSE&W, the midwife had to summon a doctor in an emergency, but there was no statutory provision for his payment.[84]

Although the Board worked with the Local Government Board for Scotland (LGBS) and LSAs on the scale of fees and mileage rates that LSAs should pay to medical practitioners in midwifery emergencies, there was widespread misunderstanding.[85] Although it was not the CMBS's responsibility, it continued to receive complaints and questions until, in 1919, the Secretary to the Board started referring these to the responsible body, the LGBS and its successor from 1919, the new Scottish Board of Health (SBH).[86] The arguments over emergency fees reflected the apprehension among many medical practitioners over the possible extension of medical benefits to cover more of the population and range of medical services provided in Scotland. Some doctors worried that this would give LAs control of medical benefit or lead to a bureaucratically controlled State medical service.[87]

The issue of maternal mortality
There was a consensus from the early 1920s that maternal mortality in England and Wales, and Scotland, was rising and that many maternal deaths were avoidable. This consensus was based on estimates of the extent of maternal mortality and on cross-national comparisons, both of which were fraught with problems. For instance there were changes in rules of registration, differences in registration in different countries of the UK and further afield, and, classification of a maternal death, including for example, questions about classification of 'associated death' and multiple causes of death.[88] To

compound the problem, different countries had varying methods of recording statistics and therefore accurate international comparisons were difficult to achieve.[89] There was also the problem of estimating the numbers of 'hidden maternal deaths'. For example, a doctor could certify a death caused by puerperal fever or post-partum haemorrhage as being caused by 'fever' or 'haemorrhage' respectively, so masking the real cause of death. Anything which could damage a late nineteenth-century doctor's name and reputation was to be avoided if possible and 'no doctor reported a death as due to sepsis if he could attribute it to another cause.'[90] The *Salvesen Report* of 1924 pin-pointed many of these issues, particularly when making inter-area and international comparisons.[91]

Nevertheless, even given allowances for inaccuracies within statistics, in the years between 1918 and 1932, there was general agreement that the MMR was rising. There was also cross-UK agreement that many of the deaths were avoidable.[92]

Puerperal Morbidity and Mortality: the *Salvesen Report*
The Salvesen Report was the result of a SBH committee inquiry into the incidence of puerperal morbidity and mortality in Scotland, and to identify the causes and to suggest any remedial measures. Although invited to make comments, the CMBS, for some unexplained reason, felt unable to co-operate fully with the Salvesen committee.[93] In contrast, the Scottish Midwives Association (SMA) responded by demonstrating its concern about unqualified midwifery practice and made suggestions for amendments to the 1915 Midwives (Scotland) Act. These included the abolition of the controversial phrase 'habitually and for gain'.[94]

The *Salvesen Report* estimated the MMR in Scotland in 1922 as 6.6 per 1000 births, an increase on the mean rate of 6.2 for the years 1915-1922.[95] The Report, emphasising that the MMR in Scotland was reducible, made fifteen main recommendations towards this aim.[96] However, although the Scottish MMR figures were poor, the Report pointed out their similarity to those in England after taking account different methods of compiling statistics:

> The puerperal mortality rate [in England] in 1918 is shown as 3.0 as against 7.0 in Scotland; but in England special tables are compiled showing deaths associated with pregnancy or the puerperium which have not been included in the computation. These include the deaths of puerperal women from influenza which prior to 1921 were shown in Scotland as puerperal mortality. If these further deaths are added for 1918 to the puerperal mortality, the English rate becomes 7.6; and the comparable figures for England and Scotland thus show no significant difference.[97]

The *Salvesen Report* recommended improved antenatal care, and condemned uncertified midwives. The Report attacked the practices of howdies and acquiescence from some medical practitioners who 'covered' for them, saying their lack of aseptic techniques and other dangerous midwifery practices resulted in risk for both mother and baby. In addition, the livelihood of certified midwives suffered from competition from howdies whose fees were lower and who did housework as well as midwifery. In a bid for wider information leading to greater knowledge, and ultimately a significantly lower MMR, the Report also recommended that LAs should investigate every death occurring within four weeks of pregnancy and report to the Scottish Board of Health (SBH).[98]

The implicit assumption within the Report was that the quality of midwives and midwifery care related to the MMR. This reinforces comments on international MMR comparisons, notably that countries with a lower MMR had well organised midwifery education.[99] However, Loudon also cited English and Scottish MMR statistics which were better for midwives than for doctors and noted the improvement in the intrapartum standard of care provided by midwives, particularly in the 1930s.[100] Responding to the Report, the CMBS pointed out to the SBH its recent steps to improve the standard of aspirant pupil midwives and the midwifery training course. The new course included extra lectures, the need for pupil midwives to witness ten births before starting to deliver babies personally, and the inclusion in the course of the hitherto low-profile antenatal care with the hope that this would have a beneficial effect in lowering the MMR.[101] The Board also agreed with the further resolve to eradicate unqualified midwifery practice.[102]

Midwives and Maternity Homes (Scotland) Act, 1927

In the five years after the *Salvesen Report*, 1925-1929, the MMR in Scotland continued to cause anxiety.[103] It remained at a minimum of 6.2 per 1000 live births reaching a peak of 7.0 in 1928.[104]

The SBH began work on a Bill to address maternal mortality in Scotland by tackling two main issues. Firstly, it agreed to an amendment to the Act in order to abolish uncertified midwives. Secondly, the requirement for more hospital maternity beds in Scotland increased in the 1920s. As hospital births slowly lost their long-standing stigma of poverty, more women saw this as an acceptable option; from a medical aspect, more women were admitted for obstetric procedures. Amongst the new maternity beds were those within privately run maternity homes which at the time were unregistered, of 'uncertain standards', and sometimes resorted to varying strategies to bend the rules.[105] More legislation was needed to regulate Maternity Homes. Amendments to the 1915 Midwives (Scotland) Act and legislation covering maternity homes came together in the 1927 Midwives and Maternity Homes (Scotland) Act.[106]

CMBS intervention assisted the Bill's passage through Parliament. It was involved with the first draft in 1925, it reminded the SBH of the urgent need for further Scottish legislation when the Government passed the equivalent Act for England and Wales in 1926, it pushed for a similar Act appropriately adjusted for Scotland, and it publicised what it was doing in its annual report.[107]

There was, however, some Parliamentary controversy over the Bill. Section 1 (2) of the 1915 Act included the phrase 'habitually and for gain'.[108] An amendment to this stated:

> If any person being either a male person or a woman not certified under this Act attends a woman in childbirth otherwise than under the direction and supervision of a duly qualified medical practitioner, that person shall, unless he or she satisfies the court that the attention was given in a case of sudden or urgent necessity, or in a case where reasonable efforts were made to obtain the services of a duly qualified medical practitioner or of a person certified under this Act, be liable to a summary conviction to a fine not exceeding ten pounds.[109]

This amendment contained two important changes, the first being the inclusion of the words 'male person'. The 1915 Act contained an anomaly in that it omitted to forbid midwifery practice by unqualified men. There is no mention in the CMBS Minutes of unqualified 'male persons' making a habit of attending women in childbirth. However, the non-inclusion of the words 'male person' in the 1915 Act was a loophole which should be closed. The Midwives and Maternity Homes Act 1926 for England and Wales made a similar amendment.[110] The second important change, and the closing of another loophole, was the exclusion of the words 'habitually and for gain', controversially included in the 1915 Act. Since 1 January 1922 it was illegal for any uncertified woman to attend a woman in childbirth 'habitually and for gain'. However, it still appeared to be quite easy to get round this obstacle by claiming that the situation was an emergency.[111]

The amendment provoked Parliamentary dissent. The words 'habitually and for gain' made the administration of the Act very difficult and it was necessary to tighten up the position. However, James Maxton (1885-1946), MP for Glasgow Bridgeton, criticised the proposed change on the grounds that the onus should be on the police rather than a neighbour to prove whether or not it was an emergency, stating:

> [T]hat woman neighbour, who has run in out of decency to lend her assistance to her neighbour in need, must prove that she acted in a case of sudden necessity... It is quite wrong that the onus of proof should be put on the woman. The onus of proof should be on the police or the authorities to say that the woman is doing this habitually and for gain and not merely as a case of emergency.[112]

Despite Maxton's argument, the Bill moved forward. The section omitting the words 'habitually and for gain' remained, although George Hardie (1874-1937), MP for Glasgow Springburn, asked for reassurance that if a neighbour went 'in to give some assistance and a fatality occurs' she would be protected. Further SBH and CMBS discussion led to another amendment making it the responsibility of LAs to provide midwives in cases where none was available.[113] As Malcolm Barclay-Harvey (1890-1969), MP for Kincardineshire & West Aberdeenshire, said, 'It was urged in Committee that...we were not doing anything to help poor people to get maternity treatment, and this Clause has been designed to meet this point... It will now be possible to arrange to give this necessary assistance in all cases.'[114]

Part 2 of the Bill dealing with the registration and inspection of maternity homes went through the Commons without difficulty. The Act received the Royal Assent on 29 July 1927 and the Board publicised it in the new issue of the Midwives' Roll.[115] Registration of maternity homes came under strict control from January 1928. The SBH had powers to make regulations regarding all record-keeping of the homes and details of employees and patients. Officers of a LSA and the SBH also had authority to enter and inspect premises used, or believed to be used, as a maternity home and inspect any relevant records. A LSA also had the power to exempt certain institutions from Part 2 of the Act.[116]

This Act kept the issue of maternal mortality in the public eye, although it was at least a decade before there was an appreciable difference in the MMR. LAs, their powers further extended with their new responsibilities towards maternity homes, worked alongside the CMBS to make improvements. In addition, the new amendment clarifying the law and practice of howdies brought the two bodies together in a joint effort to improve the MMR and improve midwifery practice.

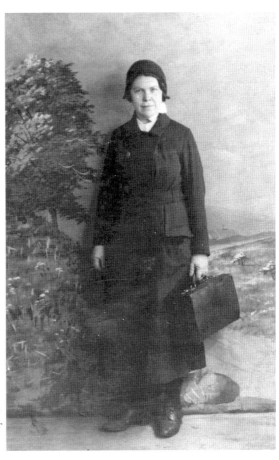

Rottenrow (GRMH) midwife 'on the district'. (Courtesy of Elizabeth Radley.)

The 1935 *Report on Maternal Morbidity and Mortality*
In 1929, the Department of Health for Scotland (DHS) replaced the SBH. The DHS, pro-active in recognising the need for further work to improve maternal morbidity and mortality, commissioned another investigation into maternal deaths in Scotland which reported in 1935. The committee, headed by Dr Charlotte Douglas and Dr Peter McKinley, inquired into reports of 2,527 maternal deaths in Scotland between October 1929 and the beginning of 1933, representing nearly all the maternal deaths in Scotland in this period.[117] Another DHS-commissioned committee, the Cathcart Committee chaired by Edward Provan Cathcart (1877-1954), met from 1933 and reported in 1936 on the serious overall health problems in Scotland which impinged on the MMR.

The Douglas and McKinley Committee also investigated midwifery practice and education. It sent a questionnaire to all practising midwives in Scotland and asked the Board about the training and system of registration of midwives in Scotland.[118] The CMBS explained the purposes of the 1915 Act, how the CMBS worked, and pointed out that a midwife was a person whose name was on the Roll, whether she was practising or not. A further point was the estimate that, of those who took and passed the CMBS examination, only ten per cent entered midwifery practice. The others were maternity nurses responsible to the doctors under whose instructions they were acting, health visitors, and those in other posts, for example, administration, who had no intention of practising as a midwife but for whom it was an advantage to have the CMBS qualification.[119] This represented considerable wastage of resources and depleted the anticipated numbers of practising midwives.

The *Douglas and McKinley Report* identified a common tendency to over-emphasise the dangers of childbearing and stressed that 'pregnancy and parturition are natural physiological processes.'[120] Nevertheless, the Report indicated the need for improvement in the maternity services in Scotland. The DHS used many of its recommendations when compiling the 1937 Maternity Services (Scotland) Bill.

While the Report emphasised the need for co-operation from childbearing women, it also criticised standards of maternity care. The authors considered antenatal care to be inadequate and recommended greater attention to detail. Twenty-eight per cent of the 2,465 maternal deaths studied for the investigation were classified as due to lack of adequate antenatal care. Of these, fifty-seven per cent of the mothers were considered to be at fault because they did not ask for antenatal care. In 143 cases, mothers started antenatal care, but either they or their relatives 'refused to follow or ignored the advice prescribed.'[121] The Report also ascribed three hundred of the maternal deaths investigated, to inadequate antenatal care on the part of doctors, midwives, or institutions, although there was evidence that the mothers had consulted one or other of these services. The authors of the Report also found fault with those providing intranatal care and concluded that many women in Scotland did not receive adequate care.[122]

An important issue was that of 'meddlesome midwifery' by GPs. The Report commented that 'it seems fairly obvious that interference during parturition is an important and preventable contributory factor in the total maternal death rate.'[123] This view was supported by Dr John Munro Kerr (1868-1960), Professor of Midwifery at the University of Glasgow, who found that in the years 1929-1931 in Glasgow, where a doctor was in charge of a delivery, which happened in many middle-class households, the MMR was 5.04. In working-class homes, where a midwife was usually in charge, the MMR was 2.6. In 1928, similar findings were found in Aberdeen. In England and Wales, findings of the Registrar General in 1931 showed that maternal mortality was higher in social classes I and II (mostly delivered by doctors), than in IV and V where midwives were in charge.[124] The difference therefore depended upon the birth attendant. Susan Williams, researching childbirth in the twentieth century, quoted a retired Welsh midwife: 'In those days on the district, the doctors didn't worry. They never waited for the mother to be fully dilated. They would just put on the forceps and try and bring out the baby. They would tear the mother to bits.'[125] However, Dr John MacLeod attempted to justify the position of the GP in midwifery practice: 'On reading various reports dealing with maternal mortality and morbidity, one feels that the General Practitioner is too often made the scapegoat.'[126] Drawing on his own experience, he refuted the suggestion that GPs were to blame:

> My own experience of 1,038 maternity cases with only one death and no deaths from sepsis, entitles me to have definite views on midwifery as conducted in the home, and on the effectiveness of the GP provided he is given proper encouragement by the administrative bodies.
>
> The tendency is to disparage his efforts, regardless of the wonderful service he has given in the past, under the most adverse conditions. Certain members...would have the practitioner replaced by a glorified midwife on the one hand, and by the specialist on the other.[127]

The *Douglas and McKinley Report* recommended that, before anticipating any instrumental delivery, the person looking after the labouring woman should obtain advice from an obstetrician. Whether doctor or midwife, that person should have direct access to the nearest hospital and, where necessary, bring help to the patient rather than transporting the patient to the hospital.[128] This recommendation was incorporated into the statutes of the 1937 Maternity Services (Scotland) Act.[129] Yet Anne Bayne, describing life as a midwife in the 1950s and 1960s, remarked that the GP still had a pivotal role. Contrary to the recommendations, in practice, the midwife still had to have the GP call for specialist help.

> It was shocking then that you couldn't on your own [as a midwife] call out a flying squad and a doctor couldn't phone from home. The doctor had to say, 'Yes, I've been to see her, [the patient] yes we need the flying squad'. He couldn't even on the midwife's say so get the flying squad. I had Kenneth Gordon - he would have gone to jail for it. He used to say, 'You're the bloody expert. You don't need me to come and stand and say "yes",' and he would do it [get the flying squad on the midwife's instruction before he saw the mother] but he was putting his nose on the line. He could have been struck off for doing it.[130]

The 1935 Report also highlighted postnatal problems, especially relating to infection, stating that these were partly the fault of the patient or relatives due to poor or neglectful care. Nevertheless, the Report attributed fifty-six puerperal deaths dominated by sepsis to lack of adequate professional care and recommended that LAs should ensure that the rule requiring notification of puerperal pyrexia was strictly obeyed, nobody suffering from an infection should be near a puerperal woman, and there should be better arrangements for six-week postnatal examinations to reduce morbidity later.[131]

Further recommendations, particularly to do with midwives, subsequently appeared in the 1937 Maternity Services (Scotland) Act which stipulated that there should be closer partnership between midwives and LAs. There were added dangers when maternity nursing was practised by non-midwives.[132] However, as well as this, to make a maternity service work, co-operation from the mothers and co-ordination between all maternity service professionals were needed.

The DHS was aware of serious overall health problems in Scotland and in 1933 gave a remit to review, investigate and report on the serious problems of Scotland's health to the Cathcart Committee which reported in 1936. The main theme was to draw all the disparate threads of current health care into one national health policy. From the aspect of the maternity services and the MMR, the *Cathcart Report* reinforced the findings of the Douglas and McKinley Report published a year earlier in 1935.[133]

The 1937 Maternity Services (Scotland) Act

When the 1936 Midwives Act for England and Wales was passed, the DHS agreed to work for a similar Scottish Act. In presenting the Maternity Services (Scotland) Bill to the Commons in January 1937, Walter Elliot (1888-1958), the Secretary of State for Scotland (SOS), said that the Bill was intended 'to deal with a stubborn and intractable problem which, for long, has preoccupied those who are engaged in the public health service in Scotland ... maternal mortality.'[134] In the debate, James Guy (1894-1972), MP for Central Edinburgh, compared the Scottish MMR of six with an English MMR of four.[135] Neither Elliot nor Guy made reference to the problems, already mentioned, in comparing the MMR between Scotland and England and how, according to the *Salvesen Report*, they were not very different.

The Scottish Bill broke new ground because the 1936 Midwives Act for England and Wales made provision for midwives only. The more comprehensive objectives of the Scottish Bill planned to provide an improved maternity service in Scotland with greater involvement of LAs.[136] Echoing the *Douglas and McKinley Report*, Elliot envisaged that mothers in Scotland having a homebirth would be entitled to the services of a midwife, doctor, and obstetrician if necessary, working together as a team.[137] The 1937 Maternity Services (Scotland) Act received the Royal Assent on 6 May 1937.

This Act laid the responsibility on LAs to make provision for certified midwives to attend women in their own homes 'before and during childbirth and from time to time thereafter during a period not less than the lying-in period.'[138] The 1936 Act for England and Wales specified fourteen days for lying-in. The Scottish Act, with no such specification, allowed the CMBS more flexibility.[139] Midwives had to be certified, but otherwise could be from any source, including employment by LAs, thus establishing a salaried midwifery service. LAs were also responsible for arranging for medical care of women having homebirths including, as well as the GP, the services of an anaesthetist and obstetrician where necessary. This also involved obtaining approval for proposed arrangements from the DHS, medical schools and midwifery training institutions.[140]

Implementation of the Act had financial implications which affected all concerned, including the issue of means-testing, and fees for maternity services. In order to provide improved maternity services for every woman, the Act authorised LAs to recover part or all of the fees if possible. Fees were payable on a scale approved by the DHS, based on a formula weighted according to the special needs of an area. Improved maternity services meant increased expenditure for LAs and the Act provided for extra parliamentary finances. This was in line with the intention of the Local Government (Scotland) Act 1929 which provided for financial help for LAs coping with additional expenditure due to the institution of a new service.[141]

The new maternity service also had an impact on midwives' working and financial arrangements. A more formal structure of payment meant that, for midwives employed by LAs, life would be more secure than hitherto when they often went without payment.[142] On the other hand, some midwives might be unable to comply with the terms and conditions of formal LA employment. For example, the Act provided recompense for a certified midwife who stopped practising within three years of the Act, or retired because her LA considered her unable to continue practising. In these cases, Parliament reimbursed LAs for half of the money paid out as compensation to midwives, and midwives had to surrender their certificate of enrolment for cancellation.[143]

The Act tackled again the old question of unqualified midwifery practice and again included the deterrent of a ten pound fine.[144] This was a further attempt to eliminate howdies in Scotland and MPs expected it to happen.[145] However, as Anne McFadden recalls, howdies were to be seen working in Fife as late as the 1950s:

> They [the howdies] would have a very...minimal training. The doctors would have taken them out with them...very often they were widows...who maybe...needed some extra money...they most definitely weren't certified midwives. They would assist him and through just being there and seeing what was done they would be able to do the normal. The only problems would be, would they know when to send for the doctor...if there was difficulty, but they did quite well and they would make a reasonable living out of it.[146]

In a further attempt to reduce the MMR by improving and maintaining midwives' skills, the Act also provided for the CMBS to frame rules for midwives' refresher courses and for LAs to arrange for midwives to attend them.[147] Refresher courses for midwives were not a new concept and were started in Scotland, first in 1927 at Govan Maternity Home and then in 1928 in Edinburgh, at the instigation of the SMA.[148] However, these were irregular and not compulsory. After the 1937 Act was passed, it became a statutory requirement for all midwives to attend refresher courses to keep up to date with current trends, although the CMBS waived this for a time during and after World War Two.

By 1939, the MMR in Scotland was reduced to just under five per 1,000 births with a further reduction from 4.4 to 2.8 in the years 1940-1945. Important factors in the reduction of the MMR included improved education and practice of midwives and doctors, greater awareness of potential problems, the development of blood transfusions, the use of sulphonamides in the control of sepsis, and, from the social aspect, improved standards of living with better nutrition.[149]

Conclusion

With new status came rules, regulations and responsibilities. Midwives and the CMBS found themselves heavily involved in the effort to improve maternity services in the inter-war years with the overall goal of making a significant reduction in the MMR in Scotland. Day-to-day work had to continue with penal cases, correspondence, reports, midwifery education and courses, and new *Rules* to conform to the 1937 Act and other Boards. This involved co-operation with others to which the CMBS gradually acclimatised. As well as work with government bodies over Reports and new legislation, the Board had to work with other CMBs while trying to maintain an element of their own independence and identity. As it developed, the Board gradually accepted its important part in influencing maternity care in Scotland. Its initial lack of help to the

Salvesen Committee was reversed after publication of the Committee's Report. Willingness to work together was repeated when it came to later reports and legislation.

Minutes, which are only a bare record of CMBS meetings, do not tell the whole story, but they suggest that the Board functioned very slowly with much of the work committee-bound and protracted. However, Government and Parliamentary proceedings also appeared to contribute to the relative delay in Scottish matters which often lagged behind their English equivalent in Parliament. For instance, the 1926 Midwives and Maternity Homes Act (for England and Wales), was passed a year before the equivalent Scottish Act which was only accelerated through the new awareness and energy of the CMBS. However, to be second could have advantages. Observation of post-1902 midwifery in England and Wales meant that the 1915 Midwives (Scotland) Act contained clauses which improved upon the 1902 Midwives Act, and the 1937 Maternity Services (Scotland) Act was more comprehensive than the 1936 Midwives Act for England and Wales. It dealt with maternity services as a whole in Scotland and not only midwives, as did the Act for England and Wales.

The CMBS found it difficult to work with other Boards, particularly the well-established CMBE&W. The Board had a recurring tendency to 'ask England' when it was unsure of how to act. It could have been a question of inexperience, or of deference to a larger neighbour – being 'in bed with an elephant'.[150] The Board frequently argued for a point of view, but then gave in under pressure. This was particularly obvious in 1934 at an inter-Board Conference to discuss extending the midwifery course curriculum to include greater antenatal care as more widely-educated midwives would help to lower the MMR. CMBS members wanted to wait for the *Douglas and McKinley Report* on maternal morbidity and mortality, to which it had contributed evidence, before deciding to extend the midwifery course in Scotland. Yet, for the sake of reciprocity, the Board eventually agreed. In the event, it was nearly five years before the new course started and new *Rules* published. So, although the Board had agreed to lengthen the course, it had time to consider the *Douglas and McKinley Report*, contribute to discussions on the Maternity Services (Scotland) Act, and convince those in midwifery training institutions in Scotland of the benefits of the changes to mothers in Scotland as well as to midwives.

1.   I shall refer to the 1915 Midwives (Scotland) Act as 'the Act' and the Central Midwives' Board for Scotland as 'the CMBS' or 'the Board', where appropriate.
2.   NAS, CMB 4/1-5, *CMBS Rules* framed under Section 5 (1) of the 1915 Midwives (Scotland) Act, (5 and 6 Geo V Ch 91), 17 April 1916.
3.   *Midwives (Scotland) Act*, 1915, [5 & 6 Geo 5 Ch. 91] 1, p 3.
4.   NAS, CMB, *Index*, p 1.
5.   See Glossary for definition of MMR.
6.   *CMBS Report*, 31 March 1963, p 2.
7.   *CMBS Report*, 31 March 1983, p 5.
8.   See Appendix 1; Midwives (Scotland) Act, 3, (1).
9.   *Ibid.*
10.   *Ibid, 3, (3).*
11.   Cowell, Wainwright, *Behind the Blue Door*, p 49.

12. The SBH was set up following the 1919 Scottish Board of Health Act and, as far as the CMBS was concerned, replaced the duties of the Privy Council.

13. NAS, CMB 1/5, *CMBS Minutes*, 27 November1936, Vol 21, p 25.

14. Ministry of Health, DHS, Ministry of Labour and National Service, *Report of the Working Party on Midwives*, (London: HMSO, 1949), para 300: the Working Party recommended that the CMBE&W and the CMBS should each have eight midwives.

15. NAS, CMB 1/7, *CMBS Minutes*, 4 November 1951, p 1.

16. *Ibid*, 14 August 1952, p 1.

17. *CMBS Report*, 31 March 1973, p 1; *CMBS Report*, 31 March 1977, p 1.

18. NAS, CMB 1/2, *CMBS Minutes*, 18 February 1916, Vol 1, p 7.

19. J D Comrie, *History of Scottish Medicine Vol 2*, (London: Baillière, Tindall and Cox, 1932), p 689.

20. H Sutherland, *A Time to Keep*, (London: Geoffrey Bles, 1934), p 81; obstetricians have probably never been the same since Halliday Croom. Orange peel ointment at 3d (old pence) per ounce is listed in *Botanic Treatment of Disease*, (Glasgow: The Botanic Medical Hall, 1912), p 91.

21. J M Munro Kerr, J Haig Ferguson, J Young, J Hendry, *A Combined Textbook of Obstetrics and Gynaecology*, (Edinburgh: E and S Livingstone, 1923), frontispiece.

22. A Oakley, *The Captured Womb*, (Oxford: Basil Blackwell Publisher, 1984), p 51.

23. NAS CMB 1/2 *CMB Minutes*, 18 February 1916, p 11.

24. *Midwives (Scotland) Act*, 3 (1).

25. NAS, CMBS 1/2, *CMBS Minutes*, 18 February 1916, Vol 1, p 8.

26. *Ibid*, 25 May 1916, p 14; *ibid*, 9 March 1916, p 11; NAS, CMB 1/2, *CMBS Report*, 22 March 1917.

27. NAS, CMB 4/2/9, Schedule: Central Midwives Board for Scotland, *Rules framed under Section 5 (1) of the Midwives (Scotland) Act*, 1915 (5 and 6 Geo V c 91), 17 April 1916; NAS, CMB 1/2, *CMBS Minutes*, 25 May 1916, Vol 1, p 14.

28. *Ibid*, p 16; *ibid*, 28 October 1916, p 31; both of these midwives originally enrolled with the CMBS for England, Alice Turnbull in October 1905 and Isabella Scrimgeour in October 1904.

29. NAS, CMB 4/2/10, Schedule, CMBS for Scotland. *Rules framed under Section 5 (1) of the Midwives (Scotland) Act*, 1915 (5 and 6 Geo V Ch 91), 26 August 1916.

30. NAS, CMB 4/2/10, *CMBS Rules* 1916; L Reid, *Scottish Midwives (1916-1983): the Central Midwives Board for Scotland and practising midwives*, unpublished PhD thesis, University of Glasgow, 2003, pp 59-64. Copies of the first and subsequent *CMBS Rules* are held in the archives at the offices of the RCM UK Board for Scotland, 37 Frederick Street, Edinburgh.

31. NAS, CMB 4/2/10, *CMBS Rules* p 5; *CMBS Rules* remained detailed until 1947.

32. NAS, CMB 4/2/10, *CMBS Rules*, p 7.

33. *CMBS Rules*, 1968, p 13; *CMBS Rules*, 1980, Approval Instrument 1980, did not specify the raised temperature rule as hitherto. However it is implicit in rule 58, p 9.

34. LR 27; L Reid, 'Midwifery in Scotland 4: postnatal care', *British Journal of Midwifery*, (2005), Vol 13, (8), pp 492-496; 'M & B' stands for May and Baker, the pharmaceutical company who produced the first sulphonamides which saved so many lives; see I Loudon, *Death in Childbirth*, (Oxford: Clarendon Press, 1992), p 260.

35. NAS, CMB 4/2/10, *CMBS Rules* p 16.

36. *Ibid*, p 18; NAS, CMB 1/3, *CMBS Minutes*, 15 December 1921, Vol 6, p 60; the six months rule was effective from 1 January 1922.

37. *Midwives (Scotland) Act*, 5 (c).

38. NAS, CMB 4/2/10, *CMBS Rules*, p 5.

39. H Bryers, *Midwifery and Maternity Services in the Gàidhealtachd and the North of Scotland, 1914-2005*, unpublished thesis, University of Aberdeen, 2010, p 41; J Towler, J Bramall , *Midwives in history and society*, (London, 1986) pp 195-196; M Van Lieburg, H Marland, 'Midwifery regulation, education and practice in the Netherlands during the nineteenth century', *Medical history*, (1989) (33), pp 296-317.

40. L Stephens, 'Midwifery-led care', in L Reid, *Midwifery: freedom to practise?* (Elsevier: Edinburgh 2007), pp 144-163.

41. Reid, *Scottish Midwives 1916-1983*, pp 43, 60, 74, 97, 104-105; McGuire M, Reid L, Hillan E, *The perceptions and experiences of newly qualified single registered midwives in Scotland*, (Glasgow: University of Glasgow, 1998), p 2.

42. The *'bona fides'* or uncertified midwives, also known as howdies, were certified by the CMBS provided they had been in practice for a minimum of one year before 1916.

43. Council Directives, (80/155/EEC), *Official Journal of the European Communities*, (1980), L 33/8.

44. Teaching or training institutions were selected from maternity hospitals and maternity departments within a general hospital.

45. *CMBS Rules*, 1940, Rules C 21 (a), (b) and (c), 20.

46. NAS, CMB 1/7, *CMBS Minutes*, 23 February 1949, p 4; .NAS, CMB 1/7, *CMBS Minutes*, 26 August 1948, p 1.

47. *CMBS Rules*, 1947, Rules B 28, 22.

48. NAS, CMB 1/7, *CMBS Minutes*, 31 May 1951, p 1; *RCM Scottish Council Minutes*, 5 May 1951.

49. *CMBS Rules*, 1968, pp 5, 18.

50. Towler, Bramall, *Midwives in History and Society*, pp 207, 227.

51. NAS, CMB 1/5, *CMBS Minutes*, 28 February 1936, Vol 20, p 38; NAS, CMB 1/5, *CMBS Minutes*, 27 March 1936, Vol 21, p 8; NAS, CMB 1/5, *CMBS Minutes*, 24 April 1936, Vol 21, p 9; NAS, CMB 1/5, *CMBS Minutes*, 28 October 1937, Vol 22, p 23; the Board and its committees worked very slowly. It is likely that this and a heavy workload combined to slow down the compilation of the first Scottish MTD course. Board Minutes do not explain why the Scottish Board of the College of Nursing was involved here. In England, the College of Midwives initially organised the course and then in collaboration with the College of Nursing. The Scottish Midwives Association, equivalent to the

English College of Midwives, probably did not have the resources to run the MTD course.

52. NAS, CMB 1/5, *CMBS Minutes*, 17 December 1937, Vol 22, p 25.
53. E F Catford, *The Royal Infirmary of Edinburgh 1929-1979*, (Edinburgh: Scottish Academic Press, 1984), pp 209-210; S Bramley, M Turner, 'Obituary: Mrs Margaret Fraser Myles 1892-1988', in *Midwifery*, (1988) (4), pp 93-94. The term 'tutor' came into use about this time, possibly to differentiate between 'teachers' who in this context were midwives without the MTD, and midwives who had passed the MTD.
54. *Maternity Services (Scotland) Act*, 1937 [I Edw 8 & I Geo 6 Ch 30], 8, (4), (a).
55. NAS, CMB 1/5, *CMBS Minutes*, 25 February 1938, Vol 22, p 32; NAS, CMB 1/6, *CMBS Minutes*, 20 February 1942, Vol 26, p 17; *ibid*, 2 April, 1942, p 31; *ibid*, 26 February 1943, p 36; *NAS, CMB* 1/7, *CMBS Minutes*, 13 April 1943, p 3.
56. NAS, CMB 1/7, *CMBS Minutes*, 25 July, 1950, p 1; NAS, CMB 1/7, *CMBS Minutes*, 20 November 1947, p 3; NAS, CMB 1/7, *CMBS Minutes*, 26 February 1953, 'Chairman's review of the Board's progress since 1915', p 4.
57. *CMBS Report*, 31 March 1967, p 2.
58. *CMBS Report*, 31 March 1971, p 2.
59. NAS, CMB 1/2, *CMBS Minutes*, 11 August 1916, Vol 1, p 23.
60. *Ibid*, 28 September 1916, p 27, 30; *Midwives (Scotland) Act*, 21.
61. NAS, CMB 1/2, *CMBS Minutes*, 28 September 1916, Vol 1, p 30.
62. *Midwives (Scotland) Act*, 13; NAS, CMB 1/2, *CMBS Minutes*, 28 September 1916, Vol 1, p 29.
63. NAS, CMB 1/2, *CMBS Minutes*, 22 March 1917, Vol 2, p 8; *ibid*, 7 February 1918, p 44.
64. NAS, CMB 1/2, *CMBS Minutes*, 17 October 1918, Vol 3, p 27; NAS, CMB 1/2, *CMBS Minutes*, 22 July 1920, Vol 5, p 28; *ibid.*, 20 January 1921, p 54.
65. NAS, CMB 1/3, *CMBS Report*, 27 July 1921, p 8.
66. NAS, CMB 1/2, *CMBS Minutes*, 25 May 1916, Vol 1, p 16; *ibid*, 7 December 1916, p 45.
67. NAS, CMB 1/2, *CMBS Report*, 27 July 1921, p 6.
68. NAS, CMB 1/2, *CMBS Report*, 17 October 1918, p 4.
69. NAS, CMB 1/2, *CMBS Minutes*, 30 September 1920, Vol 5, p 33.
70. M Uprichard, 'The Evolution of Midwifery Education', *in Midwives' Chronicle*, January 1987, p 4.
71. NAS, CMB 1/2, *CMBS Minutes*, 30 September 1920, Vol 5 p 33.
72. *Midwives (Scotland) Act*, 1 (1).
73. *Ibid*, 2; NAS, CMB 1/2, *CMBS Minutes*, 13 December 1917, Vol 2, p 40; NAS, CMB 1/2, *CMBS Minutes*, 18 July 1918, Vol 3, p 20; NAS, CMB 1/2, *CMBS Minutes*, 22 April 1920, Vol 5, p 15; NAS, CMB 1/2, *CMBS Report*, 24 July 1919, p 6.
74. *Midwives (Scotland) Act*, 16 (1).
75. *Ibid*; NAS, CMB 4/2/10, *CMBS Rules*, 1916, E (25) p 16 describes in brief the duties of an IOM.
76. LR 27; By this time the IOM was called Supervisor of Midwives (SOM).

77. NAS, CMB 1/2, *CMBS Minutes, 6 July 1916, Vol 1, p 18.*

78. *Midwives (Scotland) Act*, 16, (1); NAS, CMB 1/2, *CMBS Minutes*, 28 September 1916, Vol 1, p 28.

79. NAS, CMB 1/2, *CMBS Minutes*, 11 November 1917, Vol 2, p 32; *ibid*, 13 December 1917, p 39; *ibid*, 2 February 1918, p 45.

80. Donnison, *Midwives and Medical Men*, p 180; Towler and Bramall make the same point: Towler, Bramall, *Midwives in History and Society*, p 228.

81. *Midwives (Scotland) Act*, 22, (1).

82. NAS, CMB 1/2, *CMBS Minutes*, 28 September 1916, Vol 1, p 30; *ibid*, p 27.

83. *Ibid*, 8 February 1917, p 47.

84. Donnison, *Midwives and Medical Men*, p 182. This led to increasingly poor relationships between doctors and midwives in England and Wales. The problem of doctors' payment in England and Wales was resolved, on paper at least, when the 1918 Midwives Act brought the legislation for England and Wales into line with that of Scotland regarding the statutory obligation for LSAs to pay for medical aid in a midwifery emergency.

85. NAS, CMB 1/2, *CMBS Minutes*, 19 July 1917, Vol 2, p 22.

86. NAS, CMB 1/2, *CMBS Minutes*, 24 July 1919, Vol 4, p 14; The SBH was established in 1919 'to develop wider and more co-ordinated health services for the people of Scotland'; J Hogarth, 'General Practice', in McLachlan, (ed), *Improving the Common Weal*, p 177.

87. J Hogarth, 'General Practice', p 178.

88. Loudon, , *Death in Childbirth*, p 6; Womersley, J, 'The evolution of health information services', in McLachlan, Improving the Common Weal, p 553; G Bisset-Smith, *Vital Registration, (2nd ed),* (Edinburgh: William Green, 1907), p 5. Civil registration of births, deaths and marriages was introduced in England in 1837 but was permissive rather than compulsory; Loudon, *Death in Childbirth*, pp 23, 25, 28.

89. Loudon, *Death in Childbirth*, p 34.

90. *Ibid*, p 38; Puerperal sepsis and puerperal fever (the legal term) appear to be interchangeable. Puerperal fever was made compulsorily notifiable in Britain by the 1889 Infectious Disease (Notification) Act. Later, puerperal pyrexia was made a separate, notifiable condition in Scotland. See M Myles, *A Textbook for Midwives, (7th ed)*, (Edinburgh: Churchill Livingstone, 1971), p 478; Also, L Mackenzie, 'Notification of Puerperal Fever, II', *The Transactions of the Edinburgh Obstetrical Society*, Session LXXXVII, 1927-1928, pp 38-44. (Reproduced in *The Edinburgh Medical Journal*, New Series, Vol. XXXV, (3), March 1928).

91. Scottish Board of Health (SBH) Departmental Committee, *Report on Puerperal Morbidity and Mortality*, the *Salvesen Report*, (Edinburgh: HMSO, 1924), p 4.

92. A Oakley, *The Captured Womb* (Oxford: Basil Blackwell Publisher Ltd, 1984), p 62; *ibid*, p 65; Ministry of Health 1924, *Maternal Mortality*, (J M Campbell) Reports on public health and medical subjects No 48, (London: HMSO, 1924); *Salvesen Report*.

93. NAS, CMB 1/3, *CMBS Minutes*, 30 August 1923, Vol 8, p 32.

94. *Salvesen Report*, pp 19, 9, 37.

95. *Ibid*, p 5.

96. *Ibid*, p 8.

97. *Ibid*, p 6.

98. *Ibid*, pp 19, 21, 31.

99. Loudon, *Death in Childbirth*, pp 417, 152, 402-407. 444.

100. *Ibid*, p 251.

101. NAS, CMB 1/3, *CMBS Minutes*, 26 June 1924, Vol 9, p 26; although antenatal care was increasingly prominent in the midwifery curriculum, in practice, midwives found that their role in this field was small.

102. NAS, CMB 1/3, *CMBS Minutes*, 26 June 1924, Vol 9, pp 25, 28.

103. NAS, CMB 1/3, *CMBS Minutes*, 1 February 1923, Vol 7, p 54.

104. J M Munro Kerr, *Maternal Mortality and Morbidity: a study of their problems*, (Edinburgh: E&S Livingstone, 1933), p 59.

105. J Kinnaird, 'The Hospitals', in McLachlan, (ed), *Improving the Common Weal*, p 234; NAS, CMB 1/3; *CMBS Minutes*, 2 February 1925, Vol 9, p 50.

106. NAS, CMB 2/10-14, *CMBS Report*, 31 March 1926, p 6; *Midwives and Maternity Homes (Scotland) Act*, [17 & 18 Geo 5. Ch 17], 1927.

107. NAS, CMB 1/3, *CMBS Minutes*, 28 May 1925, Vol 10, p 17; NAS, CMB 1/3, *CMBS Minutes*, 26 August 1926, Vol 11, p 27; NAS CMB, 2/10-14, *CMBS Report*, 31 March 1926, p 9; NAS, CMB 1/3, *CMBS Minutes*, 16 December 1926, Vol 11, p 42.

108. *Midwives (Scotland) Act*, 1 (2).

109. *Midwives and Maternity Homes (Scotland) Act*, 1 (2).

110. Donnison, *Midwives and Medical Men*, p 181.

111. NAS, CMB 2/10-14, *CMBS Report*, 31 March 1926; cases of this sort probably came to light when a birth was notified which was/is a statutory requirement.

112. *Hansard*, Commons, Vol 203, 18 March 1927, col 2400.

113. NAS, CMB 1/4, *CMBS Minutes*, 16 June 1927, Vol 12, p 20; *Midwives and Maternity Homes (Scotland) Act*, 1 (2).

114. *Hansard*, Commons, Vol 207, 24 June 1927, col 2278.

115. NAS, CMB 1/4, *CMBS Minutes*, 18 August 1927, Vol 12, p 23.

116. *Midwives and Maternity Homes (Scotland) Act*, 9 (1); *ibid*, 10, 11; *ibid*, 12; *ibid*, 13 (1); *ibid*, 15, (1), (2), (3), (4).

117. DHS, *Report on Maternal Morbidity and Mortality in Scotland*, (Edinburgh: HMSO, 1935), p 5, (Douglas and McKinley Report); The authors of the Report acknowledged their gratitude to Dr James Haig Ferguson (CMBS Chairman) who studied every completed maternal death report received and who died in 1934 before the Report was published: Douglas and McKinley Report, p 29; There was a shortfall of about twenty deaths per year for which figures were not obtainable.

118. NAS, CMB 1/5, *CMBS Minutes*, 12 May 1932, Vol 17, p 18; *ibid*, 13 October 1932, p 23; NAS, CMB 1/5, *CMBS Minutes*, 22 November 1934, Vol 19, p 34.

119. *Ibid*, 20 December 1934, p 42.

120. *Douglas and McKinley Report*, p 24.

121. Ibid, p 15.

122. Ibid, pp 25, 26, 16, 27.

123. Ibid, pp 27, 10.

124. Loudon, *Death in Childbirth*, p 244.

125. A S Williams, *Women and Childbirth in the Twentieth Century*, (Stroud: Sutton Publishing, 1997), p 59.

126. J MacLeod, *Notes on Maternal Mortality and Morbidity with Special Reference to Maternity Work in General Practice*, (Unpublished MD Thesis, University of Aberdeen, 1935), p 10.

127. *Ibid*, p 2.

128. *Douglas and McKinley Report*, p 28.

129. *Maternity Services (Scotland) Act*, 1937, [1 Edw 8 & 1 Geo 6], 1, (2e).

130. LR 91.

131. *Douglas and McKinley Report*, pp 24, 28.

132. *Ibid*, p 29.

133. J Brotherston, J Brims, 'The development of public medical care: 1900-1948', in McLachlan, (ed), *Improving the Common Weal*, p 75; DHS, *Committee on Scottish Health Services Report*, Cmnd 5204, *Cathcart Report*, (Edinburgh: HMSO, 1936), Chapter XIV, *'Maternity and child welfare', pp 170-182.*

134. Hansard, Commons, Vol 319, 28 January 1937, Cols 1099-1155.

135. *Ibid.*

136. *Hansard*, Commons, Vol 317, 10 November 1936, Cols 698-699; S M Herbert, *Britain's Health*, (Harmondsworth: Penguin Books, 1939), p 138.

137. *Hansard*, Commons, Vol 319, 28 January 1937, Cols 1099-1155.

138. *Maternity Services (Scotland) Act*, 1 (1).

139. *Hansard*, Commons, Vol 319, 28 January 1937, Cols 1099-1155; NAS, CMB 1/5, *CMBS Minutes*, 19 March, 1937, Vol 22, p 8.

140. *Maternity Services (Scotland) Act*, 1 (2); *ibid*, 1 (3-11).

141. *Ibid*, 2; *Hansard*, Commons, Vol 319, 28 January 1937, cols 1099-1155; *Maternity Services (Scotland) Act*, 3 (1).

142. *Hansard*, Commons, Vol 319, 28 January 1937, cols 1099-1155.

143. *Maternity Services (Scotland) Act*, 4.

144. *Ibid*, 6 (1).

145. *Hansard*, Commons, Vol 319, 28 January 1937, cols 1099-1155.

146. LR 108.

147. *Maternity Services (Scotland) Act*, 7 (1), (2).

148. NAS, CMB 1/3, *CMBS Minutes*, 5 May 1927, Vol 11, p 15; NAS, CMB 1/3, *CMBS Minutes*, 20 September 1928, Vol 13, p 20.

149. Loudon, *Death in Childbirth*, p 255; See also Loudon, *Death in Childbirth*, pp 258-261, for a discussion on the use of antibiotics, especially prontosil rubrum in puerperal fever, firstly in hospitals and then in general practice.

150. L Kennedy, *In bed with an elephant*, (London: Bantam Press, 1995). Kennedy discusses the problems which arise when one lives next door to a much bigger neighbour. Also, P H Scott, *Still in bed with an elephant*, (Edinburgh: The Saltire Society, 1998).

Chapter 4

Antenatal: from innovation to integration

Before the beginning of the twentieth century, antenatal care as recognised today was non-existent. As pregnancy was viewed as a normal event and nature was considered to need no assistance, advice offered to pregnant women was confined to suggestions on a recommended lifestyle.[1] Since the early twentieth century, the 'normal event', pregnancy, fell increasingly under the care (or jurisdiction) of those doctors developing the specialty of obstetrics.[2] However, as women were not in the habit of attending for antenatal care, development of knowledge about pregnancy was slow. This chapter examines aspects of antenatal care in Scotland: the beginning of antenatal care and clinics; midwives' involvement (or otherwise) from 1916; how the relevant Acts and CMBS *Rules* restricted midwives' practice; antenatal care in urban and rural areas; why, for years, many mothers had no antenatal care; and, changes in care.

The dawning of organised antenatal care

In the early twentieth century, maternal and infant mortality rates were very high. For the years 1901-1905 the Infant Mortality Rate (IMR) in Scotland was 120 per 1,000 live births and the Maternal Mortality Rate (MMR) was 5.1 per 1,000 live births. The MMR rose to 6.1 in 1915 and remained around that level until the mid-1930s.[3] Correspondingly, the Boer War (1899-1902) demonstrated the low level of fitness of enlisted men. The Government's 1904 investigation and *Report on the Physical Deterioration of the Population* at last noted the importance of infant welfare: improvement should come, not from increased and better care of pregnant women, but from the less costly option of better education of pregnant women.[4]

Not everyone agreed. Edinburgh obstetrician and pioneer of antenatal care, John W Ballantyne (1861-1923) thought attention should be turned to pregnancy. 'Ballantyne's dream' saw a day when science and technology would give obstetricians the power 'to extract every fetus from the womb live and healthy' and to predict the time of birth by inducing labour. In 1901, he argued for a 'Pro-Maternity Hospital', an in-patient establishment for pregnant women, primarily for the understanding and treating of 'morbid' pregnancies, and through his influence, the first antenatal bed in Britain, soon emulated elsewhere, was opened in Edinburgh. Ballantyne's main interest was not healthy pregnant women, but pregnancy itself. Any woman in his antenatal bed could add to the knowledge of pregnancy, its physiology, pathology and effects of treatment.[5]

However, another side to caring for pregnant women put women's wellbeing first. In 1899, Dr James Haig Ferguson, also of Edinburgh, a colleague of Ballantyne's and a future CMBS chairman, helped to set up a home for unmarried mothers in late pregnancy at 4 Lauriston Place, Edinburgh. There he found 'that rest, good food, healthy surroundings and medical supervision' gave improved outcomes with fewer pre-term births, higher birthweights and lower neonatal mortality.[6] The obstetrician's first duty was to preserve maternal life and health: all pregnant women should have antenatal 'supervision'.[7] In 1915, his antenatal clinic 'for infant and prematernity consultations' began at Edinburgh Royal Maternity Hospital.[8]

The development of antenatal care
From Ballantyne and Ferguson's time, the provision of antenatal care slowly increased. It was aided after the 1915 Notification of Births (Extension) Act by the development in Scotland of 'Schemes of Maternity and Child Welfare' which allowed Local Authorities (LA) to devise antenatal clinics of varying sizes and type.[9] In addition, the 1918 Maternity and Child Welfare Act enabled municipal authorities to fund salaried midwives and health visitors, free or cheap food for mothers and children, antenatal clinics and day nurseries. The primary purpose of antenatal clinics was free medical supervision and advice for uninsured women.[10] In time, clinics also became a source of health education and 'mothercraft'. The increase in municipal clinic antenatal care eventually dominated care in pregnancy for the next forty years until hospital-based care became the controlling element of antenatal provision.[11]

Especially in towns and cities, antenatal work in municipal clinics increased in the 1920s, staffed by public health medical officers, nurses, midwives and/or health visitors.[12] To have antenatal clinics like these in highly populated areas, along with further development of hospital antenatal clinics, was in line with Government recommendations of the day. However, quality of care was an early issue and it was often inadequate and perfunctory.[13]

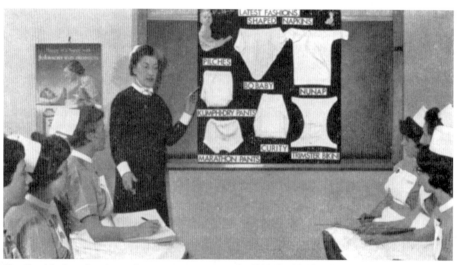

Pupil midwives having a lesson in parentcraft, GRMH 1960s. (Courtesy of Eleanor Stenhouse.) Reprinted from M Myles, A textbook for midwives (6th ed), (E&S Livingstone, 1968) p 673, fig 450.

Many mothers did not attend clinics or seek medical advice. In some areas there were no clinics within easy reach or, where they did exist, they were often inadequate. In St Andrews in 1926, poor arrangements prompted the Town Council to start a new antenatal clinic for 'necessitous and other mothers', with local doctors providing free services and midwives instructed to encourage needy mothers to attend two or three times in the pregnancy.[14] Even in areas where antenatal clinics were in operation, only a small proportion of mothers attended.[15] The first reference to antenatal care in a CMBS *Annual Report* in 1926, indicated the need and commented on the number of emergency labours where the mother had received no previous care.[16]

However, municipal clinics did not give mothers continuity of care from ante to intranatal. The 1935 *Douglas and McKinley Report* recommended more continuity or, at least, record-transfer from clinic to the midwife attending the confinement.[17] Two years later, the 1937 Maternity Services (Scotland) Act required LAs to coordinate and control maternity services professionals and to bring a spirit of team-working.[18] However, not all LAs achieved co-ordination (the Act was not adopted in Glasgow and Dundee), and LA antenatal clinics were still mainly staffed by public health doctors.[19]

The use of municipal antenatal clinics continued in urban areas of Scotland with varying levels of success until the implementation of the NHS Acts in 1948 brought further change. The NHS's tripartite structure dispelled the attempt of the 1937 Maternity Services (Scotland) Act to encourage professionals in the maternity services to work as a team. The GP, now the first point of contact for most pregnant women, had a greater part to play than ever before in antenatal care. Simultaneously, the demand for hospital births increased and the use of hospital antenatal clinics rose correspondingly, particularly as some women, to be sure of a hospital bed for delivery, by-passed the LA clinic and went directly to the hospital clinic. LA clinics, caught between GP and hospital in the competition for patients, became significantly less popular.

The demand for LA clinics fell further in the 1950s. The NHS structure left confusion in its wake and in 1956 the Government appointed the Montgomery Committee to review and report on the maternity services in Scotland.[20] The Committee's Report in 1959 recommended GP co-ordination of maternity services. If a woman went first to her LA antenatal clinic, unless she objected, the clinic staff should inform the GP. Also, LAs should instruct their midwives to urge women wishing to book their services to make arrangements with the GP.[21] The Committee also recommended more maternity beds, specifically eight antenatal hospital beds per 1,000 annual births. The LA clinics therefore declined with a drop in attendances to fifteen per cent across Britain by 1958.[22] To rectify the consequent fall in parentcraft and health education, GPs and obstetricians took over municipal clinic premises and staff in order to offer a 'comprehensive service of medical care, supervision, health education and guidance.'[23] GPs still undertook antenatal care in their surgeries and there was a rise in hospital clinics, hospital births and number of consultant obstetricians.[24]

Where did the midwife come in?
Examination of the early days of antenatal care gives little evidence of the midwife's place in this field. Although the 1915 Midwives (Scotland) Act provided for the CMBS to make Rules for certified midwives to follow, it made no reference to antenatal care. In the first complete set of CMBS *Rules* of 1916, there were no specific references to antenatal care of women, and few to pregnancy.[25] CMBS *Rules* required that a pupil midwife should be examined in:

Pregnancy
1.   Its hygiene;
2.   Its diseases and complications including abortion;
      both in relation to a) the mother and b) the unborn child.[26]

Rules E, covering midwives' practice, ordered a midwife to summon medical assistance in all cases of illness or abnormality. More specifically, during pregnancy, a midwife had to call for medical aid when there was 'any abnormality or complication, such as: deformity or stunted growth; loss of blood; abortion or threatened abortion; excessive sickness; puffiness of hands or face; fits or convulsions; dangerous varicose veins; purulent discharge; sores of the genitals'.[27] These *Rules,* therefore, acknowledged that midwives had contact with pregnant women, but did not specify how the midwife should practise and how or what pupil midwives should be taught.

      When the longer midwifery training was initiated in 1926, it included specific antenatal training and examination. This was aided by the presence of more women attending antenatal clinics.[28] A pupil midwife had to achieve the 'supervision' of at least twenty pregnant women in preparation for an examination which included 'the physiology, diagnosis, and management of normal pregnancy.'[29]

      Therefore the level of knowledge of pregnancy and antenatal care required for the CMBS examination gradually grew, although it was difficult to put this into practice. The *Rule Books* from 1918 onwards informed midwives of LA provision of 'maternity centres' and said, 'the midwife should advise the patient to avail herself of such help', thereby denying most midwives (booked to deliver the baby) the opportunity of performing normal antenatal care.[30] Some midwives did work in LA clinics, but there is no evidence that the CMBS encouraged midwives to perform antenatal care by themselves, either in clinics or in mothers' homes.

      The CMBS *Rules* did not help. Midwives had to keep a register containing details of their clients, abnormalities found, and if a mother had gone as advised to the clinic or a medical officer.[31] From 1918, midwives had to keep a form, supplied in the *Rules,* of 'Register of Cases'. However, until 1931, the only relevant antenatal details requested were 'Date of expected confinement' and 'Number of previous labours and miscarriages.' In 1931 (and only updated in 1968) the register became a two page document requiring more antenatal detail – an apparent step forward that was cancelled out in the same *Rule Book* by the Rule ordering the midwife to advise the patient to seek medical advice or attend the LA facilities and 'submit herself for medical examination' early in pregnancy.[32] If a mother did not co-operate, the midwife had to notify the LSA on the official 'Form of notification of patient's failure to follow advice.'[33]

      Therefore, in many areas midwives had little authority in antenatal care even for mothers undergoing a normal pregnancy. It was all right to co-operate by working in LA clinics, not autonomously, but under the constant surveillance of public health doctors.[34] Midwives booked for a birth could also attend clinics with women, but still under supervision.[35] They also sometimes attended lectures supplied at the clinics, particularly for the *bona fide* midwives. However, many midwives sent mothers to clinics but did not do antenatal care themselves.[36]

      In England and Wales midwives seemed to be more independent and it appeared to be the norm for a midwife to have considerable input into antenatal care. To go routinely to a doctor would encroach 'upon the duties of the midwife in the antenatal sphere.'[37] *Maternity in Great Britain* (1948), a survey of mothers who gave birth during the week 3rd to 9th March 1946, further emphasised the differences in who 'supervised' antenatal care in different parts of Britain. Mothers said that they received care from LAs including clinics, GP schemes, and midwives in clinics and at home. Some mothers received care privately from 'specialists', practitioners (GPs) and midwives. Many mothers attended one category and were sent to another. When discussing GP schemes for antenatal care, the Report stated that in Scotland medical practitioners took a much more active part in the antenatal services than in England and Wales.[38]

Variations in provision and uptake

In urban Scotland during the 1920s and 1930s, the antenatal care on offer varied widely. For differing reasons, pregnant women frequently had no professional antenatal input at all.[39] For example, Ann Lamb, who was a pupil midwife in Edinburgh, 1927-1928, said, 'There was no antenatal care. Some people didn't even know they were having a baby till they delivered. Poverty was very bad, very, very bad, but [they were] cheery people.'[40] Molly Muir, a pupil midwife in Edinburgh in the 1930s, reinforced the link between poverty and lack of antenatal care:

> Working in Gorgie at that time there were very few antenatal clinics. Sometimes when the mother went into labour you found it was a face presentation.[41] That was the worst I ever came across. Other things happened that you didn't know anything about until the mother was in labour. There was very little antenatal care.[42]

Even though mothers had little or no antenatal care, it was usual to make preparations for the birth. Molly Muir recalled:

> I think they had all made arrangements even though there were so few antenatal clinics. I think that when somebody was pregnant and they knew they were going to get the midwife in for the delivery, it was arranged quite a long time in advance. Then, when the time came she would phone the hospital [for a midwife] from a public telephone.[43]

Other reasons for non-attendance emerged. Margaret Foggie, who was a South African and a pupil midwife in Glasgow in 1934, pointed out:

> Unemployment was terrible and there was such a kind of despair about it. Glasgow Corporation produced a layette for the new baby if the woman had been to the antenatal clinic and got a form saying she was pregnant. They had to go and get this layette which was fine for the baby and very often they hadn't even bothered to go and do it. There was such a kind of feeling of I don't know what – apathy. And even in some of the new tenements that had been built where there were baths and things, they didn't use the baths. I actually have seen coal in the bath. It was very sad. I had never seen people living like that. It was awful, absolutely awful.[44]

John Martin Munro Kerr (1868-1960), the eminent obstetrician, agreed. He wrote: 'the patient herself is often her own worst enemy, whether from ignorance, apathy, ill-health, or prejudice.'[45]

Occasionally, pregnancy was considered to be a secret. This sometimes happened in Shetland where the picture of antenatal care in the 1920s and 1930s depended on location. Local historian Chrissie Sandison recollected:

> The women in the early twenties, they never had any examinations or care beforehand. I remember Jimmy's mother telling me about when she was young. When she was having her children it was kept a secret until she was sure...then the mother who was expecting would speak to some old neighbour, somebody she knew would help and they kept it a secret – although they would have been asked, they never told anybody... Lots of those expectant mothers of all those years ago...had no pre-natal examinations. An expectant mother *at da faain-fit*, which meant 'getting near to the time of delivery', would have 'spoken for' a midwife. All else was left to Mother Nature. Sometimes all went well, sometimes not.[46]

Margaret MacDonald, who was a 'Green Lady' in Glasgow from 1947 to 1952, agreed that mothers did not discuss their pregnancies and suggested this as a reason for non-attendance at clinics:

> Women in these days were different from women today. Everything today is open and above board and people talk about everything. From sex, from conception, right up to delivery. They talk about all sorts of things. In these days we didn't. It was all kept under wraps. Nothing was open and above board... They didn't trust people to know about them. They didn't want to – my mother didn't do it [go to clinics] so I'll not do it. That kind of thing. That was the attitude.[47]

Mima Sutherland, a midwife on Unst, Shetland, in the 1940s and 1950s gave a different picture, indicating continuing antenatal care:

> In my time the mothers were all supervised. You could see them and they could get their urine tested... then you would know if they needed to see the doctor. They were seen regularly. Then you would wait for them to send for you [when they went into labour].[48]

One difference between the two Shetland contributors is geographic. Chrissie Sandison was reporting the situation on the mainland of Shetland, big enough to be broken up into villages, rural communities and a capital town, Lerwick. Mima Sutherland was midwife to a more distant island community and this probably contributed to her ability to give care. Similarly, in the Outer Hebrides, the midwife (1940s-1950s) seemed to have a significant input into antenatal care:

> I did the antenatal care all the time and sometimes on the first visit the mother would say, 'There's another one on the way but don't tell the doctor yet'. I would say, 'But I must tell the doctor'. The doctor went after you notified him. They didn't book early. After that we visited fortnightly, and

weekly for the last month. We were on call when they came to term.[49]

In areas of Scotland where uncertificated midwives or howdies worked, they sometimes moved in with the family, not to provide formal antenatal care, but to help with the household work as Doddie Davidson, a howdie in Aberdeenshire, did in the 1930s and 1940s: 'I went an lived in the hoose afore the bairns were born. Usually they were needin some help especially fan there wis some little anes.'[50] Annie Kerr, a howdie in the Dumfries area in the 1940s said the same: 'I went a wee while before the baby wis born. Not as much as a couple o weeks...I wis with them and did everything that wis to be done ye know, to give her a rest. That workit in fine.'[51]

One howdie who practised in King Street, Aberdeen, in the 1930s also visited before the birth, but likewise not to give formal antenatal care. Her grand-daughter wrote, 'On her prenatal visits she instructed the mothers on what she would need regarding equipment at the time of birth and I believe that she was a stickler for having everything ready in advance wherever possible.'[52]

Therefore, in Scotland in the early decades of the twentieth century, when most babies were delivered at home by a midwife, antenatal care differed from place to place with little midwifery input. Where antenatal care existed, many mothers did not take up the opportunity unless, as happened in the smaller communities, the midwife attended them at home.

Antenatal care in urban areas
The provision of antenatal care not only differed between urban and rural communities, but also among urban areas. This is shown by examination of pupil midwives' Case Books, the 'Blue Book' that was required from 1928 for presentation at the final CMBS examination. The Blue Book contained a record, including a review of the case, of twenty women a pupil had cared for in labour (ten in hospital and ten at home), had delivered personally and looked after postnatally.[53]

The Blue Book also included a 'history of pregnancy.' This was a brief résumé of the type of care, if any, that a mother had received and how often she was seen during her pregnancy. A small survey of six Blue Books has revealed details of the pregnancy histories of 124 women from different places in Scotland from 1939 to 1946.

The 124 women were chosen by the pupil midwives for their Blue Books and therefore cannot be described as a random sample. Nevertheless, in four out of the six Blue Books, the majority of women (sixty-three per cent) attended the municipal antenatal clinic. This meant they received their antenatal care free; they were also probably seen by a public health doctor (who was not necessarily experienced in midwifery/obstetrics) and a midwife, nurse or health visitor employed at the clinic. So, when they went into labour, they would very likely be delivered by a midwife or student midwife who did not know their antenatal history. Margaret MacDonald, Green Lady, also implied that she received information about what happened at the clinic from the woman herself rather than from transfer of records.

> Antenatal care was [given] at a clinic and it wasn't always the person who was going to deliver the woman who was responsible for the antenatal care...we were responsible for giving her advice and for telling her what she

should do but she went to this clinic for any examinations... If it was a hospital emergency [we knew] nothing [about her history]. [If it was a booked case] you knew all about her [through]... what the woman would tell me. How she'd got on at the clinic... There was very little antenatal care... [Most] mothers didn't go to the clinics, definitely.[54]

Table 4.1 Antenatal Care given to mothers in urban areas

Type of ANC	Aberdeen Mat 1939-40	Glasgow Rob 1947	Edinburgh SMMP 1944	Motherwell 1945	Bellshill 1943	Glasgow SGH 1946	Total	%
ANC / municipal	16	17	6	12	8	19	78	63
Admit/ ANC	5	1	0	0	0	0	6	5
No ANC	3	1	2	2	0	0	8	6
Own GP / midwife	0	1	1	6	12/ 5	1	21/ 5	17+ 4
Hosp. Clinic	0	0	11	0	0	0	11	9
Total	24	20	20	20	20	20	124	100+4

Source: Blue Case Books 1939-1947 belonging to: LR 80, 16, 108, 2, 90, and 93.

Key:

Aberdeen Mat: Aberdeen Maternity Hospital.
Glasgow Rob: Glasgow Robroyston Hospital.
Edinburgh SMMP: Edinburgh Simpson Memorial Maternity Pavilion.
Motherwell: Motherwell Maternity Hospital.
Bellshill: County Maternity Hospital, Bellshill. Women lived in surrounding towns and villages.
Glasgow SGH: Glasgow Southern General Hospital.
ANC/Municipal: Municipal antenatal clinic run by the city or town corporation.
Admit/ANC: Mothers in this category had no antenatal care until they were admitted to the antenatal ward of their maternity hospital for a reason other than labour.
No ANC: No antenatal care at all.
Own GP/midwife: Mothers in this category went to their own GP for antenatal care. In a few instances they mentioned that they had seen a midwife there and the extra figures indicate where this has happened.
Hosp-clinic: Mothers attended the antenatal clinic at the hospital.

The Blue Book specifically mentioned in only five cases, all in Bellshill, that a midwife was involved in the antenatal care at the GP surgery. Each of these mothers had a homebirth. There is nothing in the case histories to indicate whether or not the midwife at the surgery was the midwife in attendance with the pupil midwife at the birth, reinforcing evidence of lack of continuity of care.

The difference in type of care in different towns and cities is also noticeable. For example, in the Edinburgh Blue Book the pupil midwife was training at the SMMP. Eleven out of the twenty women went to the SMMP antenatally. Therefore they would have seen midwives and doctors who were specialists or training in obstetrics.

Another type of antenatal care which is evident in the Edinburgh Blue Book was from the Cowgate Dispensary. Of the six who come into the category of 'ANC/municipal', three went to the Cowgate Dispensary and one of the women who had no antenatal care was a 'Cowgate Dispensary call' when she went into labour. Anne McFadden, whose Blue Book gives these details, explained:

> So many of the people [in] the poorer areas of Edinburgh couldn't afford to get a doctor so they went to [the Cowgate] Dispensary... The mothers could go to antenatal clinics there... But not so many of them did... The antenatal care was available at the Cowgate Dispensary... I think it's important, not all of them...made use of it... [Many more of them] could have done, but didn't. Which meant that...in the emergency of the baby's imminent arrival, they had to phone the Cowgate Dispensary which was always manned. And it was all male [medical] students... I don't remember any female... He got the information, he had the address but that was all. And he phoned [for the pupil midwife] and when you went to the house, if he was quicker than you he was there, because, remember, we were walking...and you went down and you examined – you were the one who did the rectal examination. [This is a pupil midwife] in her second part. And you examined the patient, decided, you know, how far on she was.[55]

Although pupil midwives worked with the Dispensary medical students at homebirths they did not attend their clinics. Anne McFadden continued: '[Midwives didn't work at the Dispensary], not that I know of, because, you see, we in the Simpson had our own ...antenatal clinic.' However, it seemed to be a successful combination. 'We worked hand in hand...It was really a splendid professional relationship.'[56]

As pupil midwives did not use consistent terminology when reporting in the Blue Books, it is not clear how many visits mothers paid to a clinic. The number ranged from one to twenty, and attendance was recorded as 'fairly regular', 'regular', or 'from week thirty-five', showing a lack of a systematic pattern.

Another Blue Book, belonging to Mary Findlay, who was a pupil midwife at Dunfermline Maternity Hospital in 1958-1959, revealed a change in type of antenatal care.[57] This Blue Book contained details of ten women. Of five women who had hospital births, all attended the hospital clinic. Of the five who had homebirths, one attended her own GP, two were attended by their GP and midwife probably at home, one was attended by her midwife at home, and the fifth was attended at home but the status of the attendant is not revealed.

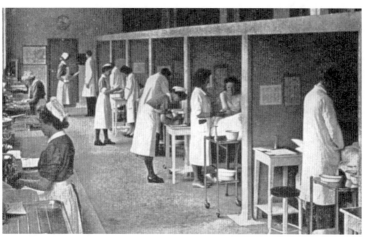

The antenatal clinic, SMMP, 1960s. Reprinted from M Myles, A textbook for midwives (6th ed), (E&S Livingstone, 1968), p 92, fig 69.

So the demise of municipal antenatal clinics was reflected in the Blue Books. Also, Mary Findlay's Blue Book shows a divide between home and hospital care in Dunfermline. This is mirrored in Bangour, West Lothian, in the early 1960s where a midwife said that mothers planning a homebirth received their antenatal care at home from the midwife.[58] The rise in hospital births in the 1950s corresponds with the rise in attendances at hospital antenatal clinics.[59] However, Ella Clelland, who was a pupil midwife in Glasgow in 1957, said of mothers planning a homebirth:

> We saw the mother antenatally, but mostly at the hospital at the clinics. She would be seen by the district midwife and student midwife and doctors once a month till thirty-two weeks, then once a fortnight and then weekly from thirty-six weeks. I don't remember much GP input at all.[60]

Sometimes midwives visited antenatally, not to give physical care but for social reasons. This was sometimes to get to know the mother before delivery and to see that she was prepared, but also to assess the premises for suitability or otherwise for homebirth. Jean Mortimer, a pupil midwife at Rottenrow in 1951-1952, wrote: 'our duties outside the hospital consisted of antenatal visits to meet the expectant mum, to assess the circumstances in the home to see if they were suitable for the delivery and to encourage attendance at the clinic.'[61]

Mary McCaskill, a pupil midwife from 1946 to 1947 in the Southern General Hospital, Glasgow, found the social antenatal visits a useful exercise and felt that they could give some continuity of care:

> During my training in the second part ... I always went out with a trained practising midwife... employed by Glasgow Corporation [a Green Lady], and carried out confinements under her supervision... And usually I had the opportunity to get to know the pregnant ladies during their antenatal period a little bit before so that I wasn't going [in] as a stranger... it was quite usual.[62]

Ella Clelland also assessed the homes and said, '[we] visited them at home to assess the situation and assess their needs and all that kind of thing.'[63] As the demand for hospital births grew and outstripped the number of beds available, the next step was early discharge home. Midwives visited, not only to assess their suitability for homebirth, but also for early discharge.

Antenatal care in rural areas

In rural Scotland antenatal care was inconsistent and depended on where a mother lived, the proximity of a clinic, her motivation, and the presence or absence of midwives and GPs. Doddie Davidson, howdie, obtained work sometimes by recommendation of the GP and often by word of mouth. She said:

> Sometimes they knew there wis a baby expectit, sometimes they didna... This wis in the thirties. They hid nae antenatal care. He [the GP] wid ken if the mother hid been ill or if some of the bairns hid been bad an he'd been up tae the hoose. Bit itherwise, no, no, they didna get ony lookin efter.[64]

Annie Kerr, also a howdie, who attended before the birth to look after the mother and run the household, saw the GP as the main player: 'He'd be attendin her an watchin her aa the time and he would know when the baby wis due.'[65] Peggy Grieve, working as a midwife in Cresswell Maternity Hospital, Dumfries, in the late 1940s, highlighted the importance given to a hospital clinic visit, and the difficulties of getting there which was also stressed in the *Montgomery Report*:[66]

> Some clinics were at the hospital and I can remember a woman coming...and she said...'Can I get away by three o'clock because I must get a bus from the White Sands at half past three?' And I said, 'I'll try, yes. Is there not another bus?' 'No,' she said, 'That's the last one... I left home at half past eight this morning.' She came from the Thornhill direction so she had to get a bus to Thornhill, from Thornhill to Dumfries and from the town centre up to Cresswell, and...back. By the time she got home it would be about half past five, six-ish... She was away all that length of time.[67]

Similarly, some mothers from Glasgow had to travel seventeen miles to get to the clinic at Lennox Castle, opened as an Emergency Maternity Hospital during World War Two. Anne Bayne, who was a pupil midwife at Lennox Castle in 1951, told of mothers' travelling problems and also how bad news was given:

> The patients used to have to travel [by bus] from Glasgow from Dundas Street, and you...had about half a mile up the avenue to come to the clinics...and the consultant saw them out there... A lot of the mothers came out to Lennox Castle...[there were] three consultants at the time that looked after the mothers. It could be hard going. The clinic that sticks in my mind very much was a young lass expecting her first baby... Tweedie Brown...examined her and he said to her, 'Oh well lass,' he said, 'I'm afraid the baby has died. Now you'll just need to go home and wait and when you go into labour, come back in.' And out she went...
>   And I thought this is terrible, this young lass. She would need to get the

bus back into Dundas Street and she could have come from the other side of Glasgow. She maybe had to wait and probably her husband wouldn't be at the bus stop waiting for her. She had still to get a bus to go somewhere else... I got her dressed and there was another woman who was expecting baby number three or four and I said to her, 'Are you going back to Glasgow?' and she said, 'Yes I am.' And I said to her, 'Do you see that lass there? Do you think you could take her under your wing? She's had a wee bit of bad news and I don't think it has sunk in and I don't know if her husband is going to be at Dundas Street to meet her.' She said, 'Dinna you worry... I'll look efter her.' So I had to depend on this woman to take her down to the bus and see her home. And then she just had to wait until she went into labour. They didn't induce labour for that at that time... It was a shame but that was just the norm then and there were high parities, eight, nine, ten was quite usual.[68]

The provision of antenatal care in rural Scotland varied on the area and also on current events. The 1937 Maternity Services (Scotland) Act provided for the development of a more cohesive maternity service in Scotland. Although World War Two began before the Act was fully in operation, in the 1940s there was more intra-professional co-operation. However, any newly-gained midwifery professional ground disappeared when the NHS started in 1948 with its tripartite system of maternity care and high GP profile. The Working Party on Midwives reporting in 1949 commented on GPs' takeover of antenatal care and subsequent diminishing of midwives' status.[69] The ideal of complementary working between midwife and GP and the acknowledgement of the midwife as an expert in all aspects of normal childbearing proved difficult to achieve, especially in the field of antenatal care. Opinions expressed by midwives were often disregarded by GPs. One midwife in the Outer Hebrides described this and how she questioned her own diagnosis:

A young girl came from the mainland to have her baby at her granny's... The first time I saw her, I thought, 'She's got a breech' and notified the doctor. We both went and he said, 'Oh no, that's not a breech. There's the head down there.' Of course I was asking myself, is the doctor right or am I?

I antenataled her [sic] twice over a fortnight and I was still convinced it was a breech. There were no phones and somebody came to my door to call me at about two in the morning... I found her very advanced in labour [with the breech presenting]. There was meconium staining and her uncle was dispatched for the doctor about eight to ten miles away. He had to go quite a bit to the next house and waken the neighbour who had a car. The baby was born and I had tidied up before the doctor arrived.[70]

Anne Bayne, practising in Tullibody in the 1950s, was usually happy with her working relationship with GPs, but described a time when she and the GP did not agree:

This was her fifth baby. She had had twins before and all along she kept saying to me, 'You know I'm haein twins. It's exactly the same as my last twins.' And I agreed wi her. I said, 'You're having twins.' So I said this to the lady doctor. Oh, nonsense, nonsense, she wasn't having twins. This GP would not agree. I said, 'She needs to go into hospital.' 'Oh no, she doesn't need to go into hospital.' So, time wore on and I still insisted that she should be going into hospital and I wrote it in her notes... Anyhow the doctor never went near her, never went to see her but still would not do anything.[71]

After both babies were born at home, with the eventual assistance of the emergency Flying Squad, the consultant obstetrician queried the homebirth in this case. Anne recalled:

I said, 'Dr Rose, it's not my wish. I've been trying since she was four months [pregnant] when I knew it was twins, to have her hospitalised. One, because of her age – she was in her early forties by then; and two, because I knew it was twins and I knew the family history. She had problems with the twins the last time.' So you had this sort of thing to contend with.[72]

Some GPs in rural areas had more input into antenatal care. One mother who had her first baby in 1963 in a small town in the north of Scotland said, 'The only professional I saw for my first pregnancy was my GP. There was no antenatal clinic. I just went to the surgery. I never saw a midwife at all until I went into hospital to have the baby.' However things were different second time round when she had a planned homebirth:

This time the midwife visited me at home the whole time. Once a month, then every two weeks and then every week. But not only that, a few days after the midwife had been, along came the doctor and did exactly the same.[73]

Such duplication of care, which has increased over time and is not cost-effective, emphasises what Cumberlege calls the 'abnormal side of pregnancy' by the constant medical presence and 'deprives the midwife of an interesting and useful side of their work' while at the same time undermines the midwife's confidence in her ability to do her job properly.[74]

So, the provision of antenatal care in rural Scotland lacked cohesion. This only gradually began to change after the reports of the Montgomery Committee in 1959 and Tennent Committee in 1973 recognised this need and made recommendations.

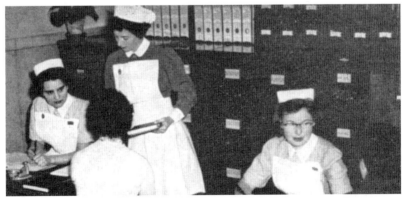

Pupil midwives taking maternal histories, SMMP 1960s. Reprinted from M Myles, A textbook for midwives (6th ed), (E&S Livingstone, 1968), p 93, fig 70.

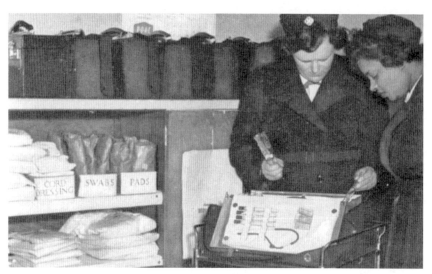

Midwife with pupil midwife setting up for antenatal visits. SMMP 1960s. Reprinted from M Myles, A textbook for midwives (6th ed), (E&S Livingstone, 1968), p 649, fig 442.

Changes in antenatal care: integration and new schemes.

Changes in the provision of antenatal care were apparent from the start of the NHS in 1948, although the varied service to women across Scotland, particularly in rural areas, continued. As far as maternity services in Scotland were concerned, the administration of the NHS was a disappointment. In 1959, the *Montgomery Report* recommended greater intra-professional co-ordination under the GP. 'Co-ordination' became 'integration', demonstrated by the 1973 *Tennent Report* together with the re-organisation of the NHS in 1974.[75] The *Tennent Report*, acknowledging that midwives were 'well on the way to integration', commented on midwifery services still divided into community and hospital.[76] Nevertheless, Agnes Morrison, who worked in Leith in the 1940s, reported some co-operation between hospital and GP:

> They would maybe go to the clinic in the Simpson and then the [doctor there] would say, 'Now we'll write to your GP and he will check on your...state of health.' It would be monthly then or something. And if he was worried he would send them back. [It was a sort of] shared care.[77]

However, on the downside, she also said 'most of ...the mothers [I delivered] I'd never seen ...before. [They had] no antenatal care.'[78]

An early attempt at integration of antenatal care of a kind (although it probably was not called that) was started in the Dumfries and Galloway area in the 1950s because of the distances to the hospital clinic. Peggy Grieve explained:

> After that, some more obstetric staff came and they started peripheral antenatal clinics and they were in Langholm, Annan, Castle Douglas, Kirkcudbright, Newton Stewart and Stranraer and Kirkconnel.... So the

doctors went out to these clinics but the clinics were run by the domiciliary midwives. Often they were treble-duty staff in those areas. The mothers' records were kept in the hospital.[79]

In a similar way, but in a city setting, peripheral or satellite clinics provided antenatal care for women in Aberdeen from the 1950s, staffed by community midwives and obstetric registrars.[80] Most subsequent new schemes involved variations of the integrated service as advocated by the *Tennent Report*, but were also a response to consumer criticisms of the 1970s. Debates on the maternity services developed rapidly in 1974-1975, firstly, because of the speed of technological change (and possibly the indiscriminate routine use of new technology). Secondly, social movements evolved, including the women's movement protesting about women's alienation from their bodies and male medical domination, the ecology movement towards things natural, and a fast-growing consumer movement desiring more control over bureaucracy and insensitivity. Thirdly, the anti-medicalisation lobby queried the causal relationship between medical advances and improved health.[81]

An innovative new scheme started in the Sighthill Health Centre, Edinburgh, in 1976, after statistics revealed a possible correlation between poor attendance rates at antenatal clinics and high Perinatal Mortality Rate (PMR).[82] A combination of community midwife, GP and/or consultant offered women antenatal care on an individual basis depending on the level of perceived risk. Once the scheme was established, consultants left most of the clinics to the midwives and GPs, giving them more time to devote to mothers at higher risk. Midwives, more able to use their initiative, arranged domiciliary visits, made decisions about hospital admissions, arranged scans, gave total prenatal care if appropriate, and worked more as team members. They also found it satisfying to give postnatal care to women they already knew well. GPs felt less sidelined as they took on more responsibility and decision-making. Women received good quality care locally with greater continuity than before. Table 4.2 shows a significant improvement in the PMR. A similar decline in the PMR took place in a corresponding scheme in the Borders.

Table 4.2 Sighthill Health Centre Antenatal Clinic: change in statistics after five years[83]

	1971-1975	1976-1980
Early attendance at clinic	63%	95%
Default rate	16%	1%
Mean antenatal bed occupancy, days/woman	8.5	4.1
Premature delivery rate	15%	7.8%
Intra-uterine growth retardation rate	15%	6.9%
PMR	27.9/1000 (1975)	8/1000 (1980)

Other innovative schemes were started. Peggy Grieve, who was Principal Nursing

Officer (Midwifery) in Fife in the 1970s, set up integration of maternity services there. It was probably a job for a diplomat:

> Dr Melville who was MOH in Kirkcaldy...approached [me] about integration, 'Would the hospital not take over the midwifery in the burgh of Kirkcaldy?' ...There were no [home] confinements...but there was [postnatal] follow up of patients... They granted me money for a full time and a part-time midwife. So that was it started in Kirkcaldy. Then Dr Riddle, who was MOH in Fife County, came and they were not prepared to give any money for staff so we had to get it through the Hospital Board... So we took over Glenrothes next. Then we...took over the district between Glenrothes and Kirkcaldy. We also did Burntisland, Auchtertool, Puddledub, which was East Fife, and then we took over North East Fife...on the first of June...it was snowing that morning. The last place was Leven and that area... As we took over we offered the GPs a midwife to go to their antenatal clinics.[84]

Some GPs were reluctant at first and Peggy Grieve found she had to go slowly.

> I remember going to the GPs and saying, 'Now she's coming to your clinic but I don't expect her just to take blood pressures and test urines... She's there as a midwife and...she can examine some of your patients.' 'Well I like to do my own,' said one GP. And I said, 'Well, OK, but,' I said, 'she can give advice to the patients on health issues and things like that.'[85]

However, Peggy Grieve had to quote the *Rule Book* to one GP who finished up happy:

> The biggest fight I had was Auchtermuchty with Dr [ ] and of course he liked to have everything his own way, and it hadn't been his idea, and when I went to see him...I said, 'Dr [ ], you were a member of the Central Midwives Board. You know what the statutory ruling is and, I said, 'not every patient is being followed up by a midwife here and it must be a practising midwife.' 'Is there a difference between a midwife and a practising midwife?' Anyway, we started it and I met him sometime later. 'That was a great invention.'[86]

There were also the professional feelings to consider, of health visitors who did some postnatal visiting:

> You had to watch very carefully with the health visitors, I could see. I had a meeting in Glenrothes with the health visitors when we were taking over and they were there with the guns and I thought if I lose this I'm finished. I hadn't been in post very long, only a year or a year and a half. And they said, 'What's wrong with us doing the visiting?' I said, 'Nothing wrong with you but what it must be, it must be a midwife for at least ten days [postnatally], longer if necessary.' ...Anyway, [we] parted with a cup of tea and a chat.[87]

The system seemed to settle down well.

> But it went well... I hand-picked the midwives... I can remember...one midwife coming into the office this day, 'I thought I would just come and tell you Miss Grieve, I was at Cardenden and Dr[ ] said to me, 'Would you like

to come and palpate this patient. I'm not sure what way she's presenting.' And she said, 'I just said to him, 'It's a breech.' And he said, 'Oh dear.' So she said, 'I'll tell you what we can do.' She [the mother] was about thirty-four weeks... She said, 'I'll get the obstetricians to get her into the clinic.' Now, you see, that was the relationship, but she was good... and they all appreciated what the integration was. What annoys me is that other places in Scotland did not push ahead with it the same way as we did.[88]

Peggy Grieve's last comment was echoed by the CMBS, showing their changing attitude: 'The Board deplore[s] the slow progress of integration of the maternity service,' emphasised the importance of the role of the midwife, and stated the necessity for the midwife's skills and ability to be used at all levels of decision making.[89]

Another example of an alteration in practice and pattern of care came from Aberdeen as a consequence of an assessment of the system in the mid-1970s. Antenatal care was routine and structured, with little room for individuality and dominated by doctors' decision-making. Midwife-involvement usually was as a doctor's assistant although occasionally community midwives saw women independently at satellite clinics. Women were disappointed with their care, and service providers were concerned that antenatal care was not up to scratch.[90]

The new system addressed issues including: 'Who provides care for whom; how often; in what location; recording what measurements and information; and, with what consequences?'[91] Three new main features emerged: 'low-risk' women would have less routine care; GPs and midwives would have more input into their care; where there were problems, diagnosis and management should improve.[92] In theory, midwives were to take more responsibility for antenatal care: running midwives' clinics at Aberdeen Maternity Hospital (AMH), peripheral clinics for low risk women, and GP antenatal clinics which performed domiciliary visits and giving home antenatal care where necessary. In practice, the redistribution of care was not as great as had been hoped. The number of low-risk women attending AMH and satellite clinics was now lower, some obstetricians might have been reluctant to refer women to midwives, some midwives were nervous, and some GPs were reluctant to take on a midwife attachment even though by 1983 many had given verbal agreement to this.[93]

Some home truths about maternity care professionals came to light. To a certain extent, each professional group involved believed that *it* was the best one to offer women information, advice and reassurance. Also, improvement in the position of one professional group would possibly lead to the detriment of another. Moreover, professionals' and pregnant women's interests did/do not always coincide: each professional group, while claiming to know 'what is best', might find it difficult to accept that a pregnant woman might not agree.[94]

Despite, or perhaps because of, the conclusions above, change continued in Aberdeen in particular and Scotland in general. Antenatal care became more community orientated with greater midwife input. Women would have a choice of maternity care co-ordinator – midwife or GP – responsible for planning with each woman, her personalised care tailored to meet her needs.[95] Alison Dale, who was a midwife in Aberdeen from the 1960s to the 2000s, described what happened in Aberdeen:

Tucker is a new system of care... The instigators were our Dr Hall and ...Dr Janet Tucker... The care...is either community care, or shared care which is hospital and community. If everything is straightforward, whether prims or parous patients, they can have their care in the community. That is midwife and GP, or just midwife...with only two visits to the hospital. That is one for a booking scan and one for a detailed anomaly scan at twenty weeks. All the rest of the care will be done in the community. They are allocated a consultant...but nine times out of ten they never need to [see her]. Shared care is any previous medical problem if they are prims or any previous obstetric or medical problem if they are parous... However they only have a first visit to see the consultant or one of the team and then if they are quite well they go back out on to the community and just referred back if there is a problem. I think mothers who are straightforward don't need to be seen at the hospital.

I do a clinic at one of the surgeries at Holburn. The midwife sees all the patients there. The GPs have very little input and even if there were a problem and you ask them, they're not really all that sure so you just quickly ferry them off.[96]

There were also other areas which demonstrated that midwives could give innovative, integrated antenatal care even while the CMBS was complaining that it was happening too slowly. Jan Fenton, a community midwife in Dundee in the 1970s, became well known in her area:

I ended up in Whitfield, which was an estate built at the back of Dundee...with 17,000 people, ...one tiny Post Office, little shoppies and ...six miles to go in the bus to...the middle of town. And they emptied the centre of Dundee and it was pathetic... Unmarried girlies, it was just so desperate...nobody liked [Whitfield]. ...I spent...half of my time visiting girls who defaulted from the clinic at Ninewells [Hospital] because...they had so far to go, they got sick on the bus [or] they couldn't afford the bus-fare... I thought, this is silly. Why don't we have a clinic in Whitfield? I desperately upset the clinic sister at Ninewells. They had tried it in Fintry and it didn't work...because the consultant who went there was a big gruff man and wouldn't be nice to them. Now these girls are very vulnerable...they didn't need somebody to be rotten to them. They needed somebody to be couthy, to be kind, to welcome them, to show an interest in them. It took me a year – eventually I [became very angry] in the hospital because nobody would listen to me – that this was what was needed... These were the girls...who needed the most care and weren't getting it. So eventually it was passed and I was told I could get on with it. That was it. Now I had never set up a clinic in my life, not a clue...but I knew all the doctors and one...had just become a consultant and he hadn't already got his niche... So I approached him. 'Would you be willing to come to Whitfield?' 'Yes,' he says. So we had a consultant. And we were given six months to establish this clinic and we started off with four patients...all we were allocated...and at the end of the six months we had twenty... We progressed from there because...I said, 'Well, why don't I book them?' because they were defaulting from booking clinics. So I booked them at Whitfield as well and of course, if they didn't come I would just appear at the house [at] five o'clock in the evening... I would knock on the door and say, 'We missed you at the clinic today. Are you OK?' One day I heard this chap [in the clinic] saying, 'Oh we thought we'd better bring her to the clinic or that wumman wid ha bin at the door again.' But then you see they began to realise that there was somebody who was thinking that it was important and they needed the care.[97]

Conclusion

In the early years of the twentieth century, pregnant women had little care from any source. For decades after the 1915 Midwives (Scotland) Act, mention of any care a midwife might give to a pregnant woman was sparse. The CMBS required the midwives that were booked for deliveries, to instruct women to attend the LA clinic or GP rather than give antenatal care themselves. As time went on they practised in a variety of areas, but mostly, especially in urban areas, in subservient roles. Continuity of care and team-working were little known concepts. Midwives helped mothers birth their babies at home, in many instances with no knowledge of the mother's history.

There was an acknowledgement that care should improve. An attempt at co-ordination of maternity services through the 1937 Maternity Services (Scotland) Act was negated by the advent of the NHS and the use of the GP as first contact for pregnant women, along with the increasing trend for hospital births and corresponding medicalisation of maternity care.

The 1970s brought open consumer criticism and debate and an eventual conscious effort to respond positively.[98] Within the 1974 re-organisation of the NHS were new schemes involving integration of the maternity services. But, midwives were still not free to perform to their full ability and the call in 1983 for shared responsibility to extend beyond arrangements between doctors and use midwifery skills to the full was only partly fulfilled: midwives could be a team player but in a subordinate role.[99]

In the early 1980s midwives began openly to challenge this position. Margaret Kitson, a senior midwife tutor in Glasgow in the 1990s, said:

Gradually midwives gained in confidence... The education of midwives improved... As the education of midwife teachers improved so the education of midwives themselves improved. Then gradually because they became more confident, because they were more able to stand beside their medical colleagues, medical domination dwindled. [Also], the generations changed and the generation of obstetricians who had seen midwives as handmaidens...gradually retired and as those people retired and the younger generation came up, there was a more equal partnership between midwives and obstetricians.[100]

However, even by 1983, the year of the CMBS's demise, midwives' talents were still being wasted as they chaperoned and acted as 'clerkess' to doctors, and endured the frustrating experience of watching doctors repeat examinations they had already performed.[101] Yet not all midwives felt themselves to be under-used and undermined. Ella Clelland, community midwife during the late 1970s in, Callander, recalled:

> I feel the input that we gave alongside the GP was much more then... To be able to go to the mother as another pair of ears and listen and see how she was as a person was worth it... We would visit one week and then we would see her at the GP's clinic maybe a fortnight later... There was much more co-operation then between the midwives and the GPs. They were very much a team then. At the clinics we worked together and both palpated and compared what we found. And the midwife was included in the plans for a woman. We were lucky here I think. We worked very well alongside the GPs. When I started, midwifery was a very normal process and it was meant to be normal until it was proved to be abnormal. Now, it's abnormal until it is proved normal. Maybe I had the best of it – I think I did. I thoroughly enjoyed all that I did.[102]

So, a midwife's ability to be an equal, respected team-player depended upon where and in what situation a midwife was working, and with whom. Jan Fenton, innovative midwife in Dundee, found she had to have a co-operative consultant before she could start her antenatal clinic and a previous clinic in Fintry failed because of the consultant's attitude. However, the degree of equality depended on everybody's attitudes: midwives, GPs and obstetricians. As long as a midwife's practice was dependent on the whims and personality of another professional, she was not practising as a respected and equal member of the team. However, gradually midwives realised that their attitude, too, needed to change. Jan Fenton and Ella Clelland succeeded not only because of the attitudes of the doctors with whom they worked, but also because of their own determination.

1.   A Oakley, *The Captured Womb*, (Oxford: Basil Blackwell, 1984), pp 13, 25.
2.   *Ibid*, p 2.
3.   H P Tait, 'Maternity and Child Welfare: The origins and progress of the maternal and child health services', in G McLachlan, (ed) *Improving the Common Weal*, (Edinburgh: Edinburgh University Press, 1987), p 416; *Hansard*, Commons, Vol 319, 28 January 1937, cols 1099-1155.
4.   Oakley, *The Captured Womb*, p 36.
5.   *Ibid*, pp 47-49, quoted from: J Ballantyne, 'Inaugural Address on the future of Obstetrics', *Trans Edin Obst Sc 32*, (1906-07) pp 3-28; M Tew, *Safer Childbirth? A critical history of maternity care, (2nd ed)*, (London: Chapman and Hall, 1995), p 88.
6.   *Ibid*, p 89.
7.   Oakley, *The Captured Womb*, p 51; J Sturrock, 'Sir James Young Simpson and his Memorial Hospital', in *Edinburgh's Infirmary*, (Edinburgh: Lammerburn Press, 1979), p 37.
8.   W L MacKenzie, *Report on the Physical Welfare of Mothers and Children, Vol.3,*

Scotland, (Dunfermline: The Carnegie United Kingdom Trust, 1917), p 51.

9. *Ibid*, p 564; see also, L Reid, 'Midwifery in Scotland 2: developing antenatal care', *British Journal of Midwifery*, (2005), Vol 13 (6), pp 392-396.

10. Oakley, *Captured Womb*, p 56; Department of Health for Scotland (DHS) and Scottish Health Services Council, *Maternity Services in Scotland*, (Montgomery Report), (Edinburgh: HMSO, 1959), para 66.

11. Oakley *Captured Womb*, pp 54-55.

12. Corporation of Glasgow Public Health Department, *Scheme for Maternity and Child Welfare*, (Glasgow: Committee on Health, 1926), pp 32, 23. Health visitors in that situation were required to have the CMBS certificate.

13. DHS, *Report on Puerperal Morbidity and Mortality, (Salvesen Report)*, (Edinburgh: HMSO, 1924), p30; Munro Kerr, Maternal Mortality and Morbidity, p 175.

14. NAS, CMB 2/10-14, *CMBS Report*, 31 March 1927, p 7.

15. Oakley *Captured Womb*, p 80.

16. NAS, CMB 2/10-14, *CMBS Report*, 31 March 1926, p 7.

17. DHS, Scientific Advisory Committee: Clinical Sub-Committee, C A Douglas, P L McKinley, *Maternal Morbidity and Mortality in Scotland*, (Edinburgh: HMSO, 1935), p 25.

18. *1937 Maternity Services (Scotland) Act*, 1, 1-11.

19. *Montgomery Report*, para 12; *ibid*, para 62.

20. J Towler and J Bramall, *Midwives in History and Society*, (London: Croom Helm, 1986), p 251; NAS, CMB, 1/7, *CMBS Minutes*, 18 October 1956, p 2; *Montgomery Report*, Edinburgh: HMSO, 1959.

21. *Montgomery Report*, paras 67-74; *ibid*, para 77.

22. Oakley, *Captured Womb*, p 138.

23. *Montgomery Report*, para 92; *ibid*, para 95.

24. Oakley, *Captured Womb*, p 218.

25. NAS, CMB 4/2/10, Schedule, CMBS for Scotland, *Rules framed under Section 5 (1) of the Midwives (Scotland) Act*, 1915 (5 and 6 Geo V c 91), 26 August, 1916.

26. NAS, *CMBS Rules*, 26 August 1916, Rules C, p 5.

27. *Ibid*, Rules E, p 10; *ibid*, Rules E (2), p 10.

28. NAS, CMB 1/3, *CMBS Minutes*, 27 June 1924, Vol 9, 27; NAS, CMB 1/3, *CMBS Minutes*, 28 May, 1925, Vol 10, 21.

29. *CMBS Rules*, 1926, 10; *ibid*, 12; *ibid*, 15. The *Rules* show how basic the antenatal care was at this time.

30. *CMBS Rules*, 1918, p 16.

31. *CMBS Rules*, 1931, p 35.

32. *Ibid*; *CMBS Rules*, 1968, 33-35; *CMBS Rules*, 1931, 17.

33. *Ibid*, p 34.

34. Munro Kerr, *Maternal Mortality and Morbidity*, p 300.

35. NAS, CMB 2/10-14, *CMBS Report*, 31 March 1927, p 6.

36. *Ibid*; NAS, CMB 2/10-14, *CMBS Report*, 31 March, 1926, p 7.

37. Towler, Bramall, *Midwives in History and Society*, 216. Discussion on CMBE&W *Rule Book* 1928.

38. G Cumberlege, *Maternity in Great Britain*, (London: Oxford University Press, 1948), pp 22-47.

39. See also, *Reid, Midwifery in Scotland 2*.

40. LR 19.

41. A face presentation, giving a long and difficult labour, could be picked up antenatally on palpation.

42. LR 46.

43. *Ibid*.

44. LR 50; Corporation of Glasgow, *Report of the Medical Officer of Health*, City of Glasgow, 1934, p 80. Layettes supplied by the Corporation were also known as 'maternity bundles'. In 1934, in Glasgow, 1,131 bundles were supplied.

45. Munro Kerr, *Maternal Mortality and Morbidity*, p 177.

46. LR 61.

47. LR 125; a Green Lady was a Glasgow Municipal Midwife.

48. LR 56.

49. LR 99.

50. LR 101.

51. LR 110.

52. Written testimony, LR 3.

53. *CMBS Rules*, 1928, p 10; See also *Reid, 'Midwifery in Scotland 2'*.

54. LR 125. The term 'hospital emergency' was used when a mother wanted a hospital delivery but had not booked and thus frequently did not obtain a hospital bed when she went into labour. These mothers often did not have antenatal care. Mothers who went to the clinics and who were booked to be delivered by choice on the district told the midwife verbally how they had fared at the clinic.

55. LR 108; see also, J Wilkinson, *The Coogate Doctors: The History of the Edinburgh Medical Missionary Society 1841-1991*, (Edinburgh: The Edinburgh Medical Missionary Society, 1991).

56. LR 108.

57. LR 82.

58. Personal communication.

59. Oakley, *Captured Womb*, p 144.

60. LR 9; the trend for hospital births in Glasgow was slower than elsewhere because of the shortage of beds. Ella Clelland's description of the timing of antenatal visits was to become a traditional pattern.

61. J Mortimer, *Tending to Care, (2nd ed)*, (Bedale: Blaisdon Publishing, 1999), p 104.

62. LR 27.

63. LR 9.

64. LR 101; see also *Reid, 'Midwifery in Scotland 2'*.

65. LR 110.

66. *Montgomery Report*, para 22.

67. LR 102.

68. LR 91.

69. Ministry of Health, DHS, Ministry of Labour and National Service, *Report of the*

Working Party on Midwives, (London: HMSO, 1949), Postscript to the
introduction, p viii.
70. LR 99.
71. LR 91.
72. *Ibid.*
73. *LR 123, personal experience.*
74. *Cumberlege, Maternity in Great Britain, p 47.*
75. *SHHD, Maternity Services: Integration of Maternity Work, (Tennent Report), (Edinburgh: HMSO, 1973).*
76. *Tennent Report*, Chapter 8, 'The Role of the Midwife in an Integrated Maternity Service', 29-31.
77. LR 35.
78. *Ibid*.
79. LR 102.
80. M Hall, S MacIntyre, M Porter, *Antenatal Care Assessed*, (Aberdeen: Aberdeen University Press, 1985), 8.
81. *Ibid, pp 2, 8, 23; Tennent Report.*
82. K Boddy, I J T Parboosingh, W C Shepherd, *A Schematic Approach to Prenatal Care*, (Edinburgh: 1976).
83. C Staines, 'Moving Forward in Antenatal Care: The Sighthill Project, Edinburgh', in *Midwives Chronicle, Supplement*, September 1983, pp 6-9.
84. LR 102.
85. *Ibid.*
86. *Ibid.*
87. LR 102; *CMBS Rules*, 1968, 12.
88. LR 102.
89. NAS, CMB 1/10, *Evidence for Royal Commission on the National Service*, December 1976.
90. Hall et al, *Antenatal Care Assessed*, Chapter 3, 'Before the Innovation', pp 21-36.
91. *Ibid*, inside dust-jacket, front.
92. *Ibid*, p 65.
93. *Ibid*, p 42; Community midwives who were already seeing women on their own at satellite clinics felt less anxious about the new system than did AMH clinic midwives who worried about the increased responsibility and that they might 'miss something important' and be blamed for it; *Ibid*, Chapter 4, 'The implementation of the innovation', pp 37-49.
94. *Ibid*, p 113.
95. The Scottish Office, CRAG/SCOTMEG Working Group on Maternity Services, *Antenatal Care*, (Edinburgh: HMSO, 1995), p 4.
96. LR 94.
97. LR 116.
98. Hall et al, *Antenatal Care Assessed*, pp 2, 8, 23.
99. Scottish Health Service Planning Council, *Shared Care in Obstetrics: A Report by the National Medical Consultative Committee*, (Edinburgh: SHHD, 1983),

para 1.6.
100. LR 120.
101. *Shared Care in Obstetrics*, paras 8.1-8.5.
102. LR 9.

Chapter 5

Events, dear girl, events: World War Two, the NHS and a midwifery shortage

From the late 1930s, midwifery in Scotland was affected by major events. These events were not specific to Scotland, yet had significant effects on maternity care and midwifery in Scotland. While connections between midwifery and war might at first glance appear to be tenuous, they exist. It was the events of World War One which precipitated the passing of the 1915 Midwives (Scotland) Act. World War Two had a major impact on recruitment and retention of enough midwives to look after mothers and deliver their babies. Circumstances brought about by the War were instrumental in changing attitudes to how and where births took place. This chapter explores these issues, their effects on midwifery practice, and post-war issues, not least of which was whether or not midwives in Scotland should be responsible for administering inhalational analgesia to labouring women.

Following World War Two, in July 1948, the National Health Service (NHS) Acts were passed and implemented. The NHS affected midwifery practice. The NHS Acts brought an administrative structure that fragmented the way childbearing women were cared for, and encouraged them to 'book' with their GP when pregnant, so by-passing the midwife as their first point of contact. The chapter considers this along with the increasing trend for births to take place in hospital instead of the home, and the consequent effect on midwifery training and practice.

World War Two: the shortage of midwives

World War Two had a major impact on the recruitment and retention of midwives. The Government anticipated these problems and instituted a form of National Service just before the war began in an effort to keep up the supply of midwives in Britain.[1] This, to begin with, was voluntary, but registration became compulsory in 1943 with the Nurses and Midwives (Registration for Employment) Order.

Midwives volunteering committed themselves to midwifery for the duration of the war. Initially, ninety-one per cent of volunteers for National Service were midwife-only trained.[2] However, by 1939, the majority of midwives were also registered nurses. Given the atmosphere of the time, it followed that many midwives who were also nurses did not want to act as midwives during the war years. It is possible that those who were nurse-trained felt they could better serve the war effort if they went into active service as nurses.[3] However Jean Woods, who was a pupil midwife in Glasgow in 1943, suggested a less altruistic reason. She said, 'You see, everybody wanted to go into the army or into the Services because you were a lieutenant, two pips up on your shoulder with a batman between two of you – well it *was* enticing.'[4]

THE NURSES AND MIDWIVES (Registration for Employment)

ORDER

1943

Persons who are or have been

NURSES (MALE or FEMALE) or MIDWIVES must REGISTER

All British subjects of either sex (whatever their period of residence in this country) **BORN AFTER 31st MARCH, 1883, and BEFORE 1st APRIL, 1926,** who fall within any of the classes or description of persons specified in Part I below, MUST register at an Employment Exchange,

on Sat. APRIL 10, 1943

PART I
PERSONS REQUIRED TO REGISTER

1. All nurses whose names appear on the General or Supplementary State Registers of the General Nursing Council for England and Wales and the General Nursing Council for Scotland.

2. Nurses not State Registered but who hold a Certificate of at least three years' training before the 30th June, 1925 in a Training School approved by the General Nursing Council for England and Wales, or before the 30th September, 1925, in a Training School approved by the General Nursing Council for Scotland.

3. State Certified Midwives whether practising or not and women whose names have been but are no longer on the Roll of Midwives except (i) those who were compulsorily retired by the local supervising authority under Section 5 (2) of the Midwives Act, 1936 or by the Local Authority under Section 4 (2) of the Maternity Services (Scotland) Act, 1937 on the ground of age or infirmity; and (ii) those whose names have been removed from the Roll by direction of the Central Midwives Board or the Central Midwives Board for Scotland acting under their Penal powers.

4. Student nurses and pupil midwives.

5. Persons who are or who have been nursing auxiliaries in the Civil Nursing Reserve, or who are or who have been V.A.D.'s or nursing members of the British Red Cross Society, St. John Ambulance Brigade or St. Andrews Ambulance Association who have had not less than six months' full time experience in nursing duties, whether or not they are now actually engaged in such duties.

6. Nursery nurses who hold a nursery nursing certificate after training at
(i) a Nursery Training College; or
(ii) a Nursery approved by the National Society of Children's Nurseries.

7. Other persons who have had at least one full year of experience in the nursing of sick persons in a hospital or similar institution.

8. All persons who, on 30th March, 1943, were employed in, or engaged for the purpose of nursing sick or injured persons.

NOTE : *Women who are in process of entering the Women's Auxiliary Services, or the Nursing Services of the Crown, but are not yet finally enrolled, and men who are in process of being called up for the Armed Forces, must nevertheless register if they have any of the qualifications listed above.*

PART II
PERSONS NOT REQUIRED TO REGISTER

1. Members of any of the Armed Forces of the Crown other than the Home Guard or Auxiliary Coastguard and other than

(i) officers holding unpaid commissions in the Royal Naval Volunteer Reserve ; (Sea Cadet Corps) ; or

(ii) officers of the Territorial Army Reserve of Officers of the Army Cadet Force ; or

(iii) commissioned officers of the Training Branch of the Royal Air Force Volunteer Reserve.

2. Women who are members of
(i) W.R.N.S., A.T.S., W.A.A.F. or
(ii) Queen Alexandra's Royal Naval Nursing Service or any reserve ; or
(iii) Queen Alexandra's Imperial Nursing Service or any Reserve : or
(iv) Members of the Territorial Army Nursing Service or any reserve ; or
(v) Princess Mary's Royal Air Force Nursing Service or any reserve ;
provided they are not women whose enrolment or other undertaking to serve was for part-time service only or for service without payment.

ALL PERSONS ATTENDING FOR REGISTRATION MUST BRING WITH THEM THEIR NATIONAL REGISTRATION IDENTITY CARDS, THEIR NATIONAL SERVICE REGISTRATION CERTIFICATES AND IF A STATE REGISTERED NURSE THEIR NUMBER ON THE STATE REGISTER AND IF A STATE CERTIFIED MIDWIFE THEIR NUMBER ON THE ROLL OF MIDWIVES.

Persons living more than six miles from an Employment Exchange, or who cannot attend in person may register by obtaining the necessary form and returning it by post duly completed not later than April 17.

Nurses and Midwives genuinely unable to register on April 10 because of their hours of duty on that date or because they are sleeping after night duty may register at a local office of the Ministry of Labour and National Service during the week April 12 to 17.

PENALTIES

Failure to comply with the Order constitutes an offence under the Defence (General) Regulations, 1939, and is punishable by fine, or imprisonment, or both.

★ AS ANNOUNCED BY THE B.B.C. ★

Issued by the Ministry of Labour and National Service

Nurses and Midwives (Registration for Employment) Order 1943.

In addition to the War affecting midwifery staffing levels, it also influenced training prospects. A close watch on the trends of practising midwives, during the War years and after, included quarterly examination of the figures for those in training, waiting lists and vacancies.[5] This could change at short notice as many pupil midwives were members of the Territorial Army Nursing Service. As they could be called up at any moment, pupil midwives worried that this would affect their training on return to civilian life. This issue led the Board to waive, for the duration of the war, the Rule which stipulated possible extra training for pupils who did not begin Part 2 within six months of passing Part 1.[6]

While some women left midwifery to join the Armed Forces, there remained pupil midwives aiming to reach the end of Part 2, albeit with difficulty. For instance, in 1941, as a result of enemy action, conditions in Greenock left pupil midwives with difficulty getting enough district cases. This was possibly due to evacuation of mothers, or because some women chose hospital as a safe haven from the blitz. However, a pupil midwife at

Rottenrow, Glasgow, seemed to contradict this when she said, 'When the bombers went over, the mothers and babies were put under the beds to give them even a little protection.'[7] In the Greenock case, the Board allowed pupil midwives, for the duration of the emergency, to have twenty-five indoor and five outdoor cases instead of twenty and ten.[8]

By April 1942 the acute shortage of trained nurses and midwives throughout Scotland left matrons of several maternity homes contemplating ceasing maternity work due to lack of staff.[9] This was exacerbated by the rising birth-rate, a trend which started in the late 1930s and continued in the 1940s.[10] As one midwife put it, 'The birth rate always went up after the men had been home on leave.'[11]

To try to improve matters, the Nurses and Midwives (Registration for Employment) Order 1943 was now rigorously upheld. It required all nurses and midwives to register with the Ministry of Labour by 10 April 1943 unless they had been compulsorily retired or had their names struck off the Roll. There was a non-compliance penalty of a maximum fine of £100, imprisonment, or both.[12] Even those who were retired were subjected to a high level of persuasion. The Ministry of Labour and National Service also decided that newly qualified midwives had to practise for a year and, as a temporary measure for the next six months, no practising midwife could take up employment other than in midwifery. Jean Woods, who served with the Queen Alexandra's Imperial Military Nursing Service (QAIMNS or QA), said, 'They were actually having to take midwives out of the QAs to staff hospitals until they had enough newly qualified ones.'[13] At the Board's behest, the DHS and the Ministry of Health negotiated with the Army Council who agreed to exempt practising midwives already waiting to be conscripted from call-up to the Army Nursing Services, and to refuse any new joining-up applications from practising midwives.[14] The new regulations did not go unchallenged and some pupil midwives protested against the compulsory one year's practice after enrolment. However, this requirement did not apply to pupil midwives who had only done Part 1. They could interrupt their training but only at that point because of the potential wastage of training places. Many did, as Anne McFadden recalled:

> Practically all of my friends decided...we'll go, and many of them went to the Armed Services as nurses...[and] actually stopped midwifery at the end of Part 1. Although they had signed on to do two parts midwifery, they couldn't be held to that now.[15]

While many women were trying to leave midwifery to join the Forces, Agnes Tillotson (now Morrison) wanted to do the opposite. She had just finished her nursing training and wanted to train as a midwife:

> I had a letter to be called up to one of the EMS [Emergency Medical Services]. [I thought I'd] be refused to go to the Simpson [in Edinburgh, to do midwifery]. So I spoke to Matron and she saw that I...got to the Simpson...and [I] loved every minute of it.[16]

Another midwife, who was training as a nurse in the early 1940s, also told how she came into midwifery during the War:

After preliminary training [in nursing] I was sent to a military hospital away up in the north of Scotland. It was full of Polish soldiers... I worked there for a wee while and I was transferred...from there to another military hospital in Dunblane... I was sent from there to Dunfermline Maternity Hospital to help [the midwives] as they were short-staffed... After I got there I said, 'This is what I want.'[17]

Alice Porter, who was a pupil midwife in Aberdeen in the 1940s, had an unforgettable experience. She was trying to finish Part 2:

During the Second World War I was instructed to go to George Street in Aberdeen. I couldn't find the place and the whole area looked deserted. I finally found a policeman who said, 'There's no-one living here. These houses have been condemned.' The windows had been blown out and the stairways were blown out and had no bannisters. We heard a noise and went up a [broken] stair to find a young woman on a couch – no blankets or sheets. Over by an empty fireplace was an old woman smoking a clay pipe and spitting into a fireplace. I asked her if there was any water in the building. She said 'No', but made no move to help me. I could not leave the young woman so I asked the policeman to come back in a couple of hours. I had to pour a bottle of Dettol on my hands before I examined the woman. I sat in a chair with a rim but no seat until it was time to deliver the child. Just before the child was born the sirens sounded and the blast blew out the sacking covering the windows and soot blew into the room from the roofs. Under these conditions I delivered the baby. The policeman arrived with an ambulance. I carried the new baby down the broken stairway to the waiting ambulance and mother and child were transported to hospital.[18]

Mima Sutherland, a midwife on Unst, Shetland, during the War also saw direct action:

My father was a policeman. He went to Unst in 1939 where the RAF garrison was... It was very busy for him. There were wrecks coming ashore and people from Norway coming and waiting for transport. Poor Dad, he just had a [bi]cycle. There were no police stations. Dad had to attend to the wrecks.

The RAF station was at Scaw. The clerk of works...and his wife had a wooden house in the centre of the camp. When she was pregnant I [used] to cycle there and get into the station to see her. She was a lovely lass and she was so brave. There were a lot of air raids here – hit and run.

The station had some narrow escapes. When this mother was in labour, doctor and I had to wait at the gate because there was an air-raid warning. Then we were allowed in. By that time her husband had gone out because of the air raid. She was very brave. She made supper and then as soon as supper was by she said, 'Mrs. Clarke, [her friend] you'll need to wash the dishes. You'll need to excuse me.' She went to her room and the baby was born almost immediately.[19]

The shortage of both midwives and nurses continued through the War although, in 1943, the problem with recruitment of pupil midwives was not so apparent. The situation changed as midwives who were nurses found that the new regulations prevented them from going on active service.[20] By 1945 the Board expressed its concern to the Department of Health for Scotland (DHS) that too few women were entering midwifery training to meet the staffing standards of maternity hospitals and training institutions.[21] The War's impact on the number of midwives was twofold. It exacerbated the already poor retention of midwives who were nurse-trained until the 1943 regulation prevented this; and, from 1943, it reduced recruitment of pupil midwives as nurses saw that, if they did midwifery, they were unlikely to be allowed to return to nursing for the duration of the conflict.

COUNTY COUNCIL OF THE COUNTY OF LANARK

COUNTY MATERNITY HOSPITAL, BELLSHILL

We hereby certify that

Margaret C Rodger

has completed her Maternity training.

The length of training has been One *year, in two periods, Parts 1 and 2.*

She has attended Lectures and received theoretical, practical, and clinical instruction, attended on and nursed not less than ten mothers and their babies during Part 1, and twenty mothers and their babies during Part 2, ten of whom were attended in the patient's own home.

Throughout her training she has been regularly engaged in the practice of the Hospital as a resident pupil midwife and during Part 2 of her training she attended five sessions at Local Authority's Maternity and Child Clinic. She has written up records of her last twenty cases and passed Part 1 and Part 2 examination of the Central Midwives Board for Scotland.

Thomson M.D, M.R.C.O.G   *Physician-Superintendent*

Janetta M Macdougall   *Matron*

Bellshill,   November   1943

Hospital Midwifery Certificate awarded to Margaret C Rodger, 1943. (Courtesy of Pat Andriou.)

World War Two also contributed to the acceleration of the trend towards hospitals for birth. The most basic reason was lack of help at home. Many women replaced men in factories, on the land and in other jobs which were usually male preserves. This meant less help in the home for newly delivered mothers and consequently greater demand for hospital births. In addition, and probably with longer term effects, there was a distinct change in maternity services from the beginning of the War. Pregnant women, evacuated to reception areas from places likely to become targets for enemy action, were provided with emergency maternity hospitals which often adapted from suitable country houses.

Although 'a drift back home set in almost immediately the scheme was launched', many mothers found that they enjoyed the break from home responsibilities and the trend for hospital births in some areas developed rapidly.[22] For example, MacGregor notes that:

> In Glasgow, the DHS commandeered Lennox Castle (125 beds) in 1943 as an emergency maternity home. When the MOH asked the mothers how they liked it, they said it was a grand idea because they could get a holiday at the same time.[23]

In the early months of the War, the proportion of institutional births in Glasgow rose by twenty per cent and the change in maternity services during the War was a contributory factor in the sharp post-war upturn in the institutional delivery rate.[24] Booking a hospital bed was strictly controlled into obstetric, medical and social categories because maternity beds were in short supply. Nevertheless, by 1948 there were almost 3,000 maternity beds in Scotland, a rise of around 2,000 since 1934.[25] Most of these came as a result of the wartime maternity policy.[26]

Refugees
While the shortage of midwives became acute, there was a source of help if the Government had been more willing to accept it. This came from medically qualified women who were refugees from other countries and willing to train as midwives. In the early 1930s, as Hitler's power grew, many people in danger of persecution by the Nazi movement left Germany to take refuge in Western European and other countries. The influx of refugees to Britain stayed at a low level until 1938 when demands from British pressure groups facilitated the immigration of a further 40,000 refugees. Many of these were known as 'transmigrants' as they had to move on when they received visas for their first choice of destination. However, for most, the outbreak of World War Two foiled these plans and they had to stay in Britain for the duration. About 80,000 refugees from Germany, Austria and Czechoslovakia lived in Britain during the war and afterwards.[27]

The British Government was reluctant to allow refugees who were medically qualified in Germany to practise in Britain, but agreed in the 1930s to accept 500 doctors although this was subsequently reduced to fifty under pressure from the British Medical Association (BMA). Many German doctors entered Britain and, despite the shortage of doctors, had no prospect of employment. Some applied to go to medical schools in Britain but then had to find money for their fees in a country where refugees were not routinely given work permits. Some found work, but well below their capabilities: 'A surgeon secretly washed corpses in a morgue, a radiologist repaired radios and a bacteriologist peddled baking powder.'[28] They found the problems of adjustment almost more than they could bear.

Some women doctors from middle European countries applied for midwifery training in Britain. This too presented problems, not least of which was the slowness of the Home Office to give its approval and of the Board to make decisions. By 1939 the CMBE&W had registered about thirty-five women refugees, most of whom had medical qualifications, as pupil midwives for the two-year course.[29] At this time the CMBS received and accepted three similar applications from medical practitioners to train as midwives in Scotland.[30] Official Home Office agreement with the midwives sub-committee of the Refugees' Joint Consultative Committee (RJCC) to allow about 200 refugees into Britain for training eventually came in September 1939.[31] Before the Board finally decided how many refugees it could accept for training in Scotland, events forced its hand. In late 1939, the management at training institutions in Greenock, Govan and Glasgow Royal Maternity Hospital (GRMH) accepted, without permission from the Board, ten women refugees from Germany, Czechoslovakia and Austria to do midwifery training. Faced with this *fait accompli*, the Board agreed to accept these applicants provided all their certificates and papers were satisfactory, but decided that no more than six refugees should be accepted as pupil midwives in any one year in Scotland.[32]

Refugees were prepared to work for less money than locals. In January 1941, three refugees applied to the Burgh Maternity Hospital, Kilmarnock for midwifery training. The CMBS discovered that the reason the refugees were attracted to this one small hospital was because the salary there was so low that few midwives from home would apply. One of those candidates was subsequently able to continue training.[33]

The Home Office and BMA had a strict policy towards medically trained refugees. Berghahn notes that, 'In spite of a shortage of doctors in some parts of Britain, only 460 foreign practitioners of all nationalities had Home Office permits to practise in July 1940.'[34] Given the shortage of midwives it would have helped if more refugee doctors had been allowed to train as midwives. The CMBS accepted a disproportionately low number of the two hundred refugees allowed to train in Britain, possibly because of a feeling of protection towards existing midwives in Scotland, or, because of a feeling of distrust of anyone who came from beyond Britain. Whatever the reason, it was to the detriment of the midwifery service at that time.

Post-war problems
The end of World War Two exacerbated the midwifery staffing problem. According to Towler and Bramall, the birth rate reached its peak in 1946, making the shortage of midwives critical. However, there were other reasons. For example, many midwives stopped practising after marriage and others returned to general nursing after midwife training, while some midwives, recalled during the war years, returned to retirement.[35] Another important element was the increased time required for their work. The 1939 CMBS Rules lengthened the lying-in period from ten to fourteen days.[36] Subsequently, midwives had to make more time-consuming postnatal visits. Also, statutory training for midwives and pupil midwives in the use of inhalational analgesia during childbirth started on 1 July 1946, increasing the time a midwife spent with a labouring woman.[37]

Government bodies and the CMBs tried different ways of handling the problem including a recruiting pamphlet sent out in 1946 and relaxation of *Rules* towards 'foreign trained' midwives.[38] Yet, recruiting midwives and nurses from beyond Scotland could not solve everything. Immediately after the War, a new two-year enrolment course for nurses was established. To begin with, nurses with enough wartime experience were enrolled without examination. Margaret Crombie was one of them and she recalled that 'when the war finished anybody who had a certain grade of nurse training...got a new certificate...*Enrolled Nurse*. So I was given one when I left because of the experience that I had.'[39] Enrolled nurses in Scotland who wanted to be midwives initially had to do the two-year course. The CMBS altered this *Rule* to eighteen months in 1961.[40]

In 1947, a Working Party (Report 1949) met to consider the UK-wide problems within midwifery. This included examination of recruitment and training, the 'proper' duties of a midwife, inter-professional relationships and how best to minimise wastage.[41] The Working Party saw conflict between GPs and midwives as a major problem and with the start of the National Health Service (NHS), GPs 'were seriously encroaching on the midwife's function by taking over the antenatal care of patients ... in some cases midwives were becoming little more than maternity nurses.'[42] The Working Party emphasised the complementary nature of the work of midwives and GPs, but recommended the retention of the role of the midwife as an expert in all aspects of normal childbearing.[43]

The Working Party also paid tribute to the midwife who was not nurse-trained. Direct entry midwives were disadvantaged as far as promotion went and the Working Party stressed the injustice of this. A greater proportion of direct entry midwives than those who were nurse-trained practised midwifery, and they appeared to be highly motivated.[44] In contrast, some nurses took midwifery training as a means to promotion in nursing. This was expensive in terms of training costs, places and time, and was only partly solved by two-part midwifery training.[45] Furthermore, the Working Party highlighted the differences in the roles of the midwife and the nurse. It stressed that the midwife was a practitioner in her own right working with women who were undergoing a significant but normal life event. By contrast, nurses worked with doctors, focussing on caring for the sick. However, the Working Party recognised the need for midwives to have a thorough grounding in nursing techniques and explored the future possibility of nurses and midwives sharing a basic training. This Report therefore marked the beginning of a move to bring students of differing disciplines together.[46] Finally, the Working Party recommended a single period of midwifery training which later came to fruition.[47]

The CMBS gave general approval to the Working Party's conclusions. They particularly highlighted that non-nurses should not be prevented from training as midwives.[48] The Board endorsed the distinction made between midwifery and nursing and agreed with the concept of complete independence for the CMBS.[49]

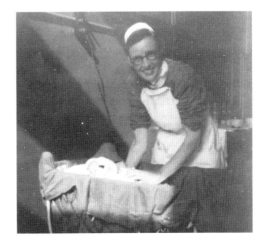

Midwife, 1946. (Courtesy of Elizabeth Radley.)

'Gas and air' and the Minnitt apparatus

While the Working Party considered midwives and their inter-professional relationships, one facet of the relationship between midwives and GPs underwent a significant change in the late 1940s: the administration of pain relief. Until 1946, the role of the midwife in Scotland in the use of inhalational analgesia in childbirth was minimal; from that year it could be administered by midwives. The CMBS was central to this change.

Up until the 1930s, the only inhalational analgesia in relatively regular use in childbirth was chloroform and its use was restricted to medical practitioners. This meant that mothers receiving chloroform for childbirth purposes at that time were only those who could afford a doctor, or who were giving birth in emergency circumstances.[50] Medical practitioners experimented with ether and nitrous oxide as analgesics in the mid-nineteenth century, but it was not until 1932 that pressure from bodies such as the National Birthday Trust stimulated the design of an apparatus for administering nitrous oxide and air, known colloquially as 'gas and air', to mothers in childbirth.[51]

The idea was that a form of inhalational analgesia should be available for midwives to use at their own discretion.[52] Dr R J Minnitt (1889-1974) of the Liverpool Maternity Hospital designed the apparatus, encased in a portable wooden box, to deliver nitrous oxide and air in a ratio of forty-five percent nitrous oxide and fifty-five per cent air, but adapted later to a fifty-fifty mix.[53] By 1936, the CMBE&W allowed midwives in England and Wales to administer gas and air to labouring mothers provided they held a certificate of proficiency. However, due to the shortage of midwives, only one in five midwives in England and Wales was qualified by 1946.[54] Furthermore, the weight of the apparatus was such that midwives could not carry it on their bicycles and although some authorities sent it in ambulances these situations were few and far between.[55]

The negative attitude of GPs also appears to have been an important factor in delaying any widespread use of gas and air by midwives until after the War. As late as 1939 the BMA debated the issue at its annual meeting. Some doctors said 'they wanted to stop midwives controlling the midwifery of the country' and the meeting ended with a resolution stating the opposition of GPs to the idea of midwives using gas and air.[56] It is probable that a suitable method could have been developed many years earlier, but the stimulus to produce it was lacking because of the low standing of midwives, historical prejudice against women in childbirth receiving pain-relief, and the attitude of members of the medical profession.[57] The attitude of GPs was particularly significant. According to Williams, GPs were being squeezed out of midwifery. This came, on one side, by pressure from obstetricians trying to consolidate their role as experts and to create a need for women to give birth in hospital, and on the other, by pressure from midwives (in England and Wales) who, helped by being allowed by the 1936 Midwives Act to use inhalational analgesia with the backing of public health officers, were increasing their share of home confinements.[58]

In Scotland, the situation was different. The 1937 Maternity Services (Scotland) Act provided for an anaesthetist to attend a woman in her home, if necessary, for the administration of chloroform.[59] There was no mention in the Act that midwives should be allowed to administer inhalational analgesia.[60] If the influence of GPs in England delayed the use of gas and air in childbirth there, the strong tradition of GPs in midwifery in Scotland was possibly even more influential in the thwarting of conferring this responsibility on midwives.[61]

Midwives in Scotland were not allowed to use inhalational analgesia for pain relief in labour until 1946. The issue was aired in 1937 when the DHS asked the Ministry of Health about midwives' use of gas and air in England and whether or not there had been any medical profession opposition.[62] Only then did the DHS consult the CMBS on this issue, by which time queries on the issue and CMBS policy were also arriving from Scottish midwifery training institutions.

The CMBS had no current policy for this in the late 1930s. Consultation with its sister CMBE&W led to a dissemination of information from England to Scotland, much discussion, and awareness of the need for the CMBS to make a decision.[63] The CMBS, with full information from the CMBE&W and awareness that facilities to run courses could be available in Scotland, declined the idea of midwives administering inhalational analgesia.[64] It pointed out to the DHS that the 1937 Maternity Services (Scotland) Act provided for an anaesthetist to be present for every woman in childbirth if necessary. The CMBS decided to establish the demand for the presence of anaesthetists before allowing midwives to administer gas and air with the Minnitt apparatus.[65]

The CMBS's decision did not appear to take into account the distinction between the use of the two substances, chloroform and inhalational analgesia. Chloroform in labour, given by an anaesthetist, was to anaesthetise mothers having difficult deliveries, while gas and air was used to alleviate the mother's pain in labour. In 1941, when the DHS asked the CMBS to reconsider, the DHS's argument centred round medical practitioners being called up for military service and the need to give greater responsibility to midwives. However, the CMBS would not alter its decision, stating that some medical practitioners might consider this as a retrograde step. Also, it stated that more change would be premature as the recommendations of the 1937 Maternity Services (Scotland) Act were still settling down. Furthermore, the CMBS pointed out to the DHS this time, that the analgesia procured from the Minnitt apparatus was only analgesia and not anaesthesia. Therefore its use could not be construed as replacing doctors who might be called up.[66]

When the War ended, the CMBS succumbed to pressure and changed its *Rules*. The CMBE&W decided to include the administration of inhalational analgesia in Part 2 midwifery training with effect from 1 July 1946, and the DHS, Glasgow Royal Maternity Hospital (GRMH), the Queen's Institute of District Nursing in Scotland (QIDNS) and the CMB Éire sent the CMBS letters in favour of this. Subsequently, to ensure the maintenance of Scottish midwifery status and qualifications, the CMBS agreed to give the same opportunity to midwives in Scotland.[67] Before long, the course for administration of inhalational analgesia became an integral part of midwifery training.[68]

The next issue was the nature of the analgesia. Trilene, the trade name for Trichlorethylene, is another form of inhalational analgesia. Although inexpensive, faster-acting than gas and air, and more portable than the Minnitt machine, Trilene was not CMBS-approved for midwives' use in the late 1940s because of its accumulative effect.[69] However, during the following six years there was a high level of discussion and negotiation on the issue and in 1955 the Board amended the *Rules* in favour of Trilene: its informed use then enjoyed a long period of acceptability.[70]

Central Midwives Board for Scotland

This is to certify that the

SOUTHERN GENERAL HOSPITAL, GLASGOW

has notified the Central Midwives Board for Scotland

that   MARY LEES MARSHALL McCASKILL

has completed the prescribed training at the institution in the administration of nitrous oxide and air by means of   Minnitts
(an apparatus recognised by the Central Midwives Board for Scotland as suitable for use by midwives under the conditions prescribed by the Board, for the purpose of producing analgesia during childbirth). In connection therewith she has received special instruction in the essentials of obstetric analgesia and in the emergencies of anæsthesia, adequate for such purpose, and has been found, after examination, to be thoroughly proficient in the use of the apparatus under the conditions prescribed by the Central Midwives Board for Scotland.

Secretary.

Date 7th November 1947.

Midwife's certificate of inhalational analgesia. (Courtesy of Mary McCaskill.)

The development of the safer fifty-fifty mixture of nitrous oxide and oxygen given by the still widely-used Entonox apparatus resulted in the end of CMBS approval of the Minnitt apparatus and nitrous oxide and air mixture in 1970.[71] However, Trilene and its inhalers remained officially sanctioned for midwives' use until1984.[72]

The CMBS's late and reluctant approval of midwives' use of inhalational analgesia reflected the influence of medical practitioners and the threat they perceived by midwives extending their skills in this way.

The National Health Service (NHS) and its aftermath
The NHS (Scotland) Act was passed in May 1947 and the NHS Acts were implemented across the UK on 5 July 1948. Health services were to be free to all as and when they were needed. Payment came from three sources: central funds, local rates and public contributions to a national insurance scheme. Administratively, the NHS was originally designed to be run on a tripartite scheme. This included: Regional Hospital Boards, which, in Scotland, included the teaching hospitals; Executive Councils, which administered general medical services, including dentistry and pharmacy, and GPs, who retained their status as independent contractors; and Local Health Authorities (LHA) responsible for providing maternity services, child welfare, midwifery, health visiting and home nursing. Maternity services provided by the local health authorities did not include hospitals.[73]

The new administrative structure fragmented maternity services, yet it did not directly alter the CMBS or its responsibilities. The CMBS Minutes make little explicit reference to the NHS, although in 1949 the CMBE&W voiced its concerns about the possibility of the midwife's role being diminished.[74] Dr R Johnstone, retiring from the CMBS Chair in 1953, called it a 'trichotomy of a single biological function' which fragmented maternity services and could lead to 'overlapping and confusion.' Strangely, he also said, 'this, however, does not directly affect the work of the Central Midwives Board and I need not dwell on it.'[75]

Nevertheless, the NHS affected midwives and their practice. Firstly, pregnant women could now go to their GP free of charge to 'book'. This meant that midwives were no longer the first point of contact. Secondly, GPs began to perform an increasing amount of antenatal care. This, exacerbated by the NHS, caused conflict between some GPs and midwives and signalled an 'unwelcome trend which could wreck the structure of the midwifery services.'[76] Extra payment for undertaking maternity care saw GPs' proportion of antenatal care rising quickly, diminishing the midwife's role and experience for pupil midwives.[77] Thirdly, the NHS brought problems from the point of view of safety and continuity of care. The Working Party reported that 'in some cases, midwives are not seeing patients until they go to deliver them.'[78] In addition, pupil midwives were not getting the opportunity to participate in antenatal care.[79] Fourthly, the NHS reinforced the existing trend towards hospital births. The new hospital boards' policy of centralisation of obstetric care matched an increasing demand for hospital births with a corresponding increase in medical involvement in normal maternity care.[80] From the mother's point of view it made economic sense and 'spared a family the extra expenses of giving birth at home, such as food, bedclothes, sanitary towels, extra washing and adequate fuel.'[81] Hospital births also gave many mothers a rest which they would not otherwise have had. Nevertheless, although the number of hospital maternity beds was increasing there were not enough to meet the rising demand. Some mothers took it for granted that a hospital bed would be available and did not book. Mary McCaskill remembers this kind of situation in Glasgow:

> At that time... it was just post-war and hospital beds weren't plentiful, a mother or a relative phoned in ...to say that Mrs A was in labour ...and could she go into hospital?... Now these telephonists...phoned round the hospitals... Rottenrow... Southern General, Stobhill, and if they couldn't obtain a bed they phoned to the night midwifery supervisor. And she got in touch with... say for instance it was me... I had to go out...as a municipal midwife...and...tell them that there was no hospital bed and the baby was going to be born in the house... [We] often got a hostile reception at first because a family was unprepared for this. They hadn't been prepared for a home confinement and they maybe didn't have a lot in the way of bed-linen and towels and even the minimum of baby clothes.[82]

Nevertheless, hospital births were becoming more common and some midwives on the district began to feel very vulnerable and to wonder what would happen to them. Mary McCaskill continued:

> Towards the end of that five years [1952]... the home deliveries had just sort of imperceptibly started to decline... Older midwives...probably in their fifties, were beginning to talk about... They didn't have so many bookings and they were wondering...what was the future and what would they be used for... Would they be maybe diversified into some other duties?[83]

Consequently, the role of the midwife on the district diminished and very nearly disappeared. The move towards full hospitalisation of birth, gathering speed in the 1950s, was virtually unstoppable.[84]

As mentioned above, there were also problems of training pupil midwives according to *Rules* because the statutory ten district deliveries required for completion of Part 2 became increasingly difficult to find. As institutional births gradually became more popular, the number of births on the district became correspondingly fewer. The Board had to decide what to do about training institutions which offered Part 2 training and yet could not provide the requisite number of mothers on the district for the pupils to deliver. The Board usually advised training institutions to continue offering Part 2 with the proviso that they should not take on more pupil midwives than they had district cases for.[85] This advice was repeated many times as training institutions in Scotland offering Part 2 endeavoured to cope or contemplated closure because of the shortage of district cases.[86]

The Board tried to consider the issue sympathetically. It even decided to accept a smaller number of domiciliary births where, due to changes in social conditions, training institutions had difficulty in providing the official number for Part 2 midwives.[87] Yet it was a long time before the Board agreed to make this reduction formal even though the issue recurred constantly through the 1950s reflecting the increasing trend of hospital births.[88] Finally, in September 1961, after receiving a formal complaint from the North East Regional Professional Committee on the Maternity Services about the issue, the Board set up an *ad hoc* committee to consider putting midwifery training on a more realistic basis and to discuss combining Parts 1 and 2 midwifery into a one year course.[89]

As Professor Johnstone said, the NHS did not directly affect the work of the CMBS. However, its effect fragmented maternity services, diminished the role of the midwife and speeded up hospitalisation and medicalisation of childbirth.

The Glasgow Royal Maternity and Women's Hospital.

——: o :——

EMERGENCY FORM

Date,.....................................

Patient's Name,...

Address,..

................Stair..............Lobby.

Age,...   ,........No. of Pregnancy,..   ....

No. of Miscarriages,..................

Presentation,...

Membranes ruptured or unruptured,...

Commencement of pains,..

Full Time or Premature,......

Size of Os,......

Fœtal Heart,.....

Cause of sending for assistance,......

Temperature,.....................Pulse,.................Resp...................

Signature,..................................... ...

Emergency form in use for homebirths in mid-1940s. Courtesy of Mary McCaskill.

Conclusion

During World War Two and afterwards, the CMBS had to cope with what, at times, must have been very difficult circumstances without guiding precedents. The shortage of midwives, exacerbated by wartime conditions, increased in the post-war years. In addition, the Working Party on Midwives highlighted problems between midwives and GPs which increased after 1948 and the implementation of the NHS Acts. The trend towards hospitalisation of childbirth affected both domiciliary and hospital midwifery practice, along with Part 2 midwifery training which depended on pupils achieving ten homebirths. Eventually the CMBS bowed to pressure and reduced this number.

Although it seemed that midwives, with improved education and greater representation on the Board, might be gaining power and strength, many limitations remained. From the top down, apart from the weighted medical presence on the Board, all changes in Board *Rules* had to be approved by the DHS to which the Board was answerable. In addition, the Board had to change the *Rules* in response to external pressures. From the bottom up, the power of midwives was limited, especially after the coming of the NHS. Within the NHS, they had the security of a salary, but because of their employee status, they relinquished what little independence they previously possessed.[90] They also lost their mothers and babies to GPs and hospitals, their practical skills through lack of practice, and their decision-making skills because many decisions were made for them.[91] Furthermore, midwives were closely governed by the CMBS which always had a statutory majority of medical practitioners.[92]

In the late 1940s and 1950s, the CMBS acknowledged an improvement in the quality of midwifery in Scotland. It had numerous opportunities to give midwives more autonomy, for instance, when it upgraded the *Rules* in 1948, and when it increased the number of midwives on the Board in 1953. It could have used its influence with the DHS during the implementation of the NHS. The Board did not grasp these opportunities. The delay in the CMBS's approval of the use of analgesia by midwives was symptomatic of the Board's desire to maintain control over midwives and their practice. Until 1977 the Chairman of the CMBS was always an obstetrician, sometimes in position for a long time. This could partly explain the Board's inability to expedite the professional progress of midwives in Scotland in the post-War decades. The attitude of both obstetricians and GPs in Scotland was highlighted by Margaret Kitson who commented:

> The tension I saw was with the medical profession who, for a very long time in Scotland...I think it wasn't so marked in England...but in Scotland, saw midwives as subservient and wanted to control midwifery. And it was only gradually that that changed.[93]

1.   J M Munro Kerr, R W Johnstone, M H Phillips, *Historical Review of British Obstetrics and Gynaecology 1800-1950* (Edinburgh, and London: Livingstone, 1954), p 345.

2.   This was not National Service in the accepted military sense. Rather, it was a form of service to the nation, where, in this instance, midwives would commit themselves to working as midwives for the duration of the war. NAS, CMB 1/6, *CMBS Minutes*, 17 February 1939, Vol 23, p 35; NAS, CMB 1/6, *CMBS*

Minutes, 24 March 1939, Vol 24, p 8; *ibid*, 5 May 1939, p 12; *ibid*, 21 July 1939, p 23.

3.   B McBryde, *A Nurse's War*, (London: Hogarth Press, 1986), p 33.

4.   LR 128; L Reid, 'Wartime midwives', *The Practising Midwife*, (2009), Vol 12 (3), p 50, See also, L Reid, 'Two pips on your shoulder', *The Scots Magazine*, (March 2009), pp 302-306.

5.   NAS, CMB 1/6, *CMBS Minutes*, 29 September 1939, Vol 24, p 25; *ibid*, 20 December 1939, p 30.1

6.   *Ibid*, 29 September 1939, p 26; *CMBS Rules*, 1940, Rule C 9, p 16.

7.   LR 2; L Reid, 'Wartime Midwives'.

8.   NAS, CMB 1/6, *CMBS Minutes*, 18 July 1941, Vol 26, p 6.

9.   NAS, CMB 1/6, *CMBS Minutes*, 2 April 1942, Vol 26, p 31.

10. Towler, Bramall, *Midwives in History and Society*, p 231.

11. Personal communication.

12. 'Editorial', *Nursing Times*, 10 April 1943, pp 229-230.

13. LR 128; Reid, 'Wartime Midwives'; the official name of the QAs changed to the Queen Alexandra's Royal Army Nursing Corps (QARANC) in 1949.

14. NAS, CMB 1/6, *CMBS Minutes*, 2 April 1942, Vol 26, p 31; *ibid*, 20 November 1942, p 32.

15. LR 108; Reid, 'Wartime Midwives'.

16. *Ibid*; LR 35.

17. LR 114; Reid, 'Wartime Midwives'.

18. *Ibid*; LR 80.

19. LR 56.

20. NAS, CMB 1/7, *CMBS Minutes*, 8 October 1943, p 1.

21. NAS, CMB 1/7, *CMBS Minutes*, 27 February 1945, p 4.

22. H P Tait, 'Maternity and child welfare', in G McLachlan, (ed), *Improving the Common Weal: Aspects of Scottish Health Services, 1900-1984*, (Edinburgh: Edinburgh University Press, 1987), p 417.

23. A MacGregor, *Public Health in Glasgow, 1905-1946*, (Edinburgh and London: Livingstone, 1967), quoted in A Oakley, *The Captured Womb*, (Oxford: Basil Blackwell Publishers, 1984), p 118.

24. Oakley, *Captured Womb*, p 118.

25. J Towler, J Bramall, *Midwives in History and Society*, (London: Croom Helm, 1986), p 229.

26. J Sturrock, 'Edinburgh Royal Maternity and Simpson Memorial Hospital', A Sir James Y Simpson Memorial Lecture delivered on 11 July 1979, reprinted from the *Journal of the Royal College of Surgeons of Edinburgh*, (May 1980), Vol 25, p 184.

27. M Berghahn, *Continental Britons*, (Oxford: Berg Publishers, 1988), p 75.

28. *Ibid*, pp 83-87.

29. NAS, CMB 1/6, *CMBS Minutes*, 24 March 1939, Vol 24, p 8.

30. NAS, CMB 1/6, *CMBS Minutes*, 9 June 1939, Vol 24, p 17; *ibid*, 21 July, 1939, p 23; *ibid*, 20 December 1939, p 31; *ibid*, 5 May 1939, pp 11, 12.

31. NAS, CMB 1/6, *CMBS Minutes*, 23 February 1940, Vol 24, p 39.

32. *Ibid*, 29 September 1939, p 26; *ibid*, 20 December 1939, p 33. At this point the current total appears to have been thirteen refugee pupil midwives in Scotland.

33. NAS, CMB 1/6, *CMBS Minutes*, 17 January 1941, Vol 25, p 21.

34. Berghahn, *Continental Britons*, p 85.

35. Towler, Bramall, *Midwives in History and Society*, p 233.

36. *CMBS Rules*, 1939, Rules D 24, p 37.

37. NAS, CMB 1/7, *CMBS Minutes*, 28 February 1946, p 3.

38. NAS, CMB 1/7, *CMBS Minutes*, 31 January 1946, p 1; NAS, CMB 1/7, *CMBS Minutes*, 31 October 1946, p 2. Rules C dealt with regulating the course of training, the conduct of examinations , the remuneration of examiners and the issue of certificates; RCS Ed 13/1/4, (CMBS), letter from Secretary CMBE&W to Secretary CMBS dated 31 October 1946, and copy of application form. RCS Ed, 13/1/1, (CMBS), Reference translated from Norwegian; NAS, CMB 1/7, *CMBS Minutes*, 31 October 1946, p 1.

39. LR 114.

40. NAS, CMB 1/8, *CMBS Minutes*, 15 June 1961, p 2; an Enrolled Nurse in Scotland was equivalent to a State Enrolled Nurse in England.

41. Ministry of Health, DHS, Ministry of Labour and National Service, *Report of the Working Party (WP) on Midwives*, (London: HMSO, 1949), Introduction, para 1; Kerr, Johnstone, Phillips, *Historical Review*, p 345; R Peters, J Kinnaird, *Health Services Administration*, (Edinburgh: Livingstone, 1965), p 316, comment on the 'Working Party on the Recruitment and Training of Nurses' (1948) recommended that midwifery should be amalgamated with the general nurses training programme.

42. Towler, Bramall, *Midwives in History and Society*, p 234.

43. *Working Party on Midwives*, paras 101, 102.

44. *Ibid*, para 116.

45. *Ibid*, paras 119-130.

46. *Ibid*, para 111-118; The 1972 *Briggs Report* made similar recommendations; Towards the end of the twentieth century, shared learning became more usual within universities, bringing students of differing disciplines together and harnessing resources.

47. Towler, Bramall, *Midwives in History and Society*, p 235; Kerr, Johnstone, Phillips, *Historical Review*, p 346.

48. A few years after this, in Professor R Johnstone's valedictory address, he implied that one of the marks of progress of midwifery in Scotland was that 'there has been a noticeable drop in the number of untrained women applying for training...and a correspondingly great increase in the number of general-trained nurses seeking to round off their practical training by studying midwifery.' NAS, CMB1/7, *CMBS Minutes*, 26 February 1953, p 3.

49. NAS, CMB 1/7, *CMBS Minutes*, 28 April, 1949, p 3; *Working Party on Midwives*, para, 291.

50. Cumberlege, *Maternity in Great Britain*, p 78.

51. D Moir, *Pain Relief in Labour, (5th ed)*, (Edinburgh: Churchill Livingstone, 1986) p 1; A S Williams, *Women and Childbirth in the Twentieth Century*

(Stroud: Sutton Publishing, 1997), pp 127-128: The National Birthday Trust responded to mothers who contacted it because of their fear of pain in childbirth.

52. Cumberlege, *Maternity in Great Britain*, p 78.

53. Williams, *Women and Childbirth in the Twentieth Century*, p 135.

54. Cumberlege, *Maternity in Great Britain*, p 79.

55. Towler, Bramall, *Midwives in History and Society*, p 237; *Working Party on Midwives*, para 105: the Minnitt apparatus in the 1940s weighed 22 lbs.

56. Williams, *Women and Childbirth in the Twentieth Century*, p 141.

57. Cumberlege, *Maternity in Great Britain*, p 78.

58. Williams, *Women and Childbirth in the Twentieth Century*, p 140.

59. *1937 Maternity Services (Scotland) Act*, 1, (2), (d).

60. *CMBS Rules*, 1948, Rules C, pp 31-33.

61. Williams, *Women and Childbirth in the Twentieth Century*, p 141.

62. *Ibid*, p 140.

63. NAS, CMB 1/6, *CMBS Minutes*, 16 December 1938, Vol 23, p 28; *ibid*, 20 January 1939, p 30; *ibid*, 17 February 1939, p 33.

64. NAS, CMB 1/6, *CMBS Minutes*, 24 March 1939, Vol 24, p 7.

65. *Ibid*, 9 June 1939, p 16.

66. NAS, CMB 1/6, *CMBS Minutes*, 17 January 1941, Vol 25, p 20. This time the Board used the anaesthesia/analgesia argument when it suited it to do so.

67. NAS, CMB 1/7, *CMBS Minutes*, 31 January 1946, p 2; NAS, CMB 1/7, *CMBS Minutes*, 28 February, 1946, p 2.

68. *Ibid*, p 3; NAS, CMB 1/7, *CMBS Minutes*, 26 August 1948, p 2.

69. Moir, *Pain Relief in Labour*, p 82; The Board also approved the Jecta gas and air apparatus in 1949. This was similar to the Minnitt apparatus in that they both delivered a 50:50 nitrous oxide and air mixture.

70. NAS, CMB 1/7, *CMBS Minutes*, 28 April 1949, p 1; 28 July 1949, p 1; 28 April 1949, p 3; 23 February 1951,p 1; 6 June 1952, p 2; 20 May 1954, p 1; 18 November 1954, p 1; 17 February 1955, p 2; 10 November 1955, p 1; H P Tait, *Trilene Analgesia*, from notes belonging to Miss Isabel Duguid, MTD, (July 1955); Moir, *Pain Relief in Labour*, p 84.

71. *Ibid*, p 67.

72. *Ibid*, p 66.

73. J Brotherston, 'The National Health Service in Scotland: 1948-1984', in McLachlan, *Improving the Common Weal*, p 106.

74. S Robinson, 'Maintaining the independence of midwives', in J Garcia, R Kilpatrick, M Richards, (eds), *The Politics of Maternity Care*, (Oxford: Clarendon Press, 1990), p 73.

75. NAS, CMB, 1/7, *CMBS Minutes*, 'Chairman's Review of the Board's Progress since 1915', 26 February 1953, pp 3-4.

76. *Working Party on Midwives*, Postscript to Introduction, p viii; Robinson, 'Maintaining the independence of midwives', p 72.

77. Robinson, *'Maintaining the independence of midwives'*, p 74.

78. *Working Party on Midwives*, Postscript to Introduction, p viii.

79. Robinson, *'Maintaining the independence of midwives'*, p 73.

80.   Tait, 'Maternity and child welfare', in McLachlan, (ed), *Improving the Common Weal*, p 420; Robinson, *'Maintaining the independence of midwives'*, p 75.

81.   Williams, *Women and Childbirth in the Twentieth Century*, p 200.

82.   LR 27.

83.   *Ibid.*

84.   For further discussion on the change in place of birth, see chapter 7.

85.   NAS, CMB 1/7, *CMBS Minutes*, 28 February 1947, p 2; NAS, CMB 1/7, *CMBS Minutes*, 26 February 1948, p 3; NAS, CMB 1/7, *CMBS Minutes*, 20 November 1947, p 3.

86.   NAS, CMB 1/7, *CMBS Minutes*, 26 February 1948, p 3.

87.   NAS, CMB 1/7, *CMBS Minutes*, 20 November 1947, p 3.

88.   NAS, CMB 1/7, *CMBS Minutes*, 28 April 1949, p 2; NAS, CMB 1/7, *CMBS Minutes*, 28 July 1949, p 1; NAS, CMB, 1/8, *CMBS Minutes*, 11 May 1961, p 1; NAS, CMB 1/7, *CMBS Minutes*, 26 February 1948, p 3.

89.   NAS, CMB, 1/8, *CMBS Minutes*, p 1; Towler, Bramall, *Midwives in History and Society*, p 235.

90.   M Cronk, *'Midwifery: a practitioner's view from within the National Health Service'*, Midwife, Health Visitor and Community Nurse, (1990), Vol 26 (3), p 58.

91.   *Ibid*, pp 58-63.

92.   NAS, CMB 1/7, *CMBS Minutes*, 14 November 1951, p 1; NAS, CMB 1/7, *CMBS Minutes*, 16 March 1953, p 1.

93.   LR 120, CMBS member 1973-1983.

Chapter 6

All change: management, education, practice and statute

The 1960s saw issues which became increasingly threatening for the future of midwifery as a profession separate from nursing, for midwifery as a career, and for the credibility of the CMBS. In Scotland, these issues centred round re-organisation of regional and hospital management along with midwifery and nursing education. The problems intensified as attempts to restructure management and education became UK-wide. This led to career problems for midwifery teachers and managers and was followed by a re-organisation of the NHS in 1974 and associated integration problems with midwifery practice. Around the same time, the UK's entry in 1973 into the European Economic Community (EEC) and discussion surrounding this, continued to be in the headlines. Further change was inevitable as the CMBS became embroiled in discussion and dispute surrounding the EEC Midwifery Directives, new midwifery courses and the parallel discussions from the Briggs Committee on nursing following its establishment in 1970. This chapter explores these issues within the context of the CMBS and the midwifery profession in Scotland.

Changes at the CMBS

By 1960, the CMBS had been in existence for forty-four years. Its main committees were those dealing with finance, penal cases and issues surrounding examinations, with other temporary committees established on an *ad hoc* basis. Sometimes it appeared to work very slowly and, in 1960, it agreed to form an Executive Committee from within its membership to make the work of the Board more expeditious and efficient.[1] This Committee quickly became essential to the Board's work and remained in place until the Board's demise in 1983.[2] One of its first tasks was to organise the appointment of an education officer to the Board.[3]

The creation of this salaried post in 1961 was an important administrative innovation. By having one person with clear duties in this field it demonstrated the serious nature of the Board's attitude to the education of midwives. The first education officer, starting on 3 April 1961, was Miss J H Beckett at a salary of £1,000 per annum rising to £1,200 with annual increments of £40.[4] On her retiral in 1973 she was succeeded by Miss Annie Grant, also a Board member, until she retired in 1982. By this time, the new United Kingdom Central Council (UKCC) and National Boards (see below) were about to take over from the current statutory nursing and midwifery bodies. To cover the intervening gap, the National Board for Scotland (NBS) appointed Miss Veronica E Pope as Professional Officer (Midwifery and Examinations) with effect from 14 September 1982, and seconded Miss Pope to the CMBS to act as its Professional Officer until the Board relinquished its statutory duties.[5]

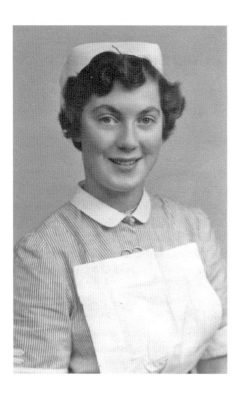

*Above: Pupil midwife Catherine
Robertson (now MacMillan), 1955,
Dunfermline Maternity Hospital.
(Courtesy of Catherine MacMillan.)*

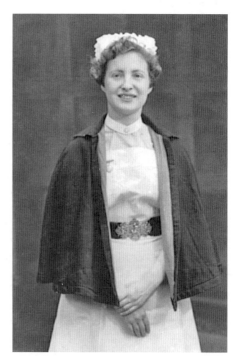

*Right: Margaret Nicol (now Ritchie),
newly qualified, SCM, 1958,
Dunfermline Maternity Hospital.
(Courtesy of Margaret Ritchie.)*

Loss of midwifery matrons, status and career prospects
The advent of the NHS had brought changes to the administration of maternity services which impinged on the place of birth, continuity of care for mothers, and midwives' practice. Across the NHS in its early years, there was a rising tide of expenditure which warranted investigation. This culminated in the *Guillebaud Report* which, in 1956, 'revealed the potentially unlimited demand for health care and the necessity of containing that demand within a finite budget.'[6] It also highlighted the confused state of the maternity services and recommended their review.[7] The Government responded, and in Scotland, also in 1956, the Montgomery Committee started to consider what the NHS should provide for the mother and child during pregnancy, confinement and lying-in, and to advise on the best way of doing this within its framework.[8] According to the *Montgomery Report*, the plan for maternity hospital and specialist services which the Regional Hospital Boards inherited, and developed under the NHS, came from the existing maternity services, together with the additions provided during the War.[9] The implementation of the NHS Acts in 1948, and the resulting changes, reinforced an earlier wartime trend towards hospital births.[10]

The CMBS, responding to an invitation to give evidence to the Committee, addressed antenatal care, care during and after confinement, and administration. The evidence lacked conviction. It mentioned the midwife as a role-player in maternity care, but missed the opportunity to highlight the midwife's role as a practitioner capable of undertaking full care of a mother in a normal child-bearing episode.[11] The CMBS emphasised that homebirths remained a satisfactory option for many women, but omitted to stress the importance of the midwife's role in homebirths, an environment where the midwife, not the doctor, delivered most of the babies. The word 'midwife' is mentioned once in this section of the submission.[12] It may be that the CMBS took this as understood. Nevertheless, it is ironic that in the last section, on administration, the Board revealed its concerns for the recruitment, retention, autonomy and career prospects of midwives in Scotland while elsewhere it failed to stress the importance of midwives and their role.[13]

Midwifery administrative problems increased. Until 1960, with a few exceptions, a midwife in charge of a maternity unit in Scotland was called 'Matron', and carried the full status that this implied. This term, although belonging to the nursing hierarchy, gave the top midwifery post in a maternity unit equal standing with senior nursing colleagues. The CMBS commented to the Montgomery Committee that administrative change was eliminating the role of the midwifery matron, but quickly found that it was powerless to prevent this loss of administrative autonomy. For instance, an early casualty of the change happened with the loss of the midwifery matron at the Vale of Leven Hospital. In 1960, a new proposal placed Vale of Leven's maternity unit under the overall authority of the hospital's Matron resulting in a lower administrative rank for the head of midwifery. The Board expressed its grave concern regarding Vale of Leven and elsewhere. In some instances, the matrons of general hospitals made themselves responsible for the recruitment and training of midwives while their major raison d'être was to recruit and train student nurses.[14] Also, as poor retention was on-going, this change imposed limitations on promotion and career-building within midwifery. This had implications for the attractiveness of a career in midwifery and consequent effect on recruitment and retention.[15]

The CMBS finally came to terms with the inevitable administrative change and turned its attention to the procedure for making appointments to senior posts.[16] It urged the Scottish Home and Health Department (SHHD), not always successfully, to recognise the importance of having a midwife on the interviewing panel for senior nursing posts involving midwifery.[17] The CMBS was making a fair point as a non-midwife assessor would not ask a candidate appropriate questions about midwifery within the hospital, and might not stipulate what was expected regarding midwifery. In time, some regard was paid to the Board's recommendations, although from the Board's point of view, the situation could never satisfactorily be resolved.[18]

Similar problems arose in midwifery education where the Board found that recruitment and training of student midwives might come under a principal who was not a midwife.[19] According to the *Rules*, approved teaching institutions had to conform to certain prescribed requirements. For example, the Board used its influence in Aberdeen in 1966 where the principal of the new College of Nursing (sic) at Foresterhill was to be a non-midwife directly in charge of recruitment and training of student midwives.[20] A compromise was reached where Aberdeen Maternity Hospital remained the approved training institution, with the matron in charge of the recruitment and training of student midwives who received theoretical training in the College.[21] In addition the North-Eastern Hospital Board invited the CMBS to nominate one of three assessors to appoint a Principal to the College.

The *Salmon Report*

Although the Foresterhill College case had a good outcome from the Board's point of view, administrative change in both management and education of nurses and midwives was inevitable and became even more apparent with the appointment of another Committee.[22] This came in the middle of what Davies and Beach describe as 'a decade of disquiet within nursing' with concerns over structure of the nursing service, its status within the NHS, and the standard and method of nurse training.[23] Inevitably, given the strong links between the two professions, midwifery was included within the Salmon Committee's remit to review and advise on the senior nursing staff structure in the hospital service (ward sister and above), the administrative function of the respective grades, and the methods of preparing staff to occupy them.

The Salmon Committee invited written and oral evidence in early 1964. The CMBS, with support from the Scottish Standing Committee of the RCOG,[24] strongly promoted the midwives' case, especially for the retention of midwife matrons.[25] Nevertheless, the Salmon Committee's Report, published in 1966, and implemented in many areas in Scotland in the 1970s, 'completely changed the management and administration of nursing [including midwifery] in hospitals.'[26] It eliminated midwifery matrons with administrative autonomy. Job descriptions for nurses and midwives were graded from the top Grade 10 to Grade 6, ward sister. Margaret Clark, Nursing Officer, SHHD, while acknowledging the need for the Salmon Committee's work, said that the Report was implemented before full evaluation of its pilot studies. The ensuing divisive hierarchy became known as 'the Salmon structure' and, when implemented across the country, thoughtlessly standardised 'an amorphous organisation'.[27]

Midwives' opinions varied. Joan Savage, Matron of the Elsie Inglis Memorial Maternity Hospital, Edinburgh, recalled:

> I enjoyed my time there until re-organisation came. Salmon came first...with all their numbers. I was a number eight. They made my tutor a number seven and I said she should be a number eight as well... It made a difference to her salary [and] she was as important... We had a number nine over us... She was floating... and we used to get directives from [her]. One included how to get the patients to write a Will. I thought this is nonsense... This is a maternity hospital. That [Salmon structuring] made a lot of difference and the change... You see, the Matron used to be in charge of everything – kitchen, domestic staff. They knew who to go to. You knew who needed help. Then the kitchens...and domestics...went into some other [management] outwith the hospital.[28]

Joan Spence, a midwife at Aberdeen Maternity Hospital in the 1970s, felt that the coming of the Salmon structure precipitated promotion upon some who were not ready.

> Salmon came in [in 1974] and very experienced ward sisters were shunted out to walk the corridors as Nursing Officers. We were told we were going to be sisters. We weren't in an interview situation where you were applying. We were told. I was going to be a relief sister between the nursery and the postnatal wards. I said to the assistant-matron, 'I don't really want a sister's post.' I was more or less told that you either did it or you would never get another one. So we were all promoted.[29]

Margaret Auld went to the Borders in 1973 as Chief Area Nursing Officer. She acknowledged the danger of over-structuring the service. However, as part of the Salmon Committee's recommendations included improvements in practice, education and career structures, the need to re-structure services in the Borders was apparent. However, she encountered some problems:

> They had not had Salmon imposed down here then, so I re-organised it when I came, with the [Health] Board's approval of course. Everything had to go to them... In retrospect, we did it too much. There was not the need for the number of nursing officers we put in here. Well... we learn by trial and error. It was just too structured. There were a number of small hospitals... in Duns, Coldstream. Kelso, Jedburgh, Hawick, Galashiels and Peebles, each with some midwifery beds. Some, I remember, [with] as little as two and some as many as twenty plus. The equipment was awful. It was...very bad...and so we decided to centralise a bit and that caused a great deal of angst.[30]

Obtaining midwives and maintaining their skills in an area with a low birth-rate was also difficult. Margaret Auld commented:

> It might have been better if we had kept some of the beds but ... you could not get the midwives. The cover was very difficult to maintain for these beds... Because there wasn't the work... The birth-rate here is...very low... The population at that time...was ninety-five thousand ...for the whole

area...and it's a very, very elderly population, the Borders... [The birth rate has] gone up a bit now because we've got more younger people coming in... So you might have a midwifery unit and one delivery a week... and you'd have a midwife sitting there and doing nothing and you were having to pay [her]. A very expensive service. And not keeping her skills up at all. So it [was] better to centralise a bit so that you could properly staff these places, make sure that everybody was up to date and we started sending ...[midwives] up to the Simpson to get updated.[31]

There were also problems and anomalies for those teaching in midwifery. There was no Salmon Committee equivalent of a principal Nurse Tutor Grade 9 for midwives. The most a senior midwife tutor could hope for was Grade 8. This would adversely affect the status of midwife tutors with a subsequent effect on midwifery teaching, practice and career prospects.[32] Yet Margaret Kitson, an exception to the trend, explained what happened to her in Glasgow:

In 1970, I came to Rottenrow as the principal tutor there... I stayed there until September '76... During that time, the Salmon Structure was introduced and I was the only Principal Nursing Officer (Midwifery Teaching) in Scotland and that was ... purely an accident of the Salmon grading. It was exactly the same as a principal tutor's job. But because there was a chief nursing officer (midwifery), a grade 10 post for the management of midwifery, there was a grade 9 post for the teacher so, if you like, there was no difference in the job, but there was a difference in the grading.[33]

The experience of others, such as Peggy Grieve, who was a midwife tutor at Cresswell Maternity Hospital, Dumfries, confirmed the CMBS's fears. Peggy Grieve found that the Salmon structure gave her a lower grading than she would otherwise have had. Because of this, she decided to move from midwifery teaching to management.

They employed another tutor and [therefore] I was the senior tutor. Then, of course, the Salmon structure came in and my grade was [reduced] because it was not a big enough hospital...for the senior person [in midwifery teaching] to be a principal nursing officer. I was only at the grade of nursing officer. Well I [appealed to] the College [the RCM] at that time and the Scottish Home and Health Department, you name it and I got nowhere. So I thought well, right, I'm not going to do this.[34]

Gelda Pryde, who was senior nursing officer in Angus in the 1970s, agreed that the Salmon structure did not favour midwife teachers. However, she felt that restructuring of management was, in the main, a good and necessary move.

It could be that [because] the Salmon structure wasn't so favourable to midwifery tutors so many of them turned to management... There were more management posts and they...were different. It wasn't a matron sitting in an office. They really had a higher pinnacle content to some of the management folk. They became nursing officers or senior nursing officers for groups of wards so they really were involved again with almost direct care if they were needed. I think it [Salmon restructuring] was a good thing... It certainly brought management and clinical practice closer together. When I came to Angus...there were matrons in every small hospital. So I had something like ...eight matrons. That would be in 1973... The Angus post [as senior nursing officer] attracted me rather than all the other senior management posts because the ones in the big hospitals were purely for general [nursing], but this one had the three maternity units and, of course, midwifery having been my main love, that was why I came here... But...[the] eight matrons... then became nursing officers of their various units, both in midwifery and in general and because my post took away a lot of the pure management... they then had the time and the remit [included] in their job to be more clinically involved... I think this was a good thing... Because I was there...with an overview of all the units, I could then begin to update the ones that really had fallen behind because they were all very isolated. They didn't really have much contact. But because my meetings brought them all together then they obviously began to discuss their ways of working in each unit. I think it made quite an impact on [them] when I did that... [They were] number seven [and I was a number] eight. I think I was perhaps more readily accepted by the midwifery nursing officers because they obviously realised that I had a lot of midwifery expertise and they were reasonably happy [although some missed the title 'matron']... And I think the doctors resented [the changes] very much. We had a lot of battles with them...[because], I think more power to the midwives probably... I think they saw me as a threat because, again, there was quite a lot of GP midwifery practice and some of it, well, didn't really come up to the standard that I would have liked.[35]

The recommendations of the *Salmon Report* included recognition of the need to look more closely at practice, to be more aware of the importance of research and continuing education, and to facilitate a clinical career structure for nurses. However, as far as midwifery was concerned, the recommendations were only partly fulfilled.[36]

Integration of midwifery services
With the enactment in 1974 of the 1972 National Health Service (Scotland) Act, the tripartite administration of the NHS in Scotland ended. It had been clumsy, disjointed and inefficient, and did little, if anything, to achieve co-operation between professionals working within the NHS. The re-organisation proposed to slim down the huge administrative network of the original NHS from five regional Boards, twenty-five executive councils, fifty-six local health committees and sixty-five boards of management to what eventually became fifteen Health Boards.[37] Re-organisation aimed, firstly, to improve patient care by integrating personal health services 'around the patient' and developing a preventative community-based health care system. Secondly, it planned to supply a unified yet supportive, flexible management system with a long-term planning process that would have a building-block effect upon future developments.[38]

Integration of the maternity services in Scotland from 1974 was part of the wider plan for change. The *Montgomery Report* of 1959 had recommended greater co-ordination of the maternity services under the GP to reduce confusion and increase continuity of care. Yet, by the mid-1960s, the service remained disjointed. For instance, if a woman planned a hospital birth, hospital staff usually accepted antenatal responsibility for her. Thus, the booking GP handed over her care. The domiciliary/district midwife employed by the LA often did not see the mother before the birth. The midwife had nothing to do with the birth and first saw the mother and baby postnatally on discharge. Discharge became increasingly early to accommodate the demand for maternity beds. So, the domiciliary midwife did little antenatal and intranatal care and did not practise holistically, leading to loss of both skills and job satisfaction. From the mother's point of view, she did not receive continuity of care as she saw different doctors and midwives at the clinics, had an unknown midwife to deliver her, and did not become acquainted with her district midwife until post-delivery.

One proposed answer to the problem that gained favour in the 1960s was integration.[39] Even before Government reports in the 1970s, this was happening on a pragmatic basis between the three branches of the maternity services. Formalisation came in 1971 with the formation of the Tennent Committee which reported in 1973.[40] Its remit was: 'to examine the integration of the maternity and midwifery work of the hospital and the specialist, general medical and local health authority services in Scotland and to make recommendations.'[41]

The CMBS considered total integration of the maternity services in Scotland to be essential and made recommendations to the Tennent Committee. Firstly, ultimate clinical responsibility for women in each childbearing episode should lie with a consultant obstetrician. Secondly, the place of birth for all would be hospital, either consultant or GP unit, selected according to an agreed policy. Thirdly, midwives should be essential members of the team, ante, intra, and postnatally, but, in the labour ward particularly, the midwife should 'carry out measures of treatment as delegated by the medical staff,' making it clear that to be a team player did not mean parity of status.[42]

Obstetricians had been influential in the production of the *Peel Report* which preceded the *Tennent Report* by three years.[43] Although there was no supporting evidence, for the first time a Government Report advocated 100% hospital delivery on the grounds of safety.[44] Although the *Peel Report* did not apply to Scotland, the *Tennent Report*, while acknowledging geographical and demographical differences, agreed with Peel's main conclusions and recommendations.[45] The term '100% hospital confinement' is implicit in the *Tennent Report's* text recommending further integration of the maternity services in Scotland. The recommendations highlighted the midwife's role as a team-member while acknowledging updating and career problems. Greater co-ordination between community and hospital would improve midwifery care for mothers and enhance the professional development of midwives within a district.[46]

So, the *Tennent Report* and its recommendations for an integrated maternity service fitted in with NHS re-organisation plans. But it did not seem to offer real progress for the midwifery profession.

The European Economic Community (EEC): The Midwifery Directives
In 1973, the UK became a member of the EEC, joining existing members, France, Italy,

Germany, the Netherlands, Luxembourg and Belgium, and two other new members, Denmark and Ireland. This long-talked-about step resulted in changes for everyone, including the profession of midwifery. The CMBS was in the thick of the changes brought about by the UK's entry into the EEC and subsequent new EEC rules for the education of midwives. These new problems centred on old issues: firstly the solipsistic attitude of others who ignored the Board or did not realise that the Board existed; and secondly, the question of who might enter training in midwifery and how long were courses to be. For a long time, the CMBs of Scotland, and England and Wales had held varying opinions, one of the most recent being the cessation of direct-entry midwifery training in Scotland in 1968.[47] In the 1970s, because of the UK's entry to the EEC, the CMBs had to try to resolve their differences and speak with one voice while negotiating the EEC Midwifery Directives.

CMBS Minutes first mention the EEC in December 1970.[48] It was important that the CMBS should have a voice in any UK-wide discussion on midwifery, firstly because it was an independent Board, equal in status to the CMBE&W, and secondly because midwifery in Scotland varied considerably from England and Wales, particularly when it came to training. But, until September 1971, all discussions on the EEC had been conducted by the Secretary of the CMBE&W and 'England was apparently recognised as synonymous with Britain.'[49] The CMBS was concerned about its exclusion. A joint meeting proved difficult to arrange and, to compound the Board's feeling of omission, the Department of Health & Social Security (DHSS) compiled the publication, *The Common Market and the Nursing Profession*, in consultation with the CMBE&W but not with the CMBS.[50] The CMBS could not accept that the CMBE&W was in any position to speak for midwifery in the UK as a whole.

The first draft of the EEC Midwifery Directives was published in 1972. They stated that a person could become a midwife in two ways: firstly after three years midwifery training (direct entry) and secondly after two years midwifery training, following general nurse training.[51] This required in-depth consultation which was not happening inside the UK until the UK countries set up a liaison committee to establish a common and constructive approach. This committee finally met on 7 December 1972. [52]

Finding common ground within the UK Liaison Committee proved to be difficult.[53] The members could not agree on a joint approach, particularly in regard to non-nurses being trained as midwives.[54] At the CMBS's instigation, the SHHD agreed to consult further with the DHSS.[55] The Executive Committee wanted to ensure that there was no wide assumption that the views expressed by the CMBE&W were the agreed views of the UK Midwifery Boards.[56] Further trouble came in January 1975 when the CMBS heard by chance about an EEC sub-committee meeting at the House of Lords. CMBS representative, Miss Sheelagh Bramley, and CMBS Secretary, Miss Dorothy S Young attended. At the meeting they found the Sub-Committee under the impression that the CMBE&W was the statutory body responsible for midwifery in the UK, and had been sending information about the Directives to the CMBE&W, but not to the CMBS. Prior to the meeting, Miss Bramley and Miss Young were called to meet the Chairman of the CMBE&W so that they could speak with one voice, 'namely the English voice'. However, Miss Bramley would not agree to this and the incident led to a CMBS complaint to the Scottish Office and the CMBE&W.[57]

The UK Liaison Committee struggled on. The members were surprised to hear that all the EEC countries would have to conform to the types of training in the Directives once acceptance was reached. The CMBS also had a problem accepting the idea of a direct-entry midwifery course.[58] Nevertheless, realising that agreement must be reached the Boards gradually began to come together, although the next argument regarding the extension of the midwifery course for registered nurses to eighteen months rumbled on until the CMBS acquiesced.[59]

By 1979, agreement was in sight. The other EEC countries agreed to a two-year post-nursing midwifery training programme. The UK, now speaking with 'one voice', wanted an eighteen-month training programme with an additional period of six months post-enrolment experience for midwives planning to practise in other EEC countries. The negotiators agreed the eighteen-month training, but stipulated a year's additional experience as a condition of free movement within the EEC. Finally, the EEC Midwifery Directives were agreed and signed on 21 January 1980 and Member States were required to conform to their requirements within three years.[60]

There were other issues. The EEC Midwifery Directives stated that those doing the eighteen-month midwifery course should be qualified in general nursing.[61] The only other way of becoming a midwife was by completing a three year course. The issue of registered nurses who were not Registered General Nurses (RGN) becoming midwives was one over which the CMBS and the CMBE&W had disagreed for many years. In Scotland, registered nurses were allowed to do the shorter midwifery course.[62] Although the CMBE&W eventually conceded that Registered Sick Children's Nurses (RSCN) could do the shorter course, all others in England and Wales had to do a longer course. This would put registered nurses in Scotland, who were not RGNs and who wished to become midwives, at a disadvantage after the Directives came into operation; there was no way around the problem.[63] Also, since 1968, there was no direct entry midwifery course in Scotland. By the time the EEC Midwives' Directives came into effect on 23 January 1983 a solution had not been found.

The Briggs Committee and beyond
During the 1960s, the 'decade of disquiet', the need for change in the health services became increasingly apparent with an integrated rather than a fragmented structure of health care.[64] This need was partly fulfilled by the recommendations of the 1959 *Montgomery* and 1973 *Tennent Reports* and integration of the health service in the 1970s. However, implementation of the *Salmon Report* did little to alleviate the unrest and insecurity over education and practice within the nursing and midwifery professions. Against this background the cross-UK Committee on Nursing commenced its work:

> To review the role of the nurse and the midwife in the hospital and the community and the education and training required for that role, so that the best use is made of available manpower to meet present needs and the needs of an integrated health service.[65]

The Committee on Nursing comprised twenty members, three of whom were from Scotland: Ivor Batchelor, Professor of Psychiatry, University of Dundee, Margaret Scott

Wright, Professor of Nursing at the University of Edinburgh, and Margaret Auld, midwife, Matron of the SMMP and CMBS member, who commented:

> [The Committee's] remit was huge... [It had] to look at the way in which nurse/midwifery training was carried out and health visiting and district nursing and to decide the appropriate way that this should be organised and monitored.[66]

Although the Committee was concerned about the different professions within its remit, because of requirements to work within existing resource levels it had to focus on the needs of the service rather than those of the professions.[67] Margaret Auld observed that, 'It grew out of the fact that there had been...endless committees before us who said that there were shortages of nurses and midwives.'[68]

The Briggs Committee also focussed on the existing statutory arrangements and what it saw as many inflexible failings.[69] Margaret Auld commented:

> There was a feeling that the way in which nursing was structured was wrong... You kept repeating bits of courses... If you wanted to take an additional qualification you found yourself repeating...work and this was...misuse of time. There [were]...far too many registering bodies all overlapping...health visitors, the district nurses, nursing, midwifery.[70]

Committee members were put under great pressure to complete their Report within the agreed timescale. Margaret Auld said, 'The Chairman, Asa Briggs, ...promised the Government they'd have it in two years and the Report was actually written and prepared and presented in the two years.'[71] Because of the heavy workload, the Briggs Committee also had five sub-committees most of which Margaret Auld attended. 'I was on a lot of them because I was the only [practising] midwife in the whole committee.'[72] This highlights the issue of 'balance' which remained sensitive during the Committee's lifetime. Nurses were concerned that the Committee did not sufficiently represent 'junior nursing staff from the provinces' and 'midwives were uncomfortable with the inclusion of only one practising midwife.'[73]

The CMBS was one of the bodies to present written evidence to the Briggs Committee.[74] It covered the role of the midwife in all areas of practice, the problems of recruitment to midwifery, the importance of both tutors and clinical instructors, midwifery training, and made a strong statement on a career structure for midwives particularly after the implementation of the *Salmon Report*:

> It has become apparent that midwifery is taking a subservient place to general and psychiatric nursing... The midwife is an important and valued member of the obstetric team... The Salmon structure does not give credit for [the] special responsibilities and status of the midwife and...the only solution would be to have a separate structure for midwives...without losing status, prospects or salary.[75]

However, this did not match the Board's earlier evidence that 'the midwifery service should be based on 100% hospitalisation...with ultimately 100% consultant responsibility,' and that integration of midwifery services was essential for 'bringing together the consultant, the GP and the midwife as a team with the consultant accepting ultimate clinical responsibility.'[76] While integration was important and necessary in light of the re-organisation of NHS administration, the Board's comments potentially took autonomy from the midwife. Yet, later in the evidence, the Board emphasised the midwife's 'statutory authority'.

The Briggs Committee faced controversial issues from nurses, including district nurses, and health visitors as well as midwives. Nevertheless, specific arguments from midwifery bodies required particular attention. These included the issue of professional identity and the 'distinctiveness of midwifery' which the Committee affirmed, the midwife's role as educator of medical students as well as student midwives, her history of independent practice (although only a vestige of real independent midwifery practice was left by the 1970s), and the strength of the development of midwifery separate from nursing.[77] These special features were arguments for continuing separate statutory regulation. The Briggs Committee did not agree. This was partly to do with its decision to bring nursing and midwifery education closer together to develop the hitherto relatively poor communication between nurses and midwives. In addition, the *Briggs Report* recommended that 'in future all midwives should be nurses.'[78] It saw this as an added incentive to fuse the separate structures and argued that statutory amalgamation of nurses and midwives would help them to be seen as a stronger body when it came to negotiating policy. The committee saw this as a particularly important point in the light of the EEC draft proposals.[79] Margaret Kitson, CMBS member, commented:

> The reason for the setting up of the UKCC [United Kingdom Central Council] was really quite simple...that because we were part of the United Kingdom and because the United Kingdom had to speak with a single voice in Europe we had to have a single statutory body. End of story. We had to have it.[80]

Nevertheless, it is worth noting that neither the Scottish Church nor Scottish Law were required to amalgamate with their English counterparts when the UK joined the EEC. They were protected by articles laid down in the 1707 Act of Union between the Scottish and English Parliaments and national differences were preserved.[81]

Another important midwifery issue was that distinct national differences between the CMBs compounded professional sensitivities. Written evidence of both CMBs to the Briggs Committee conflicted on some fundamental points to the extent that the Committee required each body to supply oral evidence which highlighted national differences.[82] Although CMBS representatives hoped to liaise further with the General Nursing Council (GNC) for Scotland, they did not want changes which included amalgamation with other UK bodies. They argued that gains already made in integrating maternity services in Scotland, because of its smaller population and fewer training schools, might be lost if this were to happen.[83]

The 1972 *Briggs Report* contained seventy-five recommendations. The first five recommended extensive changes to the new statutory framework for midwifery and nursing. In particular was the plan for the formation of what became the UKCC and four National Boards.[84] This plan effectively signalled the end of the existing statutory bodies.

For midwifery, apart from the predicted end of the current statutory bodies, including the CMBS, one recommendation in the first section was of particular importance, namely that, 'Midwifery interests should be represented by a statutory Standing Midwifery Committee of the Council...which would advise the Council and Boards on midwifery education and have direct control of midwifery practice.'[85] Margaret Auld, as the only practising midwife on the Briggs Committee, was heavily involved with this. She said:

> I fought very hard to get a midwifery committee because I felt that midwives were different in their preparation...their work and...responsibilities... There needed to be a committee... composed mostly of midwives from the four countries... [to] decide the appropriateness of preparation and so on. The committee, with some reluctance from some members, agreed to this – some members thought this was a divisive solution and favoured unification. I had thought we'd won the argument because we'd written papers about the role and function of midwives and talked about her work and that we'd agreed that a statutory committee would be set up... It was almost at the penultimate meeting in London. We went down to the meeting on the Friday... There was a paper tabled which suggested that there would be a unified structure and I understood this to mean no separate midwifery committee. The UKCC would be a unified body composed of midwives, health visitors, nurses, district nurses and so on. The work required on behalf of these professions would be through the Council. I felt that everyone looked at me for a response. I was so angry I said I could not make a decision now – the paper was tabled, that I'd have to take it away and think about it.
>
> Everyone else managed to leave the hotel that night. I could not get on the night sleeper so had to stay. I flew up to Edinburgh on the Saturday morning and thought about it – and I thought, well, what are the implications of this? So I had an informal discussion with a lawyer and tackled it anew with him – the implications and differences of being a unified body, or working through a statutory committee. It became clear in my mind what I needed to do. I got in touch with the secretariat in London and said that I just couldn't go along with this and if they persisted, I would consider writing a minority report which of course nobody wants because it polarises opinion so much. So, for whatever reason, the Statutory Committee for midwives was back in again.[86]

The Standing Midwifery Committee, with a majority of midwives, 'should include expert midwife and other members in addition to those belonging to the main Council.' It would advise the Council and Boards on midwifery education and act as the national statutory body concerned with the control of practice in midwifery.[87] This was implemented in the Act (see Table 6.1).

The *Briggs Report* recommended controversial changes for midwifery education. In Scotland, instead of the one year midwifery training for registered nurses, or eighteen months for enrolled nurses, the Report recommended two routes, both following Registration as a nurse. Firstly, after a three year nursing course, a twelve month course

Table 6.1 New Committee Structure of the UKCC and National Boards in 1983

**United Kingdom Central Council for
Nurses, Midwives and Health Visitors**

Statutory Committees

| Finance Committee * (FC) | | | Midwifery Committee* (MC) |

Non statutory committees

Training Clinical	Nursing Studies	Mental Nursing Occupational	Health Nursing

National Boards

National Board for Scotland	English National Board	Welsh National Board	National Board for Northern Ireland
FC* MC*	FC* MC*	FC* MC*	FC* MC*
Local Training Committee	Local Training Committee	Local Training Committee	Local Training Committee

In addition there were Joint Committees of the UKCC and the National Boards including Health Visiting JC*, and other Joint Committees to do with training, clinical nursing studies, mental nursing, occupational health nursing and district nursing. * indicates statutory committees of the UKCC and NBs.

Source: 1979 Nurses, Midwives and Health Visitors Act, Chapter 36, sections 7, 8 and 9.

leading to registration as a midwife. Secondly, following an eighteen month Certificate in Nursing Practice (which the Briggs Committee recommended all student nurses and midwives should complete), an eighteen month course leading to Registration as a midwife. Each course, four or three years, would merit the award of a higher certificate.[88] These recommendations, coinciding with discussions on the EEC Midwifery Directives, were not fulfilled completely. Yet they paved the way for further discussion after the 1979 Nurses, Midwives and Health Visitors Act.[89]

The publication of the *Briggs Report* was not the end of the controversy: it could be seen as the end of the beginning. Six years passed before the introduction of the Nurses, Midwives and Health Visitors Bill to the House of Commons. Many differences of opinion within the professions in the UK emerged. The CMBS opposed the Report mainly because of its recommendation for a central UK body. It was unconvinced about this, especially as midwifery in Scotland would then be in a minority position.[90] Also, the CMBS suggested that the Briggs Committee had reached this recommendation without sufficient evidence and so could not justify such a change in the statutory framework.[91] In addition, the Board opposed the recommended two routes to becoming a midwife. It said that this would lead to two grades of midwife (although this was not what the Briggs Committee intended), which would be divisive, and reduce career prospects for the three-year midwives. Scottish midwives, responding to a referendum on the issue in 1973, supported the Board's opinions but with no effect.[92]

The Board was disappointed, if not surprised when the Government accepted the main recommendations of the Report in May 1974.[93] Nevertheless, the effort to modify the recommendations went on. Now that a UKCC was to become a reality, the next step was to press for maximum decentralisation of the proposed National Boards. In this the CMBS worked with the GNC for Scotland which was now anxious to present a united Scottish front to enlarge the functions of the National Boards with a corresponding increase in autonomy.[94] The National Boards, it was argued, should include education, finance, discipline and practice. This much wider set of responsibilities than originally envisaged would give the Boards maximum autonomy. In spite of some opposition from English statutory bodies, the CMBS drew hope from a Government statement recommending maximum de-centralisation to the Boards for appropriate issues.[95]

It became evident that it was not widely known what midwives and the CMBs did. Government Department officials were surprised to learn of the responsibilities of the CMBs and thought that a Standing Midwifery Committee might not be enough to cope with the midwives' situation in the statutory structure.[96] The CMBS argued that there should also be a Standing Midwifery Committee at National Board level to address the particular features of midwifery in each UK country, and at the same time increase the potential power of the National Boards.[97] This eventually came to fruition as shown in Table 6.1.

A significant number of meetings degenerated into wrangles between English and Scottish representatives because of the degree of de-centralisation and delegation of function to the Boards at national level.[98] Margaret Kitson, who was a midwife and CMBS member, looked at reasons why she thought these arguments occurred:

> There was still this very strong Scottish feeling...that, right or wrong, north of the border we were better in terms of education and health service. I mean, the services to the patient, that we were better than they were in England and we really didn't want to get tagged on to that lot down there. That was one thing... The other very trenchant thing was that we didn't want to be taken over. And we felt that with the formation of a UKCC, Scotland would just get lost and its identity would get lost...
>
> Going to meetings in England was a very salutary experience...and not necessarily a happy one because no matter which meeting, Scottish representation was always numerically smaller than English. Scottish views...seemed always to be viewed by the English as inferior and we were just troublemakers. There was no support from Welsh or Irish delegations who, certainly in the view of Scots, seemed just to accept what the English said and 'it would be all right'. So we always felt isolated and on the defensive...
>
> It wasn't just the Board...the forum didn't matter. We did feel that we

were ignored and that forced us on to the defensive. There was no doubt about it...

This is really an aside. One person to whom Scotland, Wales and Ireland [have] great need to be grateful in the setting up of the UKCC, was Enoch Powell. He said, 'If you have a Council, you have to have equal representation.' And he fought for it... I think that a lot of the agonising that went on with the setting up of the UKCC was because of the fear of being taken over. I don't think that that would happen now. I think people [who are] the leaders of nursing and midwifery in Scotland now are much more confident than we were. They're much more confident and they're more confident of a Scottish identity.[99]

The issue of Scottish, along with professional, identity was therefore important. It influenced the argument and was intensified by the contemporary political debate on devolution. The 1970s was a decade of increasing discussion of legislation about devolution for Scotland and Wales. It seemed inappropriate for the Government to be discussing devolving power while at the same time the recommendations of the Briggs Committee were to centralise power. Ian Sharp of the SHHD presented another argument in favour of de-centralising power from the proposed Central Council. He noted that if the Briggs legislation came before Parliament about the same time as legislation on Scottish devolution 'it would be well-nigh impossible for Scottish ministers to defend' the handing over 'to a Great Britain body functions over which Scotland has exercised its own statutory control for so long.'[100]

Before the 1979 Nurses, Midwives and Health Visitors Act was passed representatives of the CMBS took part in the Briggs Co-ordinating Committee and Working Groups, drafting the 'Briggs Bill' and deciding on the committee structure of the Central Council and the National Boards. This included statutory midwifery committees at both Council and Board levels and very much stronger National Boards than first envisaged.[101] Lobbying by professional groups continued right through the legislative process, with midwives 'arguably, the most successful, gaining increased authority for the Central Council's Standing Midwifery Committee.'[102]

The Nurses, Midwives and Health Visitors Act received the Royal Assent on 4 April 1979 and established the UKCC and four National Boards which took over the functions of nine bodies including the CMBs, firstly in 'shadow' form and then officially, on 1 July 1983.[103] The principal functions of the UKCC were to prepare and maintain a register; and to establish and improve standards of training and professional conduct.[104] Each country of the UK had a National Board comprising thirty-five members in Northern Ireland and forty-five members in the other countries. The functions of the National Boards covered: the provision of educational courses and their examinations; collaboration with the UKCC in the promotion of improved training methods; and investigation of alleged misconduct before recourse to the UKCC for further proceedings.[105] As far as the CMBS was concerned, the UKCC and the NBS took over all of its functions. As shown in Table 6.1, each body had a statutory Midwifery Committee. This committee, with a majority of midwives, had to be consulted on all matters pertaining to midwifery.

The Government's original desire to delay the introduction of any necessary subordinate legislation for twelve months was set aside in view of the strength of feeling against this proposal. In consequence, it agreed to set up the National Boards on 15 September 1980, and the Central Council on 1 November 1981, with the existing statutory bodies continuing for two or three years after the new bodies were established.[106] The CMBS therefore maintained a high profile, liaising with the new bodies, attending meetings and ensuring that midwifery interests in Scotland continued to be heard at the highest level.[107]

Statutory care for midwifery in Scotland moved from the CMBS into the hands of the UKCC and the NBS on 1 July 1983. The move from the old statutory bodies to the new was not trouble free. The events of the previous thirteen years, since the setting up of the Briggs Committee, precluded that. After the implementation of the 1979 Act, it was clear that there was conflict, insecurity and mistrust between the different professions, with varying nationalities and traditions now pulled together under one Act. Overcoming these divisions was one of the biggest challenges to face the UKCC and the National Boards.[108]

Conclusion

The last years of the CMBS saw the Board, on the whole, increasing its effectiveness both administratively and in its ability to promote the interests of midwifery. Its Executive Committee expedited decision-making, raised efficiency, and appointed an Education Officer to the Board. This new post had wide responsibilities which publicised the work of the Board and raised its status amongst midwives and other professionals.

At the same time, the CMBS struggled with what must have seemed like one-sided battles over loss of midwifery matrons, perceived loss of midwifery status and diminishing career prospects. These events conspired inadvertently to reduce the autonomy and status of midwives and the Board found there was no going back. Yet the Board's views could be ambiguous. For instance, on the issue of integration of midwifery, the CMBS appeared to recommend that midwives should have the authority that was theirs by statute, yet under the overall control of a consultant obstetrician. The CMBS wanted midwives to be in the team, but not with equal status.

During its last years, the CMBS, facing extinction, appeared to champion midwives more than ever before. From 1977 to 1983, it had two dedicated midwife Chairmen, Sheelagh Bramley and Mary Turner. Margaret Kitson, remembered working with them both:

> Miss Bramley was a great champion of midwives. She upheld what she saw as the rights of the profession against all odds and against all opposition and she was determined that midwifery should be seen, not only a profession in its own right, but as a profession that could produce managers and teachers who could stand beside their nursing colleagues and not in any inferior capacity to them. And she...really tried...very hard to ensure that midwives would always remain independent and [would] not be subservient to nursing, ever.[109]

Latterly, midwife members of the CMBS increased in number due to electing bodies choosing them instead of lay members. Earlier, being a midwife on the CMBS dominated by non-midwives was not easy for new members. Margaret Kitson remembered how Mary Turner in the Chair changed things:

> I was elected by the midwives [in 1973]... I felt then I had a great responsibility to speak for the midwives, but it was really very difficult because there was a patronising attitude amongst the people who had been on the Board for a long time. There was a very definite, 'we know best'. There wasn't encouragement to speak up and only gradually did that change. And the change really came when Mary Turner...became the Chairman of the Board [in 1978]... She changed it in the most professional...way, without being abrasive, without being confrontational, but by being very positive and just always stating her case very clearly, listening to argument, but by, just in a very gentle way, changing the whole atmosphere in the Board so that it became much more possible for people to express their views.[110]

The CMBS lost the battle for its existence and therefore for the independence of midwives in Scotland, for what it saw as the right education for midwives, and for midwives' right to manage themselves clinically and educationally without interference. Yet the UKCC Midwifery Committee for which Margaret Auld fought became a reality. Through the intervention of the CMBS and others, the planned National Boards were made stronger for all the professions involved. Particularly for midwifery, the NBS, like the other National Boards, was strengthened by a statutory Midwifery Committee to consult and advise before any changes in midwifery could be made.

1. NAS, CMB 1/8, *CMBS Minutes*, 11 February 1960, p 2.
2. The Board originally planned to meet monthly. In 1947 this Rule was officially reduced to quarterly unless otherwise decided at a previous meeting.
3. NAS, CMB 1/8, *CMBS Minutes*, 14 April 1960, p 1.
4. NAS, CMB 1/8, *CMBS Minutes*, 27 July 1960, p 1; NAS, CMB 1/8, *CMBS Minutes*, 7 December 1960, p 1.
5. The NBS was set up in September 1980; *CMBS Report*, 31 March 1983, p 4; NAS, CMB 1/9, *CMBS Minutes*, 18 March 1982, p 3; NAS, CMB 1/9, *CMBS Minutes*, 17 June 1982, p 1.
6. DH, Report of the committee of enquiry into the cost of the National Health Service, (*Guillebaud Report*) Cmnd 9663: (London: HMSO, 1956); J Brotherston, 'The National Health Service in Scotland: 1948-1984', in McLachlan, (ed), *Improving the Common Weal*, p 148.
7. *Ibid*, p 260; Towler, Bramall, *Midwives in History and Society*, p 251.
8. NAS, CMB, 1/7, *CMBS Minutes*, 18 October 1956, p 2.
9. DHS, Scottish Health Services Council, *Maternity Services in Scotland*, (*Montgomery Report*), (Edinburgh: HMSO, 1959), p 7.
10. The 1946 NHS Act for England and Wales, the 1946 Health Services Act (Northern Ireland) and the 1947 NHS (Scotland) Act were all implemented on the same day, 5 July 1948.

11. *Montgomery Report*, Chapter 5, paras 57-102; NAS, CMB, 1/7, *CMBS Minutes*, 14 February 1957, Statement by the CMB to the Scottish maternity services review committee, pp 1-3.
12. NAS, CMB 1/7, *CMBS Minutes*, 14 February 1957, Statement, pp 1-3.
13. *Ibid.*
14. NAS, CMB 1/8, *CMBS Minutes*, 7 December 1960, p 2; 21 September 1961, p 5.
15. R Mander, 'Who needs midwifery?' *in Nursing Times*, (1987), Vol 83 (26), pp 34-35.
16. NAS, CMB 1/8, *CMBS Minutes*, 16 March 1961, p 3.
17. Previously the DHS.
18. NAS, CMB 1/8, *CMBS Minutes*, 20 February 1964, p 2; NAS, CMB 1/8, *CMBS Minutes*, 17 September 1964, p 2; NAS, CMB 1/8, *CMBS Minutes*, 17 December 1964, p 1.
19. The term 'student midwife' gradually superseded 'pupil midwife' in the 1960s. It was made official in the *CMBS Rules*, 31 March 1968, p 5; *CMBS Report*, 31 March 1968, p 2.
20. *CMBS Report*, 31 March 1967, p 3.
21. After the RCM Scottish Council drew the CMBS's attention to this case, the Board appears to have acted very speedily; NAS, CMB 1/8, *CMBS Minutes*, 21 July 1966, p 2.
22. Ministry of Health and Scottish Home and Health Department, *Report of the Committee on Senior Nursing Staff Structure*, (London: HMSO, 1966).
23. C Davies, A Beach, *Interpreting Professional Self-Regulation: A History of the United Kingdom Central Council for Nursing, Midwifery and Health Visiting*, (London: Routledge, 2000), p 3.
24. NAS, CMB 1/8, *CMBS Minutes*, 15 July 1965, p 1.
25. NAS, CMB 1/8, *CMBS Minutes*, 16 December 1965, p 5.
26. J Main, 'Nursing: Nursing, Midwifery and Health Visiting', in McLachlan, (ed), *Improving the Common Weal*, p 477.
27. M Clark, 'Changing clinical practice in nursing', in A Duncan, G McLachlan, (eds), *Hospital Medicine and Nursing in the 1980s: Interaction between the Professions of Medicine and Nursing*, pp 50-51.
28. LR 109.
29. LR 95.
30. LR 105.
31. *Ibid.*
32. *CMBS Report*, 31 March 1969, p 4.
33. LR 120.
34. LR 102.
35. LR 69.
36. Clark, *'Changing clinical practice in nursing'*, pp 50-51.
37. D Hunter, 'The Re-organised Health Service', in M G Clarke, H M Drucker, (eds), *Our Changing Scotland: A Yearbook of Scottish Government, 1976-77*, (Edinburgh: EUSPB, 1976), p 32.
38. *Ibid*, p 32; Brotherston, *'The National Health Service in Scotland: 1948-1984'*,

pp 130-133.

39. R Peters, 'Nursing and midwifery services' in R Peters, J Kinnaird, in *Health Services Administration*, (Edinburgh: Livingstone, 1965), p 318.

40. SHHD, *Maternity Services: Integration of Maternity Work, (Tennent Report)*, (Edinburgh: HMSO, 1973).

41. *Tennent Report*, p 1.

42. NAS, CMB 1/9, *CMBS Minutes* 16 December 1971, Appendix IV, 'Comments on the integration of maternity services', pp 1-2.

43. Department of Health, *Report of the standing maternity and midwifery advisory committee, (Peel Report)*, (London: HMSO, 1970),); R Campbell, A Macfarlane, 'Recent debate on the place of birth', in J Garcia, R Kilpatrick, M Richards, *The Politics of Maternity Care*, (Oxford: Clarendon Press, 1990), p 217.

44. *Ibid*, p 218.

45. *Tennent Report*, p 2.

46. *Ibid*, p 13; *ibid*, Chapter 8, 'The role of the midwife in an integrated maternity service', pp 29-31.

47. *CMBS Rules*, 1968, p 5; *CMBS Report*, 31 March 1968, p 2. This development slipped through with little comment.

48. NAS, CMB 1/8, *CMBS Minutes*, 17 December 1970, p 3.

49. NAS, CMB 1/9, *CMBS Minutes*, 16 September 1971, p 2.

50. NAS, CMB 1/9, *CMBS Minutes*, 16 December 1971, p 2.

51. The Draft Directives conceded that eighteen month training could be substituted provided a longer period of nursing had been achieved.

52. NAS, CMB 1/9, *CMBS Minutes*, 17 February 1972, p 1; NAS, CMB 1/9, *CMBS Minutes*, 20 April, 1972, p 1; Officials from the relevant countries set up a Midwifery Liaison Committee (MLC) to discuss the draft Directives in Brussels. UK Health Department officials could attend this meeting, but not representatives of the UK Boards as the MLC comprised professional rather than statutory bodies. Miss Annie Grant (CMBS member) was invited to be representative for the RCM Scottish Council on this Committee; NAS, CMB 1/9, *CMBS Minutes*, 21 December, 1972, p 1; see also Reid, *Scottish Midwives 1916-1983*, pp 160-166.

53. NAS, CMB 1/9, *CMBS Minutes*, 19 April 1973, p 1.

54. *CMBS Report*, 31 March 1974, p 2; NAS, CMB 1/9, *CMBS Minutes*, 19 July 1973, p 1.

55. NAS, CMB 1/9, *CMBS Minutes*, 20 December 1973, p 2.

56. *Ibid*, Appendix 2, p 2.

57. NAS, CMB 1/9, *CMBS Minutes*, 20 February 1975, p 2; the CMBS chairman informed the Chairman CMBE&W that it did not have authority to speak for the UK.

58. NAS, CMB 1/9, *CMBS Minutes*, 17 April 1975, p 1; *CMBS Report*, 31 March 1975, pp 2-3.

59. NAS, CMB 1/9, *CMBS Minutes*, 17 July 1975, p 1; also, see *CMBS Report*, 31 March 1976, p 2. To extend the course to eighteen months would conform with part of the draft Directives; NAS, CMB 1/9, *CMBS Minutes*, 18 December 1975,

p 3; ibid, 16 December 1976, p 2; *CMBS Report*, 31 March 1977, p 4; The course was finally introduced with effect from 31 August 1981.

60. NAS, CMB 1/9, *CMBS Minutes*, 13 December 1979, p 1; *CMBS Report*, 31 March 1980 p 3.

61. EEC Council Directives, (80/154/EEC), *Official Journal of the European Communities*, 11 February 1980, No L 33/3.

62. By this time the Registered Fever Nurse (RFN) course was no longer obtainable in Scotland.

63. NAS, CMB 1/9, *CMBS Minutes*, 18 December 1980, p 1.

64. Brotherston, *'National Health Service in Scotland'*, pp 130-133.

65. DHSS, SHHD, Welsh Office, *Report of the Committee on Nursing, (Briggs Report)*, Cmnd. 5115, (London: HMSO, 1972), p 1; author's comment: it would have been good to have seen the words '...and midwifery' in the title.

66. LR 105.

67. Davies, Beach, *Interpreting Professional Self-Regulation*, p 5.

68. LR105.

69. Davies, Beach, *Interpreting Professional Self-Regulation*, p 5.

70. LR 105.

71. *Ibid.*

72. *Ibid.*

73. Davies, Beach, *Interpreting Professional Self-Regulation*, p 5.

74. NAS, CMB 1/8, *CMBS Minutes*, 16 July 1970, p 2.

75. NAS, CMB 1/8, *CMBS Minutes*, 17 September 1970, 'Evidence for the committee on nursing', (Briggs Committee), Appendix II, pp 1-5.

76. *Ibid.*

77. R Dingwall, A M Rafferty, C Webster, *An Introduction to the Social History of Nursing*, (London: Routledge, 1988), p 172.

78. *Briggs Report*, para 626.

79. Davies, Beach, *Interpreting Professional Self-Regulation*, p 8; *Briggs Report*, para 307.

80. LR 120.

81. D Daiches, *Scotland and the Union*, (London: John Murray, 1977) p 132.

82. Davies and Beach, *Interpreting Professional Self-Regulation*, p 8; NAS, CMB 1/9, *CMBS Minutes*, 18 February 1971, p 1; *CMBS Report*, 31 March 1971, p 3.

83. Davies, Beach, *Interpreting Professional Self-Regulation*, p 9; The GNC for Scotland was also against a single statutory body, because of the differences between Scottish and English law.

84. *Briggs Report*, pp 212, 1, 2.

85. *Ibid*, p 212, 3.

86. LR 105.

87. *Briggs Report*, pp 187 and 188, paras 627 and 629.

88. *Ibid*, p 213, paras 16, 18-21.

89. M Uprichard, 'The evolution of midwifery education', in *Midwives' Chronicle*, January 1987, p 6.

90. NAS, CMB 1/9, *CMBS Minutes*, 21 December 1972, Appendix 1, p 2; *CMBS*

Report, 31 March, 1973, p 2; NAS, CMB 1/9, *CMBS Minutes*, 21 December 1972, (Report of meeting of executive committee with representatives of the RCM Scottish Board and the Scottish Midwives Teachers' Club), p 1.
91. *CMBS Report*, 31 March 1973, p 2.
92. Uprichard, *'The evolution of midwifery education'*, p 6; NAS, CMB 1/9, *CMBS Minutes*, 15 February 1973, p 1-2; *CMBS Report*, 31 March 1973, p 3; *CMBS Report*, 31 March 1974, p 2; NAS, CMB 1/9, *CMBS Minutes*, 15 February 1973 pp 1-2.
93. *CMBS Report*, 31 March 1975, p 2.
94. NAS, CMB 1/9, *CMBS Minutes*, 19 September 1974, p 2.
95. NAS, CMB 1/9, *CMBS Minutes*, 19 December 1974, p 1.
96. NAS, CMB 1/9, *CMBS Minutes*, 18 July 1974, p 3.
97. *CMBS Report*, 31 March 1975, p 2.
98. NAS, CMB 1/9, *CMBS Minutes*, 17 April 1975, p 1.
99. LR 120.
100. Letter from I Sharp, SHHD, to R B Hodgetts, DHSS, quoted in Davies, Beach, *Interpreting Professional Self-Regulation*, p 14.
101. *CMBS Report*, 31 March 1978, p 3.
102. Davies, Beach, *Interpreting Professional Self-Regulation*, p 17.
103. *Ibid*, p 24.
104. *1979 Nurses, Midwives and Health Visitors Act*, Chapter 36, Section 2; Davies, Beach, *Interpreting Professional Self-Regulation*, p 25.
105. *1979 Act*, Section 6.
106. NAS, CMB 1/9, *CMBS Minutes*, 20 September 1979, p 4; *CMBS Report*, 31 March 1981, p 3; *CMBS Report*, 31 March 1980, p 3.
107. *CMBS Report*, 31 March 1981, p 4; NAS, CMB 1/9, *CMBS Minutes*, 19 March 1981, p 2; NAS, CMB 1/9, *CMBS Minutes*, 18 June 1981, p 1; NAS, CMB 1/9, *CMBS Minutes*, 24 April 1980, p 1; NAS, CMB 1/9, *CMBS Minutes*, 18 September 1980, p 1; *CMBS Report*, 31 March 1982, p 3; NAS, CMB 1/9, *CMBS Minutes*, 29 April 1982, p 1.
108. Davies, Beach, *Interpreting Professional Self-Regulation*, p 18.
109. LR 120.
110. *Ibid.*

Chapter 7

From home to hospital: birth gets on the conveyor belt

During the twentieth century many aspects of midwifery practice changed beyond all previous recognition. One aspect which did not change was the mechanism or process of normal birth. Yet during this time, the shift from an estimated ninety-five percent homebirths to 99.5 per cent hospital births (see Appendix 2), along with increasing medicalisation of childbirth, took the 'normality' out of many births and had a negative impact on midwifery. Ella Clelland, who was a midwife from the 1950s to the 1980s, commented:

> When I came [to Callander] the home delivery levels had dropped and midwifery didn't have the same feel. I missed it...but people were so full of fear of litigation that it made you stand back from it and that took joy away from the things I had enjoyed in the past. I suppose we didn't stop to worry too much – we just got on with it. You did as good a job as you could... I feel that midwifery now is all abnormal until it is proved normal, which is not how it is intended to be and which is very sad. I think when I saw the beginning of abnormal practices, which is probably too strong a term to use, was when I saw them starting this induction of labour and people knew that they were going to be put into labour. That, for me, was the beginning of abnormality. And including midwives as a part of it.[1]

With the change in place of birth, midwives' relationships with mothers also underwent change. At home, the mother retained a significant identity. Even though she was in labour and requiring help, she remained the host in her own home. When a woman came into hospital she was no longer in control of her environment. Circumstances dictated a weaker, more subservient role for her and her significant identity was diminished. The midwife's identity in hospital was also lessened as she now had to adhere to emerging hospital policies. Some midwives were therefore no longer able to give mothers the complete care, emotional as well as physical, to which many of them believed mothers were entitled. One midwife said:

> I always feel that women, when they are pregnant, when they are in labour and just after, need to be mothered themselves in order to help them to mother, even if they have got a mother-figure in their own family. They need the caring that goes along with midwifery. There was no caring. The women were delivered – it was just like a sausage factory.[2]

Who delivered the babies?
Unlike her role in antenatal care, from 1915 the midwife's statutory role as a person

allowed to care for a woman throughout normal labour has never been in doubt. The 1915 Midwives (Scotland) Act, and the first set of CMBS *Rules* in 1916, specified the demonstration of competence in intranatal care through a required number of deliveries in order for a midwife to be certified.[3] Later in 1916, the CMBS, complete with two midwife members, published a more detailed set of *Rules*, including those dealing with midwifery practice and, specifically, midwives' duties towards women in labour. Nevertheless, although midwives and medical practitioners were (and are) the only people in Scotland permitted legally to help a woman give birth, the role of the midwife in intranatal care, although enshrined in statute, was, in practice, subordinate to medical practitioners. Midwives were not educated in the same way as medical practitioners and, within the CMBS-approved training institutions, medical practitioners initially supplied the lectures and, through the CMBS, had a large say in what midwives should be taught.

The power of LAs over midwives and their practice in Scotland developed in the early twentieth century. The 1915 Notification of Births (Extension) Act, governed 'solely by the need for preserving the health of expectant mothers, nursing mothers, and children up to the age of five,' gave LAs wide powers.[4] Although these powers were supposed to be adoptive, not obligatory, the obligation that the Government and the Local Government Board for Scotland (LGBS) placed on LAs was considerable. An important part of this was the initiation of 'Schemes of Maternity Service and Child Welfare' which the LGBS invited each LA to submit. As a result, the Maternity Services Schemes in Scotland gave power to LAs and their MOHs to organise maternity care.[5] Also, through the 1915 Midwives (Scotland) Act, LAs were empowered and obliged to supervise midwives closely as Local Supervising Authorities (LSA). Dr Leslie MacKenzie, Public Health expert and medical member of the LGBS, considered the Midwives Act and the power it gave to the LAs to be central to the success of the Maternity Schemes.[6]

Under the Maternity Schemes, Scottish medical practitioners continued to take a more active part in the care of childbearing women than their English counterparts and supervised (nominally) all home confinements, although they were not necessarily present at the birth.[7] Cumberlege's survey of maternity in Great Britain showed that doctors carried out twenty-six per cent of rural and eighteen per cent of urban home deliveries in Scotland. The comparable figures for England and Wales were twenty and twelve per cent.[8] It was difficult to gauge the extent of GPs' active participation in midwifery care at home because, Cumberlege noted, 'when a doctor has been in charge of a confinement, the delivery will in all probability be accredited to him even if it has actually been undertaken by a midwife.'[9] This survey made a distinction between the person in charge of the confinement and the person actually delivering the baby. It emphasised that although a doctor was in charge of a confinement this did not necessarily mean that he carried out the delivery of the baby.[10] Ann Lamb, who practised midwifery from the 1920s said, 'I delivered most of my babies at home without a doctor. I felt kind of safer with a doctor but I would still deliver the baby. Oh, yes, the doctor was just there to look on.'[11] The 1959 *Montgomery Report* on maternity services in Scotland said that a doctor's presence at a delivery 'was scarcely a matter that could be made obligatory' and added that doctors were not usually present at a hospital delivery either.[12]

It is likely that more than half of the births in Britain in the nineteenth century were undertaken by midwives.[13] These were mostly uncertified women, the howdies, or 'handywomen' as they were termed in England. However, this estimate was not consistent throughout the country. In Glasgow in 1870, seventy-five per cent of mothers were delivered by midwives, contrasting with areas of Edinburgh where midwife deliveries were fewer.[14] These inconsistencies were further highlighted in 1895. Dr R Buist, a future CMBS Chairman, said that 'within three hundred yards of his house there were eight or nine midwives in actual practice.'[15] However, GP Dr S Maevie, said that 'in Berwickshire he had not heard of a midwife and...[when he was in practice] in Strathavon, near Tomintoul, he had no dealings with midwives at all. He had heard of an occasional attendance by a midwife, but never came in contact with them.'[16] Table 7.1 breaks down the numbers of delivering professionals in Glasgow Cowcaddens and shows the extent of midwives' involvement there at the beginning of the twentieth century.[17]

Table 7.1 Number of deliveries per category of professional:

Category	Number of deliveries	Percentage by profession
Doctors	79	25.5
Maternity Hospital Nurses [sic]	12	3.9
Nurses from other training schools	77	25.0
Handywomen/howdies	126	40.7
Delivered in poorhouses	3	1.0
Not found when visited	12	3.9
Totals	309	100.0

Table 7.1 shows that of the 309 sample total, 215 or 69.6 percent were delivered by midwives at some level. Fifteen or 4.9 percent were probably delivered by midwives and it is probable that there would have been some kind of semi-experienced person, for example a neighbour or howdie, present at the seventy-nine doctor-attended births. Cowcaddens was considered one of the poorer parts of Glasgow and it was in villages and working-class areas of towns and cities where midwife deliveries predominated. On the other hand, in the small non-manufacturing towns, suburbs and affluent areas of large towns and cities, GPs delivered many of the babies.[18] This echoes the 1948 *Report on Maternity in Great Britain* which said that GPs were more likely to deliver the baby if the mother was the wife of a professional, salaried worker and having her first confinement. Lower down the social scale the figures for GP deliveries become correspondingly less.[19]

The change in place of birth
The shift from home to hospital as the place where most women give birth was one of the major changes in maternity care in the twentieth century. The movement in Scotland from nearly all homebirths to nearly all hospital births began slowly in the early

twentieth century and peaked in 1981 when 99.5 per cent of babies in Scotland were born in hospital.[20]

Reasons for the change particularly involved the growing medicalisation of childbirth through the twentieth century. An important issue was that of pain relief in labour, unknown to most early twentieth century women. Chloroform, first used as an anaesthetic in obstetrics in Edinburgh in 1847 by Sir James Young Simpson (1811-1870), and still used in Scotland in the first half of the twentieth century along with 'twilight sleep' (morphine and scopolamine), had to be administered by, or under the supervision of, a medical practitioner.[21] Most women receiving these drugs were those who could afford to pay a doctor as well as a midwife. A mother receiving these drugs required constant observation and, as private maternity homes and maternity beds in ordinary nursing homes also came into vogue in the 1920s, it was much easier to admit a mother to one of those if she requested analgesic drugs. Soon, affluent mothers began to go to maternity homes for their confinement whether they felt they required analgesia or not.[22] Conditions in maternity homes and hospitals advanced and there was greater attention given to reduction of cross-infection.[23] As the reputations of nursing homes grew, more women prepared to go to them. Advances in medicine, instrumental in reducing maternal mortality in the 1930s and 1940s, added to the increase in hospitalisation. These included: the use of the first antibiotics for puerperal sepsis, particularly Prontosil; the development of blood transfusions; and better education of doctors and midwives leading to greater awareness of problems prompting admission to hospital when necessary.[24]

The 1935 *Douglas and McKinley Report* highlighted the issue of maternal mortality and the care given to mothers by midwives and doctors. The Report, emphasising normality, was not directly instrumental in increasing hospitalisation for childbirth. Nevertheless, its conclusion reflected the need for improvement in the maternity services in Scotland.[25] The statutes of the 1937 Maternity Services (Scotland) Act echoed many of this Report's recommendations, in particular the provision of midwives in the home, along with GPs, specialist obstetricians and anaesthetists where necessary. In 1939, before these arrangements were fully in place, World War Two intervened, bringing with it an acceleration of the trend towards the hospital for birth.

By 1959, the homebirth rate was dropping sharply. In 1957 it was twenty-nine per cent, a drop of fifteen per cent since the start of the NHS in 1948.[26] Further reasons for the trend away from homebirths included women's demands for hospital confinement because of media suggestions that it was safer, women following fashion, and also women asking for a 'definite booking' as they feared being discharged too quickly if they were admitted in an emergency. The Queen's Institute of District Nursing, which included many practising midwives, summed up the reasons as being,

> due to excessive propaganda from hospital specialists stressing greater safety, lack of suitable housing in certain areas, insufficiently developed or insufficiently flexible home help services, economy to the mother...in spite of the increase in the home confinement grant, and encouragement by GPs [to have a hospital birth], sometimes irrespective of medical, obstetric or social need.[27]

However, by this time there was insufficient hospital accommodation for all women who requested hospital births and a form of selection was necessary. To 'encourage a new trend towards domiciliary confinement' there was even a suggestion to reduce the cost of home helps for maternity cases.[28] Yet, to counter this, further medicalisation in the 1950s and 1960s resulted in increasingly detailed selection criteria for conditions requiring care in hospital.[29] This included an assessment of 'risk factors' associated with an increase in antenatal care, and testing – including ultrasonic scanning. In the 1970s and 1980s, medicalisation and the use of technology developed further, for example, induction and augmentation of labour, the growing trend for epidural anaesthesia, the rise in instrumental vaginal deliveries and Caesarean section rates. Selection shifted from selection for hospital delivery, to selection for homebirths.[30]

The *Peel Report* (1970) arose from the perceived need to consider the future of the domiciliary midwifery service and the question of bed needs for maternity patients.[31] The Report was not officially an expression of Government policy, but its recommendation of 100% hospital deliveries on the grounds of safety (without supporting evidence) received wide attention.[32] The *Peel Report* did not apply to Scotland. Nevertheless, Scotland's *Tennent Report* (1973) agreed with the *Peel Report*'s main conclusions and recommendations.[33] The hospital birth rate, which stood at 98.5% in 1973, was set to rise even further.[34] In the space of fourteen years, the trend for hospital births, already escalating as a result of World War Two, the creation of the NHS, and women's demands, was accelerated by the recommendations of these Reports

The change in place of birth also affected the intranatal practice and morale of domiciliary midwives. Mary McCaskill recalled:

> Towards the end of [1952], the home deliveries had just sort of imperceptibly started to decline... Older midwives,...probably in their fifties, were beginning to [say] they didn't have so many bookings and they were wondering...what was the future and what would they be used for... Would they be maybe diversified into some other duties?'[35]

Furthermore, as the number of homebirths declined, so did the job-satisfaction of district midwives. Experienced district midwives expressed frustration at what they saw as a lack of domiciliary midwifery. Their remit had moved from giving full intranatal and postnatal care to some antenatal visits, and postnatal visits to women who had been confined in hospital. Also, the lack of intranatal practice could result in a loss of skills for both district midwives and GPs, and would lead to difficulties in arranging for intrapartum training for pupil midwives.[36] Wilma Coleman, who was a senior midwife in Perth from the 1970s, agreed that 'once the home confinements went down and women came into hospital, the community midwives very quickly lost their intrapartum skills and their antenatal skills.'[37]

The CMBS Minutes highlighted this problem many times. As the number of hospital births rose, few student midwives delivered a baby at home, although much depended upon the area and the number of maternity beds there. For example, one district midwife in Govan recalled:

> I was appointed as a district midwifery sister from 1957 to 1964. Govan was densely populated at that time...the birth rate extremely high. Because of the

shortage of beds in the maternity unit of the Southern General Hospital, home confinements were essential and during my seven years in the community, I delivered 1,322 babies.[38]

This situation in Glasgow continued for some years and any pupil midwives working there would have had no problem obtaining deliveries. Ella Clelland, a pupil midwife at Rottenrow (GRMH) in 1957, recalled: 'I think we had to deliver ten in the hospital in the beginning and twenty out[side]. We never had any difficulty getting cases.'[39] Twelve years later, in 1969, Maureen Hamilton, in Glasgow had a similar level of experience. She said, 'We had quite a few home deliveries and no problem getting them. I think probably after that...they were beginning to go down a bit in numbers. But certainly none of our crowd had any problem.'[40] Yet Alison Dale, who also trained in 1969, but in Aberdeen, said, 'Only one girl in our set...saw a home delivery and there were very few by the time that we were training.'[41] Sooner or later, homebirths were phased out as a compulsory part of the midwifery training syllabus and community midwives quickly lost their intrapartum skills.[42] One solution was for domiciliary midwifery to become a hospital responsibility allowing some interchange of midwives between domiciliary and hospital services.[43] This early suggestion on integration of the maternity services was to come to fruition in future years.

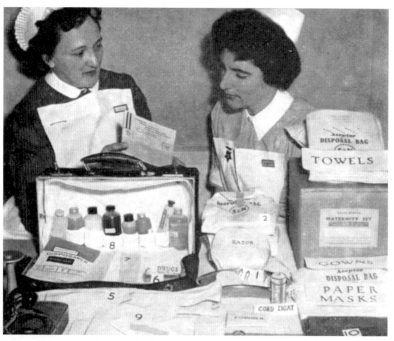

Sister showing student midwife notification of birth form and requirements for homebirth, SMMP Reprinted from M Myles, A textbook for midwives (6th ed), (E&S Livingstone, 1968), p 650, fig 443.

Another suggestion was the DOMINO scheme.[44] This was designed to provide more continuity of care for mothers while helping community midwives maintain their skills. The first reported use of this scheme was in West Middlesex in 1971, although ideas for similar schemes were mooted in the early 1960s. Mothers having a DOMINO delivery were looked after antenatally by their community midwife and escorted into hospital in labour by the community midwife on call, who then delivered the baby and looked after the mother and baby for a few hours afterwards before escorting them home. Postnatal care continued as usual. For midwives, DOMINO deliveries had the added bonus that they could give intranatal as well as antenatal care.[45] Jan Fenton, in Dundee in the 1970s, had many DOMINO deliveries. She said:

> We started the DOMINOS in the 1970s. A lot of the girls...were frightened of hospitals. [There was] a little lass...and she wanted the baby at home... This was very much frowned on. She was determined. She discovered that she was having twins...but we went into hospital with her... Dr Smith [the consultant] got out of his bed at two o'clock in the morning and sat beside the bed so that there was no interference from the staff... This is the rapport...that we had. I delivered the twins...it was marvellous. And then eventually I was delivering babies from all over the town... They'd obviously had a bad experience the first time. I got up in the middle of the night, went in, delivered a baby and came home. But you see I was using my expertise in the hospital and this was one way of keeping it up... These were all DOMINOS... It was brilliant... Eventually I think I did about twenty-four in a year. Now that was two a month and it's quite a lot when you consider getting up during the night or at weekends. And I've even done it on my day off...if they were frightened.[46]

Challenges of homebirths: pests and poverty
Discussions on home and hospital births tend to centre on safety and its statistics. But most midwives' recollections focus on other challenges, such as dealing with body-vermin and poverty, as well as their reaction to acute situations.

One constant feature, significant by the number of midwives who spoke about it, was the presence in many homes of bugs, fleas and lice. They had different ways of handling these. Anne Bayne, working in Glasgow in the early 1950s, said:

> We lived our lives with fleas. In fact we got a chemist to mix DDT with our talcum powder to try and control fleas because I used to just come up in great welts with fleas. Montrose Street itself, where we sat and waited to be called out for deliveries, it was just hoatching with fleas. So we dusted everything we could with this DDT-talcum powder to try and keep the fleas at bay.[47]

Mollie Muir, pupil midwife at the 'old Simpson' in 1934, like other pupil midwives, had to take medical students to homebirths as part of their training. Normally she took the bugs as a matter of course but recalled intervening on one occasion, when one landed on her student:

> The night that I was at this thirteenth baby, the student who was with me, ooh

he was spotless, and he had on a lovely forget-me-not blue shirt, just stiff with being well-washed and well-ironed, and suddenly a great fat bug jumped on to his sleeve. I took it with my fingers and threw it down and stood on it. But apart from that, of course, we had a lot of lice and fleas. We didn't have to de-louse ourselves. We wore caps and the whole idea of the cap was to keep the lice from your hair.[48]

Bugs, fleas and lice were so commonplace that it was standard practice for pupil midwives to be taught what to do with their coats when they were in someone's house. Betty Smith who was a pupil-midwife in Glasgow in the 1940s said, '...we were taught...never to put our coats over a bed or a soft chair. We always had to hang them on a hard chair because of bed-bugs....'[49] But Margaret Foggie, a South African pupil-midwife in Glasgow in 1934 found many uses for newspapers. She said:

I remember seeing bugs...various things, on the wall... I didn't know quite where to hang my coat in the houses. I would wrap it up in some of the newspaper. We went bulging with newspapers. It was used for everything.[50]

If all precautions failed, Agnes Morrison, who was a pupil-midwife and midwife in Leith in 1946, described what she had to do once she returned home:

If I'd been down there [Leith Walk] I can remember what I really had to do... Take my apron off, go into the bathroom, stand and strip [and have] a piece of soap in my hand to catch the fleas...to get them to go against the white and, you know, getting them... Fleas seemed to like me. I'd be covered in fleas at night... Those houses must be riddled.[51]

The poverty epitomised by these quotations was echoed over and over again by midwives. The problem of lack of equipment arose frequently, and the solutions demonstrated midwives' ingenuity and versatility. Ann Lamb, who was a pupil-midwife in Edinburgh in 1927, managed to take a positive attitude:

They were very poor, and by poor, I mean *poor*. There was only one sheet to deliver the mother on, so a firm was very good and gave us paper, white wallpaper, and we made a sheet of that. We never had any sepsis, don't forget, and we had nothing much to work on, but I never remember a case of sepsis or anything wrong with the mother or baby. They were very happy, but, oh, they had nothing.[52]

Many midwives used newspapers to put under the mother. Margaret Foggie said:

We delivered the baby...straight on to newspapers. The other children and the father would all...have been turfed out. I did hear from somebody later that very often the father was still in the bed. He was working during the day so he had to have his sleep and you would have to get him out at the last moment. I never quite had to do that. I always managed that earlier to give me a clear run. The poor mothers, after they had had nine or ten children, they didn't really want another baby. It was awfully sad.[53]

Mima Sutherland, pupil-midwife in Aberdeen in 1931, had a similar experience with poverty, but also found herself helping out the medical student:

> Some of the homes were very poor. One woman had nothing but a pile of *Radio Times*, and when I went downstairs the wifie gave me some clothes for the baby. I had a [medical] student with me too. We often had them, sometimes from abroad. Usually a midwife there supervised the student and also had to subsidise the student's bus fares. They didn't have a maik [ha'penny].[54]

Molly Muir in Edinburgh in 1934 wondered about lack of neighbours in one particular instance. She said:

> I went to a case one night, in the middle of the night in the High Street, and it was their thirteenth child and they had one room. He was unemployed... They had two double beds in that one room and they all slept [there], and while I was dealing with the birth the father got the others up and took them out just to walk the streets... I often wondered since then why they didn't have neighbours who might have helped them at a time like that.[55]

Yet she showed how equipment could be supplied:

> We took...a rubber draw sheet and we put that under the mother to deliver the baby and then, in this particular house, they only had one [bentwood] chair... I bathed the baby in a baking-bowl... Next morning I had to go up from Simpson's and take clothes for the baby. We used to get clothes handed into the Simpson's from people who were finished with them. We could always draw on that.[56]

Agnes Morrison said that she 'loved every minute of it'. But that did not blind her to the conditions she encountered and the ability to use whatever came in useful in an emergency:

> There was an army technicians' hut in Granton...a camp that had been invaded by squatters and we delivered babies there. It was really terrible conditions... People had just squatted up and got themselves organised in their rooms... There was a communal bath... I remember [being] called to a case in this camp and you went into the room where they lived and everything was happening in there and there was a mother in labour. In the cot were two little ones and here was this third one. And she was twenty-something. She looked like forty-something, poor woman. I can see father yet, sitting over the far end, and I remember he was a painter on the Forth Bridge. You know, I was getting so annoyed with him. I felt this... What a situation to be in. She had her baby and they were all right. Then...she haemorrhaged...and I was giving ergometrine and trying to get the uterus [to contract] and she was going into shock, and I said, 'Could you get me some heat...hot water bottles?' 'Oh no,' [he replied]. I said, 'Any beer bottles?' 'Oh yes.' I said, 'Well fill them up with hot water, as much as it will stand and bring as many to me.' I can see me packing beer bottles round this woman to

give her heat... [I was there] by myself. It was a terrible situation until I could get her stabilised. Again, we were just called at the last minute... I'd never seen her before... No antenatal care, here she was struggling with two other little ones and...she had about two army blankets I think – you know, those grey things. Nothing, no comforts.[57]

Agnes Morrison also remembered happier homes:

And then further on in Newhaven, a lovely little fishing village, and I remember a baby there and still the little old cottage-type house with the brasses absolutely shining on the fire, the mantlepiece and all the baby's clothes being aired over the brass thing above the range. That was lovely. There was something very nice about that – a wild night outside and the cosy little cottage you were in, and the baby.[58]

She also remembered very clearly the one stillbirth she had on the district, probably resulting from no antenatal care and an inexperienced doctor sent out to help.

I lost one baby on district... The pupil midwife...had called somebody and I was... sent. It was a breech presentation. So immediately I phoned into the Simpson to get medical help. Unfortunately they sent such a junior little person who did what we were never taught to do. He got on to the feet and the arms shot up...and therefore we had the head and two arms to pass through the birth canal. And he, he was getting into a [state]. You know, I hate to tell you, but I said, 'Would you mind just letting me...' – because strangely enough one of the consultants at the Simpson had been conducting a breech presentation and he never turned the babies... I was doing my training and happened to be in the labour ward and he said, 'Would you just come...and I'll show you. Never rush a breech presentation.' And I'll never forget, step by step he showed me what to do and how to go up and bring the arm down one at a time and gently. But too much time had been lost. It was dead. I knew I was going to deliver a dead baby...but we were more concerned about getting the baby delivered by that time... But when I think of all the situations we were in, to lose only one, I was amazed.[59]

Midwives and doctors were bound within a hospital hierarchy no matter how junior the doctor was. By taking over from the doctor, Agnes Morrison's concern at what was happening broke the boundaries of convention. Yet by saying 'I hate to tell you...', all those years later she still felt that she had to excuse her breach of etiquette. However, in doing so, she also displayed the confidence of midwives on the district at that time.

Anne Chapman practised in Glasgow in the early part of World War Two and also worked with women in very poor circumstances. She described life in 'the dunnies':

These people were travelling people and they would travel around in caravans. Most of them had quite big families and they couldn't get a place to stay in the winter. They came back to Glasgow and their caravans would probably be put on Glasgow Green or wherever, and they got the dunny down underneath the tenements. You went in the tenement building and instead of going up you went down. The dunnies were mostly empty in the summertime. Every tenement had them. The dunny was the whole stretch of the tenement underneath with no division, just long areas under the tenements with trodden earth floors. The people would just move in. Some of them had sacking and they could put up sacks or whatever they had to curtain it off a bit. It made it a wee bit more private. There would be one family on one side and another family on the other side. When you went to deliver them you just used any thing you could get. Sometimes the babies were delivered on to a heap of rags. If they had a camp bed they were considered posh.[60]

Some travelling people were not so overtly poor. Anne Chapman commented:

And then you had the caravans on Glasgow Green. We were often there. They were in a different street of course and oh they were clean, my goodness I used to wonder how they kept them so clean. But I think the particular caravan you delivered the mother in was just kept special.[61]

Whatever midwives carried with them in the way of equipment, when it came to their working environment, they had to accept and make the best of what was there.

Midwives' equipment
Midwives on the district carried most of their equipment with them. In the days before midwives had cars, this involved carrying what they could while walking, cycling or using trams and buses. Their loads were often heavy and awkward.

The standard piece of equipment was/is the midwife's bag. Myles indicated the need for two bags particularly for a confinement, identified as 'separate delivery and puerperal bags of metal or leather.'[62] With variations, a midwife's bag for delivery in the early twentieth century contained an enema syringe, catheter, bath and clinical thermometers, disinfectant soap, nail-brush, biniodide of mercury, lubricant, safety-pins, scissors, tape-measure, cord-thread/tape, ergometrine, chloral hydrate, sal volatile, measuring-glass, syringe and needles, cotton-wool, lint, permanganate of potash, suturing materials, clean aprons, mackintosh sheeting and apron, note-book and copying-ink pencil, four-hourly charts, and scales for infant weighing.[63]

Nearly every midwife interviewed for oral history purposes mentioned her bag. No midwife on the district then, or now, went without it. Ann Lamb spoke about her 'brown bag' and Moira Michie from Aberdeen stressed the importance of her howdie grandmother's bag.[64] When James Tweedie's grandmother, who was a howdie in Douglas (later Happendon), from 1877 to 1923 was called out to a tinkers' camp, the bag was the first thing she picked up. He wrote:

In case the lass was in distress,
Gran took her black bag from the press
And off on that frosty morn she went,
To help the wife in the tinker's tent.
And there in the moonlight's fleeting beam,
The bairn was born and washed in the stream.[65]

Bags, used every day, had to be re-packed every day. Agnes Morrison, working in Leith in the 1940s, said:

> We had our...bags which we picked up...[when] we came in... We had to do them all up and sterilise stuff and pack them all again...every day. We took it whether we were doing postnatal or whatever and then it was up to us to have it all cleaned out, things sterilised [and] boiled up... We might have to do it mid-day [as well].[66]

Pupil midwives on the district had to have their bags inspected before they went out as Linda Stamp, pupil midwife at Rottenrow in the 1940s, recalled:

> The sister there was pretty old and supervised what we took out with us. She inspected our bags before we went out. She was very fussy. We took all that was essential. We had our sterile things in little packs. They weren't really sterile packs of course at all but they were washed and clean, and clean towels and the umbilical cords. To make the umbilical cords we had very fine thread just like string. It was very white and it had to be a certain length and we had so many taped together...[67]

But certified midwives also had their bags inspected by the Supervisor of Midwives (SOM). Mary McCaskill, in Glasgow in the 1940s, said, 'You had your bags inspected regularly...not more than three months between each...'[68]

The bag was looked upon as a passport, for instance to the top of the queue for the Glasgow trams. Margaret Dearnley, who was a midwife in Glasgow in the 1940s, recalled:

> You wore your uniform, you're carrying your bag. And if you went to stand in the tramcar line...they would say, 'Oh,' – great big queues of people of course – 'Here's the nurse, some puir sowel's waitin on her comin.' And you were pushed up the line and they let you on. And the driver would say, 'Where are you going? ...They would stop at the close that you wanted to go to. Wasn't that fantastic?[69]

Anne McFadden, who was a pupil-midwife in Edinburgh in the 1940s, remembered how her midwife's bag gave her a clear passage:

> The whole culture was quite difficult. You could call them the drug addicts but it wasn't the kind of drugs we know about... They used the gas fittings [from lamps] and the methylated spirits and they were lying asleep down the Vennel Steps down into the Grassmarket. But, they were so respectful, whenever they saw a black bag, up they got...and said...'Sorry, let you pass'... And you had your black bag with you.[70]

Also important was the delivery pack or box. One midwife in the late 1930s said:

> First of all...we made up these packs and I had a gown and masks and bonnet and cotton wool and swabs, but then latterly the boxes came all ready and you just opened it in the house. But, you know, it was amazing, you had children there and we wrapped this up in brown paper and put it up on top of

the cupboard. Nothing was ever touched. Nothing.[71]

Sterile delivery packs were supplied free to mothers, at a cost in 1951 to the LA of 18/6 (eighteen shillings and six pence) (92 1/2 pence) each on condition the pack was opened only by the midwife or doctor and if not used, returned unopened.[72] The administration differed from place to place. Mary McCaskill recalled:

> If the mother was booked to have a home confinement, she got the pack...from the central office...at about thirty-six weeks. She'd go with a chitty from me and collect that pack. She didn't have to pay for it... [I carried it to the house]...if it was an unbooked or emergency delivery. You kept say four, or maybe six packs, in your own home so that you could produce them during the night when the central office would be closed... There would be a sterile sheet for delivery, swabs and sanitary towels... The midwife carried the Dettol.[73]

However Anne Bayne, in 1950s Glasgow, had a different story:

> The most common thing that happened everywhere, after thirty-six weeks [of pregnancy], you went in and collected your brown box [and took it to the mother]. This was the delivery box and in it was waterproof paper, cotton wool, sanitary towels and so on – and a bottle of Dettol. Well, the Dettol in Glasgow was always white! 'We got it like that. That was how it came.' Of course they had used the Dettol and filled it up with water and of course when you put water into Dettol it turns white. So all we finished up with was this white Dettol.[74]

When the baby was born the midwife delivered the placenta which had to be disposed of. In most areas, the midwife examined the placenta and, if it appeared complete, wrapped it in newspaper and burnt it on the fire. However Rottenrow pupil midwives had to take the placenta back to the hospital for examination. Ella Banks recalled an unusual piece of equipment:

> We had to have a sponge bag and in that sponge bag, you had to put the placenta and bring it back to the hospital to be checked to see that it was complete and healthy. The sponge bag had strings that you pulled across. And you put your placenta in there and took it back to the hospital.[75]

Linda Stamp added:

> I don't know of anyone leaving it on the tram but one time the cat ran off with the placenta – this was my friend's placenta. She ran after the cat and she did get some of it, but not very much.[76]

However Anne Bayne remembered someone using another type of receptacle. She found herself helping a Rottenrow pupil midwife who had left her placenta on a bus in a *National Dried Milk* tin. They had to go to the bus depot and retrieve it.[77]

In 1946, the CMB allowed midwives to administer gas and air on their own responsibility. This meant that there was now often another piece of equipment, the

Minnitt apparatus, for midwives to carry as well as everything else. Mary McCaskill recalled:

> We had a portable Minnitt machine. [The cylinder and the machine] were all in the box together. It was quite heavy even although it was portable... Quite often we would ask the husband if he would carry [it].[78]

However bulky, heavy and awkward the equipment, it was necessary for successful domiciliary midwifery. In 1959, the CMBS responded to a complaint about the weight of equipment a midwife had to carry by justifying the need for everything but calling for employing authorities to provide adequate transport.[79] Before this, some LAs supplied taxis and Mary McCaskill described what happened there:

> Somewhere between eight and nine at night till six o'clock in the morning, Glasgow Corporation provided a car and a driver... If it was during the hours of darkness he would come to my house and take me to where the confinement was and then he would come to the house and bring me [home].[80]

Margaret Dearnley agreed:

> If you were beyond the tram route, or very far away, or it was very early in the morning you got the green car, the town car... You phoned in to say you were leaving, where you were and it was two o'clock in the morning [and] you had to go back to Rottenrow. So they sent a 'green caur' as they talked about which was the...town limousine.[81]

This did not always solve the problem. Many midwives walked, cycled or used public transport when it was available, or, as Anne Chapman in Glasgow in the 1940s recalled, they were glad of some memorable very early-morning lifts:

> We had to walk everywhere... We used to stand up on the back of a refuse cart and get a lift... If the driver saw us he would stop and yell, 'Where are ye goin?' and he would take us...'Jump on.' And there we were clutching on the back, the student and I, rattling away and then he would shout, 'What street are ye goin to?' These men were great.[82]

Anne Bayne in 1950s Edinburgh used a hazardous sounding bicycle:

> [My bicycle] had nae brakes. The policeman stood at point duty at the Haymarket where five roads meet and I never knew whether he knew I had nae brakes or if it was just, 'Here comes the nurse.' But he always stopped the traffic for me and I sailed through.[83]

However, later, when she went to Tullibody, she graduated from her push-bike to another method of two-wheeled transport:

> [The LA] had one little Vespa scooter...and they decided [they would] give it to me... There were no instructions with it... The first night I had it ...we couldn't even start it.[84]

Anne Bayne spoke about wee boys putting stones into her petrol tank, but also remembered:

> The Vespa took a mixture of two star petrol plus...oil. Between Stirling and Tullibody was the Black Grange Petrol Pump...the man was a blacksmith. 'That's OK,' he said. 'We'll just get this wee drum,' and he wrote *NURSE* in big writing on it. And he said, 'Now, we'll measure in the gallon, we'll add 2/3 pint of oil...and we'll gie it a good shake and we'll fill up your tank.' Any extra he kept for me. 'Nobody will touch it and next time we'll do the same.'
>
> This went on for three years. I would say to the man, 'Now I need to pay my petrol bill.' And he always put it off. So I never paid for petrol until it came to the time that I was getting married and I said to him one day, 'Now I must get this bill.' When I returned, he said, 'Now nurse, your bill. I kent you werna runnin up a bill... Yer bill's been peyed.' That was the local miners.[85]

The 1949 Working Party on Midwives highlighted midwives' transport problems and recommended the provision of a car for every midwife, financial help to run it and assistance with driving lessons.[86] Eventually, it was a condition of the job that community midwives should be able to drive and LAs either supplied a car or assisted midwives either to buy or lease cars, helping to solve both transport and equipment problems.

Relationships and policies

An important difference between caring for labouring mothers at home or in hospital is the contrast in relationship between midwife and mother. Until at least the 1980s, when a mother went to hospital she entered an environment in which she had to relinquish authority. At home, the mother and her relatives retained, and still do, the status of host and all pupil/student midwives were and are taught to respect this before going into the community. This contrast has become less marked since the 1990s when maternity services were reviewed and findings published. The Scottish *Policy Review* recognised that some aspects of maternity care were unacceptable, and advocated more informed choice for mothers and woman-centred care leading to different professional attitudes, collectively through changed policy and individually through personal actions.[87]

Anne Chapman clearly demonstrated the respect required when home visiting:

> I used to go to lots of gypsies' tents and caravans out in the rural areas. They always had dogs... Once I went to a quarry... There was just one entrance into it and they had tents all round. There was a dog's kennel at one side of the entrance and a dog's kennel at the other and two of the most ferocious Alsatians I have ever seen in my life... They were tied so they couldn't meet each other, but you could never have passed through this small space between them. I was terrified. The first time I went I was on my bicycle... I called and I shouted. Somebody was supposed to be in labour.[88]

Finally Anne sent some children for their granny. She said:

> The granny appeared and one word fae her and these dogs went slinking into

their kennels. I couldn't believe it. And then she said, 'Noo nurse come on, bring yer bike. Somebody might lift it leavin it there.' This was me on my own in this old, old quarry...and a big fire in the middle where they did their cooking. These dogs were really ugly. They were still howling and barking...but one word from her and they were away.[89]

Through controlling the dogs, the granny retained control of the situation. The second reminder of who was host came after the baby was born:

When the baby was born and everything was grand the granny said, 'Ye'll need tae get a cup o tea.' And it was out of a tin can. But you never said 'no' because you wouldn't want anyone to think you were feeling a bit uppity. They were always so grateful and always wanted to give you tea or whatever they had. And there was always the camp fire...with the kettle or tinnie on the boil. One time I had delivered the baby...the mother had been given a syrup tin of tea and the grandfather who was really proud of the bairn, turned and said to me, 'A drink o tea. Ye'll tak it.' Well I couldn't refuse. 'Hae a seat.' I sat down on the ground and was handed a tinnie of tea with a handle. But the tinnie had been on the fire and my mouth was badly burnt. Well, I never said a word. But by the next day I had to report to Sister. I couldn't go out because of my sore mouth.[90]

Here, Anne Chapman conformed to the rules of being a guest in someone's home even though she was there professionally.

Anne Bayne, when a pupil midwife in Lennox Castle and Glasgow in 1951, had another unusual experience which would be unlikely to have happened in hospital and which demonstrated the need to fit in with the customs of the home. She had been looking for this woman in labour for some time:

Eventually I knocked on a door and when...I went in I could hear definite labour pain... There she was on the bed ...in the corner. There was the most amazing mat on the floor. It had strange signs on it and round it were all these men... Their turbans were off and they all had long hair and they were praying. I stood at the door...and I thought, she's going to deliver...what do I do here? ...they must have known that I had come in. So I...just went for it. I got half way across this mat and they whipped it from under me and I landed on my back with my feet up. One of them was leaning over me. I can see his long hair yet... He was saying, 'You damned, you go to hell. You damned you go to hell'... At that point I would have quite liked to have been in hell... However I picked myself up with what dignity I could and I went across to her. She didn't speak. Well, they all just stayed there. I thought, if anything goes wrong with this delivery, I am for it...the Green Lady hadn't arrived. I prepared as best I could. I can't remember that much. A woman appeared at the door with water. They knew the drill. I delivered this baby. As soon as I delivered the baby, these men took the baby from me... I came out of there shaking like a leaf.[91]

Anne Bayne, by crossing the prayer mat (with the best of intentions) to get to the labouring mother, transgressed the cultural mores of the home she was in and paid the price by undergoing a frightening experience. In contrast, Anne Chapman conformed by drinking tea out of a hot tinnie, burning her mouth and having the grace not to mention it to her host.

When a woman went to hospital to have her baby she had to conform to the mores and policies of the hospital. One example of this was the use in some hospitals of what was known as 'the slab'. Professor R W Johnstone, describing the 'new Simpson' in 1939, made clear the passivity expected of the mother on the slab: 'She [the mother] is taken up by ...a lift to the first floor where the main delivery suite is situated. She goes first to a reception room where her clothing is removed; thence to a bathroom where she receives a warm spray bath on a shallow porcelain slab.'[92] Washing mothers on 'the slab' on admission was one way of preventing cross-infection. However, the way that hospital policy decreed staff should perform this task took authority from the mother and put it into the hands of, not an individual, but the policy-makers. Collectively, members of staff appeared to obey policy. Individually, they had doubts about what they were doing. Margaret Foggie remembered the slab in Rottenrow in 1934:

> Another thing they had at Rottenrow... when they [the mothers] were admitted to the first place and it was called the slab... They undressed them and hosed them down on this concrete slab before they were allowed further. It was awful... having a woman undressed and being hosed down. They would then have a clean nightie put on.[93]

Twelve years later the slab was still there. Peggy Grieve who was a pupil-midwife in Rottenrow in 1946, described what happened:

> The slab was the admission room and there was...this old ... midwife... in charge... She was a tartar. Very often she would...have a student with her and the patients would come in there... Some of them had had no antenatal care... They just arrived and they were stripped of their clothes.... And they would be washed. I think some of them needed it, but that was it. It was called the slab because there was just a slab...of formica, you know, like a work surface... I think there were two of them, two slabs...[in this]...square room. They were literally put on to the slab. There was a sheet on it, but that was all... They used to whip the sheet off it if somebody came in pretty dirty... This was them coming in, in labour. Even if they came in pushing, they didn't bypass the slab. Sometimes they had a delivery in the slab. They put them into these hospital gowns...that opened down the back and they had red dressing gowns and they could have a red sort of cape thing when they were sitting up in bed. They got that in the slab.[94]

The use of the slab exemplifies the way hospital policy, made for a good reason (in this case the reduction of infection), put midwives and student-midwives into the difficult position of subjecting women to prescribed procedures.

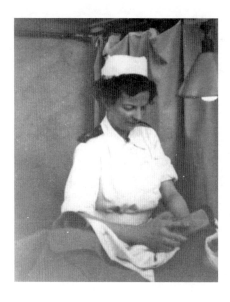

Elizabeth Harrison (née Radley),
working in the slab, Rottenrow
(GRMH) 1950.
(Courtesy of Elizabeth Radley.)

As the ratio of home to hospital births changed, more midwives were employed in the hospitals, and correspondingly fewer on the district or 'in the community'. More midwives therefore found themselves having to conform to policies which took away their decision-making abilities as well as practical skills. Working inside an institution played a part in midwives' loss of confidence in themselves, and in women's ability to give birth. The concept of an institution's representation of illness and pathology with its policies and procedures seemed to encourage midwives working within it to behave differently from outside the hospital. This put their expertise and decision-making skills in jeopardy.[95]

Mary Cronk, a midwife, stressed the rapid change in midwifery practice in the 1960s, the impact of the *Peel Report* (1970) and the corresponding 'growth in number, strength and power of the emerging profession of obstetrics.' She wrote:

> By 1975 I was not practising as a midwife. I was delivering babies according to a preset series of instructions. I was not exercising clinical judgement, and as long as I did what I was told, I was 'covered'. It was easier to just accept it, and get on with it, trying not to think too hard about what I was doing to women.[96]

One pupil-midwife in the 1970s nearly gave up. She explained:

> At this time all the women had...to have artificial rupture of membranes (ARM) and syntocinon on the due day... I remember...working with these women... Induction was always by ARM... I remember women queuing up to go into a labour room to have their legs put up in stirrups, to have ARM done. I remember some women screaming because...the cervix was not ready... After this they were taken back to their four-bedded rooms and they were attached to a syntocinon drip right away and it was turned up at regular intervals, so it was increasingly painful, with minimal pain relief... They

were all on their beds...not allowed to walk around. [They were] all either crying quietly...moaning and groaning. We just had to do the clinical observations and move on to the next woman. You didn't have time to do the caring that is part of midwifery. It was awful...

[There were]...four single rooms and one double delivery room and by two o'clock in the afternoon, you were delivering without even gloves on because the babies were popping out all over the place and there just wasn't enough staff to deal with this... You were not allowed to take the women to the labour room until they were actually in the second stage of labour which meant that they got minimal pain relief. It also meant that when they were wishing to push you had to say, 'Don't push! Get off the bed and on to the trolley'...then through at least three or four sets of double doors having previously phoned the labour ward to make sure that there was a labour bed available... You had to get them into the labour ward before they delivered their baby, and woe betide you if they delivered on the bed or on the trolley...

It was such a nightmare that by the end of three months I thought of giving up. Then I thought, No, I don't give up that easily. I'll get to the end of this. I just felt that this wasn't the way to treat women and I really didn't want any part of this... There was no caring.[97]

Professor Sir Malcolm MacNaughton (b.1925) offered some justification for increased induction of labour (IOL) rates in the 1970s. One of the major causes of perinatal mortality in Glasgow, which in 1970 was 28/1000, was explained as, 'Mature unknown deaths which were usually those between thirty-eight and forty-two weeks. We therefore made some changes in policy such as more IOL, and in 1974 there had been a reduction in the number of those late deaths.'[98] However, this justification does not explain the indiscriminate policy described above.

Another example of sweeping use of hospital policy was the performance of episiotomy. From 1968, the CMBS *Rules* permitted midwives to perform episiotomies and revised the syllabus appropriately.[99] Initially, obstetricians did not approve of this move. However, by the mid-1970s in some maternity units, it was policy that many women should have an episiotomy.[100] The midwife quoted above said:

Every woman, whether they needed it or not, had to have an episiotomy. Some of the time I would not have recognised that there was a need, but it was what had to be done and even if you were delivering unsupervised it had to be done. You weren't allowed to say, 'No I'm not going to do it.'[101]

Mary Cronk epitomised the feelings of many midwives, many of whom were afraid to 'rock the boat', when she disliked doing routine 'policy-led' episiotomies. She recognised that midwives were in danger of losing their right to practise and to make clinical judgements for which they were accountable. One day, in 1976, she did not make the routine expected episiotomy and challenged the consultant to complain. This he did not do.[102] Progress since then has been marked. Mary Cronk wrote of how terrified she was, but how, 'It seems ridiculous now when we have fought and won so many battles over our rights to practise.'[103]

Two midwives who practised in England before returning to Scotland commented on their experiences. Both remarked on the difference in midwife-doctor relationships between Scotland and England with a subsequent impact on midwifery practice. Margaret Kitson practising in 1965 used the specific example of episiotomy to illustrate a general attitude:

> There seemed to me south of the border to be a much more relaxed attitude. And there was also a greater willingness to allow midwives to be, this famous phrase, 'independent practitioners'. When I first came to Scotland to work as a midwife...one of [my first births] resulted in sudden and serious fetal distress just at the end of the second stage... I made an episiotomy because I had been trained to do it. That is what I would have done in England. And the furore there was about that. How had I dared to do that? ...I had actually immediately sent for the doctor. But why had I not waited until the doctor appeared? My reason was very simply that I did not want that baby to die and I knew what I was doing and I simply went ahead... Now, in England that was perfectly acceptable and up here I felt as if my hands were tied.[104]

Margaret Kitson commented on the attitude of midwives in Scotland to their own profession and said:

> There was an unwillingness at that time, amongst the middle and senior managers in midwifery, to accept that midwives could form judgements based on knowledge and experience which could lead to action which was perfectly acceptable.[105]

She described their deferential attitude to members of the medical profession:

> The doctor was the next thing to God... I respected my medical colleagues...and they had skills and experience I certainly didn't have and I didn't want to usurp them, but I had skills too... And not just me, the midwives round about me. But they were terrified to use them because somebody was going to come down on their head and say, 'You're not supposed to do that.'[106]

She felt there was a distinct difference between midwifery practice in Scotland and England and suggested why this might be:

> I think it was partly cultural. I think there is, or was a greater deference to medical staff in Scotland. Not just obstetricians, but all medical staff in Scotland than there was in England. So I think it was partly cultural...and partly historical.[107]

Gelda Pryde, who practised in Nottingham in the 1960s, also spoke about Scottish midwives' attitude to doctors:

> I had been doing all these things [extended midwifery procedures] in England and then I came back to [Scotland]...and I just couldn't believe the difference because the midwives were very much ruled by the medical staff

there and it took me a long time to make myself stand back.[108]

She suggested that a cultural lack of confidence affected their practice and emphasised the difference in attitudes she had noted.

> I don't know whether it's something to do with the midwifery training but they certainly lacked, when I came back ... the confidence to discuss patients on an equal with doctors. Something would start to go wrong and they would call the GP in and ten minutes later, the GP would be away...and they would phone me saying, 'I'm so worried because doctor says such and such and I don't think that's right.' 'Well, did you say that you weren't happy?' 'Well, but the doctor said...' And that was something I couldn't come to terms with... It was very much...'The doctor said,' in Scotland and you didn't...say, 'Well I'm sorry I don't agree with you and I'm here observing the patient twenty-four hours a day and you're only paying a flying visit so I think my opinion is as valid as yours, if not more so.' I don't know if it was anything to do with their training or whether Scots are just naturally a bit more reluctant to stand up and be counted. Even when...we went to Nottingham to start our training...we were the only two Scots there, and the girls in our group were all from English hospitals... And they all seemed to have much more self-confidence than we had. We sort of stood back whereas they were always in there.[109]

Margaret Kitson offered another explanation that might have added to the growing medical domination in the 1950s and 1960s.

> There had been in the fifties and...into the sixties a recruitment difficulty in nursing and midwifery. The result...was that there were some nurses and midwives whose basic education...[was] not...as good as it might have been. The big training schools in Scotland were still able to recruit students who had good...scholastic education qualifications, but some...hadn't been able to do that. ...It was easy then for medical domination to take over... I really do think that that was a factor. It was something we suffered from again in the seventies and there is always a temptation when recruitment is difficult, to reduce standards and it's a mistake. It just does not work. And...the profession is left with the results of that for a very long time, for the working lives of the people who have been recruited. Now some...whose initial deficit was the result of lack of opportunity not ability...did well... But it was very difficult for others and anyone... trying to pull these souls up. I think that was a big factor and one that tends to be forgotten.[110]

These cross-border testimonies show that within the practical business of caring for a woman as she birthed her baby, midwives had to cope with many inter-twining strands of relationships, policy, culture and history.

Conclusion
The issue of the place of normal birth is a continuing one. This chapter has attempted to

show differing situations in which mothers gave birth and the midwife's role within these. It has also revealed LAs' power and control over maternity care from an early stage under the peculiarly Scottish 'Maternity Services Schemes'. Doctors had official control over births in Scotland, even though they were not necessarily present at the delivery of the baby. This put midwives into an uncomfortable position. On the one hand, they were legally autonomous practitioners. On the other, they were subservient to the medical profession and, as some have argued, deference to doctors was greater in Scotland than in England.

As the trend towards hospital births grew, the midwife's position became more tenuous. In the home situation, her position was more clearly defined. In hospital, even though midwives delivered most of the babies, there was a blurring of midwifery and medical roles. The accounts of midwives in this chapter confirm that while midwives saw themselves as autonomous in the area of normal childbirth, medical staff saw the overall responsibility and its exercise as theirs.[111] Sometimes, doctors took over entirely. One midwife said: 'a great emphasis was put on what the doctor said, what the doctors wanted and how it was going to be. The women themselves were not considered and what they wanted wasn't considered. Nobody said they did not want to be induced.'[112]

The change from homebirths to hospital meant that the bugs and fleas were washed off at 'the slab' and clean sheets replaced newspapers. Women welcomed the respite from household chores which the hospital provided. At the same time the judgement and autonomy of midwives who demonstrated their skill and resourcefulness in the conditions of extreme poverty they faced in providing domiciliary care, was limited and frustrated. Women were subject to procedures like indiscriminate induction of labour and episiotomy to conform to hospital policy. As the effects of medicalisation of childbirth became more evident, midwives found themselves in the dilemma of obeying hospital policy and protocols rather than being autonomous midwives and advocates to mothers.

1.   LR 9.
2.   LR 85.
3.   NAS, CMB 4/2/9, *CMBS Rules*, 17 April 1916, p 4, paras 2, 3, 4.
4.   W L MacKenzie, *Report on the Physical Welfare of Mothers and Children. Vol 3. Scotland.* (Dunfermline: The Carnegie United Kingdom Trust, 1917), Chapter 49, 'Schemes of maternity and child welfare', pp 535-561.
5.   *Ibid*, p 535.
6.   *Ibid*, p 545.
7.   G Cumberlege, *Maternity in Great Britain*, (London: Oxford University Press, 1948), p 28; The word 'supervised' here is not used in the same context as official 'supervision of midwifery' which the IOMs did. Here it means 'in overall control'.
8.   Cumberlege, *Maternity in Great Britain*, p 68; in 1946 48% of babies in Scotland were delivered at home, Cumberlege p 53.
9.   *Ibid*, p 65.
10.   *Ibid*, p 67.
11.   LR 47; see also, L Reid, 'Midwifery in Scotland 3: intranatal practices', *British*

Journal of Midwifery, (2005), Vol 13 (7), pp 426-431.

12. DHS, Scottish Health Services Council, *Maternity Services in Scotland, (Montgomery Report)*, (Edinburgh: HMSO, 1959), p 18.

13. I Loudon, *Death in Childbirth*, (Oxford: Clarendon Press, 1992), p 177.

14. *Ibid*, p 176.

15. *The Transactions of the Edinburgh Obstetrical Society*, Vol 20, Session 1894-95, (Edinburgh: Oliver and Boyd, 1895), pp 169. Discussion: 'Should midwives be registered in Scotland?'

16. *Ibid*, p172.

17. T Ferguson, *Scottish Social Welfare: 1864-1914*, (Edinburgh: E &S Livingstone, 1958), p 510. Statistics collected by Dr A K Chalmers, (MOH for Glasgow) for three months of 1906.

18. Loudon, *Death in Childbirth*, p 176.

19. Cumberlege, *Maternity in Great Britain*, p 66.

20. *GRO* Scotland; see Appendix 2.

21. D Moir, *Pain Relief in Labour, (5th ed)*, (Edinburgh: Churchill Livingstone, 1986), p 1; *ibid*, p 5. Twilight sleep was first used in Germany in 1902.

22. Registration and inspection of maternity homes was made statutory in the 1927 *Midwives and Maternity Homes (Scotland) Act*, [17 &18 Geo 5 Ch 17], Part II, pp 5-9.

23. E F Murray, 'Some observations on puerperal sepsis with special reference to its occurrence in maternity hospitals', *Transactions of Edinburgh Obstetrical Society*, Session LXXXIX, in Edinburgh Medical Journal, New Series, (1930), Vol. XXXVII, (10), p 149, discussion following this paper; R W Johnstone, 'The Simpson Memorial Maternity Pavilion, Royal Infirmary, Edinburgh', (Manchester: Sherratt and Hughes 1939), reprinted from the *Journal of Obstetrics and Gynaecology of the British Empire*, Vol 46 (6) pp 1020-1028.

24. Loudon, *Death in Childbirth*, pp 258-261.

25. *Douglas and McKinley Report*, p 27.

26. Figures taken from statistical information in the *Montgomery Report*, 1959, Appendix III, p 56.

27. *Montgomery Report*, pp 14-16.

28. *Ibid*, p 39-40.

29. SHHD, *Provision of Maternity Services in Scotland: A Policy Review*, (Edinburgh: Her Majesty's Stationery Office, 1993).

30. S Kitzinger, *Birth at Home*, (Oxford: Oxford University Press, 1979), p 47. Kitzinger noted that a contrasting form of selection happened in the Netherlands where 'women, instead of being 'selected' for homebirth, as in the UK, are selected for hospital birth.

31. R Campbell, A Macfarlane, 'Recent debate on the place of birth', in J Garcia, R Kilpatrick, M Richards, *The Politics of Maternity Care* (Oxford: Clarendon Press, 1990), p 217.

32. *Ibid*, p 218.

33. *Tennent Report*, pp 2, 13.

34. *GRO*, Scotland.

35. LR 27.
36. *Montgomery Report*, p 20.
37. LR 74.
38. *Written communication*, LR 34; Reid, 'Midwifery in Scotland 3'.
39. LR 9.
40. LR 112.
41. LR 94; Reid, 'Midwifery in Scotland 3'.
42. LR 74.
43. *Montgomery Report*, p 20.
44. DOMINO stands for DOMiciliary IN and OUT.
45. T Murphy-Black, 'Systems of midwifery care in use in Scotland', in *Midwifery*, 1992, (8), p 115; R Campbell, A Macfarlane, *Where to be born? The debate and the evidence, (2nd ed)*, (National Perinatal Epidemiology Unit: Oxford, 1994), p 93.
46. LR 116; L Reid, 'Midwifery in Scotland 3'.
47. LR 91; L Reid, 'Starting from scratch', *The Practising Midwife*, (2010), Vol 13 (4), p 42.
48. LR 46; Reid, 'Starting from scratch'.
49. *Ibid*; LR 93.
50. LR 50; Reid, 'Starting from scratch'.
51. *Ibid*; LR 35.
52. LR 47.
53. LR 50.
54. LR 56.
55. LR 46.
56. *Ibid*.
57. LR 35.
58. *Ibid*.
59. *Ibid*.
60. LR 11; L Reid, 'Homebirths in the dunny', *The Practising Midwife*, (2008), Vol 11, (4), p 50.
61. *Ibid*; LR 11.
62. M Myles, *A Textbook for Midwives, (4th ed)*, (Edinburgh: E and S Livingstone, 1962), p 654; L Reid, 'Bearing the load for women', *The Practising Midwife*, (2008), Vol 11, (7), p 50.
63. J K Watson, *A Complete Handbook of Midwifery for Midwives and Nurses, (3rd ed)*, (London: The Scientific Press Limited, 1914), pp 139-141.
64. LR 47; *Written communication*, LR 3; Reid, 'Bearing the load for women'.
65. *Ibid; Written communication*, LR 42.
66. LR 35.
67. LR 115.
68. LR 27.
69. LR 20; Reid, 'Bearing the load for women'.
70. *Ibid*; LR 108.
71. LR 99.

72. *Dressings for confinement and lying-in period*, DHS Circular no 84/1951, 8 August 1951, notes belonging to Miss Isobel Duguid, RGN, SCM, MTD; Myles, *Textbook for Midwives, (4th ed)*, p 653.

73. LR 27.

74. LR 91.

75. LR 2; Reid, 'Bearing the load for women'.

76. *Ibid*; LR 115.

77. LR 91; Reid, 'Bearing the load for women'.

78. LR 27; Myles, *A Textbook for Midwives, (4th ed)*, p 270. The Minnitt-minor apparatus for nitrous oxide-air analgesia in domiciliary midwifery practice weighed 12.5 lbs; Reid, 'Bearing the load for women'.

79. NAS, CMB 1/7, *CMBS Minutes*, 12 March 1959, p 1.

80. LR 27; L Reid, 'Shanks's pony to Council 'caur'', *The Practising Midwife*, (2008), Vol 11 (5), p 74.

81. LR 20; Reid, 'Shanks's pony to Council 'caur''.

82. LR 11; Reid, 'Shanks's pony to Council 'caur''.

83. *Ibid*; LR 91.

84. *Ibid*; Reid, 'Shanks's pony to Council 'caur''.

85. Ibid; LR 91.

86. *Working Party on Midwives*, p 57.

87. SHHD, *Provision of Maternity Services in Scotland: A Policy Review*, (Edinburgh: HMSO, 1993); E Hillan, M McGuire, L Reid, *Midwives and woman-centred care*, (Edinburgh: RCM Scottish Board, and University of Glasgow, 1997).

88. LR 11; Reid, 'Homebirths in the dunny'.

89. *Ibid*; LR 11.

90. *Ibid; Reid*, 'Homebirths in the dunny'.

91. LR 91.

92. R W Johnstone, *'The Simpson Memorial Maternity Pavilion'*, pp 1022; Reid, 'Midwifery in Scotland, 3'.

93. *Ibid*; LR 50; 'Reid, Starting from scratch'.

94. *Ibid*; LR 102.

95. C Flint, *Sensitive Midwifery*, (London: Heinmann Midwifery, 1986), pp 131-132.

96. M Cronk, 'Midwifery: A practitioner's view from within the National Health Service', in *Midwife, Health Visitor and Community Nurse*, (1990), Vol 6 (3), p 61.

97. LR 85; Reid, 'Midwifery in Scotland 3'.

98. M MacNaughton, Mabel Liddiard Memorial Lecture: 'Perinatal mortality in Scotland', in *Midwives Chronicle*, (March 1992), p 47.

99. *CMB Rules*, 31 March, 1968, p 11; M Myles, *A Textbook for Midwives, (7th ed)*, (Edinburgh: Churchill Livingstone, 1971) p 618; *CMBS Report* 31 March 1969, pp 3-4; The CMBS did not make hospital policy, although there was often vigorous interchange of views between maternity unit management committees and the CMBS.

100. NAS, CMB 1/8, *CMBS Minutes*, 20 February 1969, pp 1, 4.

101. LR 85.
102. Cronk, *'Midwifery: A practitioner's view from within the National Health Service'*, p 61; there is nothing in the relevant CMBS *Rules* to say that midwives should obey hospital policy without question.
103. *Ibid.*
104. LR 120.
105. *Ibid.*
106. *Ibid.*
107. *Ibid.*
108. LR 69.
109. *Ibid.*
110. LR 120.
111. R Mander, 'Autonomy in midwifery and maternity care', *in Midwives Chronicle, (October 1993), pp 369-374.*
112. LR 85; Reid, 'Midwifery in Scotland 3'.

Chapter 8
Postnatal policies: 'not paid to think'

Care of the mother and baby in the postnatal period has been a long-standing and important part of a midwife's work and has been recognised officially in Scotland since the first complete set of CMBS *Rules*.[1] Two terms which may be used to describe the time immediately after birth are the 'lying-in period' and the 'postnatal period'. 'Lying-in' used to mean 'the time occupied by the labour and a period of ten days thereafter.'[2] Later, the term 'lying-in' was used separately from 'labour'. In this chapter the terms 'lying-in' and 'postnatal' are interchangeable.[3]

This chapter explores aspects of midwifery practice during the postnatal period surrounding care of mother and baby, reflected by changing customs over the years. It includes an overview of CMBS *Rules* on postnatal care and why some midwives found it difficult to adhere to them. It also examines the custom of keeping mothers in bed for ten days postnatally and how this changed. With early ambulation of mothers coinciding chronologically with rising hospital birth rates and a shortage of hospital beds, the next step was early discharge home for mothers and their babies and the chapter shows some midwives' views of this plan. Midwives' voices are also used to demonstrate contrasts in the homes and lifestyles of the people with whom they worked. Examination of these features of midwives' postnatal practice gives an idea of how much autonomy midwives maintained in an area of great importance to mothers and their babies.

Midwives and the postnatal period: an overview
From the publication of the first complete set of CMBS *Rules* in August 1916, there was a statutory requirement in Scotland for midwives to attend upon and examine a mother and her infant for the ten-day postnatal period.[4] The only exception to the ten-day rule was between 1939 and 1965 when the statutory period increased to fourteen days, with a similar increase in England and Wales.[5] This occurred as a result of a change in the CMBE&W and CMBS *Rules* after the 1936 Midwives Act, which applied to England and Wales, and the 1937 Maternity Services (Scotland) Act. Although the Acts had different wording, both entitled every woman having a baby in England, Wales and Scotland to free home visits by a midwife for fourteen days.[6] The Acts were framed as a response to anxiety surrounding the maternal mortality rate (MMR). During the lying-in period, the CMBS expected midwives 'to visit the patient twice a day for the first three days following delivery and at least daily thereafter for a minimum period of ten days, or for as long as her expertise is required.'[7] The equivalent CMBE&W Rule was the same except for intermittent attendance of a midwife from the tenth day up to the twenty-eighth day postnatally.[8] In Scotland, the midwife decided whether or not it was necessary to carry on visiting after the tenth day. Reasons for continuing visits could include excessive or offensive lochia in the mother, in which case the midwife called in the GP, feeding problems, and non-separation of the umbilical cord. Fay MacLeod, practising in Glasgow in the 1960s said, 'Yes, ten days or you visited them till the cord

came off. Or if there wis any complications like breastfeeding and [problems] like that.'[9] Where necessary, the midwife continued to visit until the problem was resolved.

As the place of birth changed, most women, often in hospital for up to ten days postnatally, did not see the district midwife. More midwives were employed in maternity units and fewer on the district. The role of the midwife on the district, already eroded by having fewer homebirths and little or no antenatal care to give, was diminished and very nearly extinguished by the late 1960s. At the same time the rising number of hospital births and corresponding requirement for antenatal beds contributed to a shortage of institutional maternity beds.[10] This led to a change in the postnatal care of mothers, with increasingly early ambulation and self-care. To cope with these changes, 'early discharge home' emerged in the 1950s and gradually became an accepted part of postnatal care. The need for the district or community midwife slowly re-appeared, but not usually to give full midwifery care. Yet, the number of district midwives had declined to a level too low to cope with the increasing number of postnatal mothers discharged early. In 1965, the CMBS reluctantly agreed to an amendment to the 1947 NHS (Scotland) Act allowing health visitors and home nurses to attend mothers in the lying-in period. With the trend for early discharge, this was happening already and the CMBS felt that, under the circumstances, however unhappy it was over the concession, it could not oppose the amendment.[11]

The CMBS tried to retrieve the position in 1973. The 1965 decision was never included in the *Rules* and by 1973 only four members of the 1965 Board remained. It is probable that the newer members were unaware of any change. In 1973, the CMBS noted that health visitors were visiting postnatal mothers discharged early from hospital and it appeared fairly common 'in many areas' for the health visitor to take over from the midwife after the sixth day.[12] LAs' arrangements for the postnatal care of mother and baby up to the tenth day varied considerably and therefore some mothers did not have the services of a midwife for the full postnatal period.[13] In some areas, LA midwives were attached to maternity hospitals enabling them to follow up mothers and babies in the hospital catchment area according to the *Rules*. The Board, in line with the 1973 *Tennent Report*, recommended the initiation of this across Scotland and used the integration policy of the NHS re-organisation of 1974 to expedite the move.[14] To dispel any doubt, in 1975 the Board reiterated the requirement for a midwife to attend for the whole of the ten days postnatal period.[15]

By 1980, 99.5% of babies in Scotland were born in hospital, and community midwives' primary remit was to give postnatal care. However, their workforce was reduced because of the lowered homebirth rate and they were attending to increasing numbers of mothers discharged early from hospital. This resulted in many more visits to make but with less midwife-time for each woman.[16] In addition, overall, there was a lack of continuity of care for women. Most antenatal care was performed by GPs and obstetricians, most births were conducted by hospital midwives, and midwives on the community gave postnatal care. Therefore postnatal care was the only area where community midwives were able to maintain their skills.

Rules on giving postnatal care
Whether a woman gave birth at home or in hospital, the basic postnatal *Rules* for

midwives were the same. In the early days of the CMBS, the emphasis was on physical recovery of the mother, cleanliness of both mother and baby, establishment of breastfeeding (ideally), and close observance of both mother and baby for any signs of abnormalities in which circumstance the midwife was obligated to call for medical assistance. Abnormalities included in the case of a lying-in woman:

Fits or convulsions
Abdominal swelling and tenderness
Offensive lochia, if persistent
Rigor with raised temperature
Rise of temperature above 100 degrees Fahrenheit with quickening of the pulse for more than twenty-four hours
Unusual swelling of the breasts with local tenderness or pain
Secondary postpartum haemorrhage
White leg (*Phlegmasia alba dolens*)

In the case of the child, abnormalities or complications included:

Injuries received during birth
Any malformation or deformity endangering the child's life
Dangerous feebleness
Inflammation of, or discharge from the eyes, however slight
Serious skin eruptions, especially those marked by the formation of watery blisters
Inflammation about, or haemorrhage from, the navel.[17]

These *Rules* did not mention other less tangible aspects of postnatal care. Midwives' responsibilities in the postnatal period include the educational, psychosocial and physical.[18] To fulfil educational responsibilities, from the 1930s the CMBS included the teaching of mothercraft, infant care and the principles of nutrition in the Part 2 syllabus. The need for midwives to teach 'the constructive hygiene of mothercraft' was one of the arguments for increasing the training time in 1939.[19] This aspect developed until, by the end of the CMBS's existence, teaching parentcraft antenatally had become an important part of the midwife's role.

The importance of psychosocial and emotional aspects of postnatal care did not receive full acknowledgement until the later decades of the twentieth century.[20] Early editions (1-10) of Myles' *A Textbook for Midwives* discussed briefly the psychology of the puerperium. However it was only when *Myles Textbook for Midwives* was given a whole new look that the authors gave prominence to the psychology of the puerperium and included chapters on sociology related to midwifery and counselling skills in midwifery practice.[21]

During a postnatal visit, the midwife's duty was to perform a full physical examination of mother and baby. Prevention of infection was of primary importance. As the mother was officially confined to bed for ten days (although as shown below this was a rule virtually impossible to keep), the midwife's duties included monitoring the temperature, pulse and respirations, bed-bathing, performing vulval swabbings, abdominal palpation to check for uterine involution, examination of the lochia and perineal area, and examination of the legs for signs of swellings indicative of possible deep venous thrombosis (DVT). In addition, the administration of an enema and assistance in putting the baby to the breast could be part of a postnatal visit. During the same visit, the midwife had to take the baby's temperature, perform a top-to-toe examination paying particular attention to the eyes and skin, bath and dress the baby, attend to the cord/umbilical area depending on the custom of the day, and make sure the baby was feeding and sleeping well. The midwife had to record all her observations and if there was any problem, the *Rules* required her to send for medical aid. Midwives practising in hospital also performed and recorded these postnatal examinations and observations. This gives some idea of the amount of work involved in a full postnatal visit, particularly when mothers were kept in bed for ten days. Midwives visited mothers twice daily for the first three days and daily thereafter.

As well as their postnatal visits, midwives on the district were on call for mothers in labour most of the time. Mary McCaskill, working in Glasgow in the late 1940s said, 'We were on...twenty-four hour call [for deliveries]... We would have anything between...eight...to about fourteen, fifteen postnatal visits to do.'[22] By the 1960s, LAs realised that to be out all night looking after a mother in labour followed by a day of postnatal visits and perhaps another mother in labour did not make for the best midwifery and they started to employ more part-time married midwives. Fay McLeod was one of them. She explained:

> We were relieving the full time midwives. Say somebody had been up all night delivering, then you were sent there to do their calls while they caught up on their sleep. So you could be in Possilpark one day, and Easterhouse the next, Drumchapel the next and then Silverburn the next. You could be anywhere. All over Glasgow.[23]

Having part-time relief midwives presented a problem of lack of continuity of care for mothers, which affected the midwife/mother relationship. Fay McLeod said, 'If you were in one place for the whole week it was heaven... You actually got to know the people.'[24] However, most of the time they could be anywhere and in every type of home:

> ...from a [house] in Pollokshields to a wee single-end somewhere, where they didn't have a basin to bath the baby. And in those days you had to bath every baby in every house. When the cord came off you would say, 'You could just bath baby yourself tomorrow.'[25]

However Margaret McInally, also in Glasgow, argued that this was not always so, citing the mother's apprehension as a reason. She said, 'At the first bath you had to say, "now, I'll supervise you the first bath," because they were very frightened, you know.'[26]

Not every mother received full postnatal care which meant that the CMB *Rules* were not always kept. Ann Lamb, working privately in Inverurie in the 1940s, said, 'I just stayed in the house for a week. That was after the birth for the postnatal care, but there wasn't really much postnatal care in my day – just a wee look.'[27] Care was also less defined when howdies were in charge. Occasionally, in rural areas, there was no midwife to give postnatal care. Doddie Davidson, who was a howdie in 1940s Aberdeenshire, said:

> There wis nae midwife... I looked after the mother after the baby was born...

I washed the Mam and saw that she wis [all right]... And the bairn too. I bathed the bairns. An then ye stayed, sometimes a wik, sometimes mair. Sometimes ye didna hae time ti spare, but ye aye hid aboot a wik wi them or ten days.'[28]

Another howdie, Annie Kerr, also in the 1940s but at the other end of the country, said:

I took care of the baby afterwards until she wis fit. I wid mebbe be there a fortnight... When I was staying with the women having their babies, I did everything. The washing, cleaning, into Castle Douglas for the messages. The mother would see to herself – by that time she was fit. I took care of her when she was in bed. I didna let her work while I was there. That's what I was there to dae. I was there to work. And save her, till she gathered her own strength again. I gave her a basin to wash herself. I never took nowt tae dae wi the washin. I looked after the baby and everything for her and did aa the housework.[29]

Yet one howdie, Johann Roberton, working in Aberdeen in the early decades of the twentieth century, did things differently, even though still not conforming to CMB *Rules*. According to her granddaughter:

Postnatally, she had a strict routine and according to my late mother, Grandma would clean up the patient first after expulsion of the afterbirth and immediately wrap her up in a supporting binder round the stomach to prevent sagging of the abdominal muscles. My mother felt the benefit of this in later years! The binders were usually made of flannelette sheets torn to the required strip for size. She also collected old sheets from neighbours and made the bandages herself. If the mother had insufficient milk she too was 'binded' to prevent drooping.[30]

One district midwife, in the 1960s, had a set routine immediately after a homebirth. She said:

One of the joys I had was this lovely feeling of warmth and a lovely feeling from everyone. It used to be my great joy once we had got the baby and I used to wrap it up all nice and cosy and give everybody a wee quick look and then I'd have lovely warm sheets and a warm nightie and bath towels ready – things for the mother and the baby, and after everyone had seen the baby...I used to put some oil on it to get the vernix off and I used to wrap it up in warm towels and leave it there resting. Then I would bed-bath the mother from top to bottom, give her her tooth-mug, into her clean sheets and warm nightie, offer her her cosmetic bag, get the hair brushed and then I used to say to usually the [grand]mother, 'I think your daughter would just love a cup of tea,' and she would go and do that and I would bath the baby, dress him in nice warm things, put him in a warm cot and then they were allowed to come in and I used to go away and go to the bathroom and do all the cleaning out, all the slungeing, getting rid of everything that had to be got rid of and assessing the afterbirth. I did that on my own to give them time together and

I would leave that house and there wouldn't be a speck of blood anywhere. That was my great joy of home confinements. Probably I was lucky. I had a lot of lovely home confinements. Any difficulties that I had I would know when to call the doctor.[31]

Occasionally a mother would not allow the midwife in to do postnatal care. In Glasgow, for instance, a pupil midwife could deliver the baby with a midwife and never see the mother again. Anne Bayne said, 'Often when the Green Lady went [to do a postnatal visit] she did not get in.'[32] Therefore, the CMBS's ideal of postnatal care was not always performed according to the book.

It was easier to keep to the *Rules* when mothers were in hospital and under a watchful eye. Ella Clelland, in her first midwifery post at the Vert Hospital, Haddington, in the 1950s recalled:

We kept the mothers ten days and with a first baby sometimes fourteen. We had them in bed for five days and we swabbed them by douching them with Dettol water. We used to have a big trolley and all these jugs of Dettol douche water and pans underneath it and you went along and put them on the bedpan, and you had the douche and swabbing equipment, turned them on to their side, examined their stitches and made sure that that was well healing.[33]

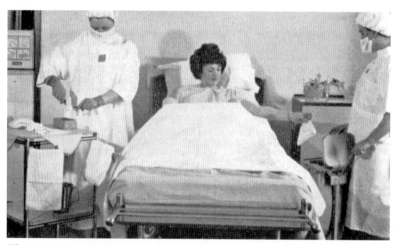

The way it was then. Perineal toilet, Bellshill Maternity Hospital, 1960s. Courtesy of Susan Stewart and reprinted from M Myles, A textbook for midwives (6th ed), (E & S Livingstone, 1968) p 458, fig 315.

On the district, even though midwives worked on their own, the LSA checked that they obeyed the *Rules*. Mary McCaskill, a Green Lady in Glasgow in the late 1940s, said, 'You had to have your *Rule* book and that had to be produced at all times and ... we were subject to inspection [at home] of uniform and equipment – the bag.' She also said that, when an inspection was pending, midwives collaborated to demonstrate that their equipment appeared complete.[34]

If the midwife found a problem beyond her remit when visiting postnatally, she was required to call for medical assistance. This was particularly important if the mother had a raised temperature signifying the possibility of an infection. Mary McCaskill's description of what she personally had to do in this situation shows the importance afforded to the dangers of infection.[35]

CMBS *Rules* for midwives to follow therefore emphasised the physical care of mother and baby. They were not always kept to the letter, especially early in the century, and where howdies were practising. Yet even after the discovery of the first antibiotics, the CMB *Rules* regarding suspected infection and LA supervision of midwives on this issue were for many years clearly stated and strictly kept.

Keeping the postnatal mother in bed

At the beginning of the twentieth century, medical practitioners, not unlike their nineteenth century predecessors, considered that a necessary lying-in period should last for at least ten days.[36] In 1914, Watson had urged that 'The patient is to be kept in bed for at least ten days and in her bedroom for a fortnight.'[37] This was so that the mother could recover from the birth in a peaceful atmosphere with few visitors and establish breastfeeding. This midwifery textbook, like others, demonstrated, at least on paper, the authority that medical practitioners had over midwives.[38] In practice, this rule was difficult for a midwife to achieve and left a mother weak and often debilitated through lack of exercise. Mima Sutherland, practising in Unst, Shetland, in the 1930s and 1940s, said:

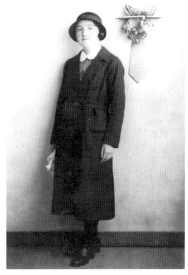

> After the birth, I used to see them twice in the day. We were supposed to see them [for] fourteen days. By the time they put their legs oot ower the side of the bed they would say, 'Look at my legs. What are they like?' They were wasted.[39]

Mima Sutherland, midwife, circa 1937-1940. (Courtesy of Janet Bayne, and The Museum, Fetlar, Shetland.)

Mothers often pretended to midwives that they had stayed in bed when in reality they had not. One midwife described how she always knew if the mother had been out of bed by the state of her feet.[40] Molly Muir, in Edinburgh in the 1930s, recalled:

> My district was Gorgie where I went every morning to bath my babies and deal with the mother for about two weeks. Most of them had a neighbour who was very good to them. I remember one time calling at this house. I did

the mother and bathed the baby and then I said, 'You know you've got on awfully well. I think you could get up this afternoon for an hour.' I carried on further up the street to another lady and she said, 'Hasn't Mrs. S. done well. She was up having tea with me yesterday afternoon.' You never knew what was happening when your back was turned. They weren't ill. She was pretending that she was doing all that she was supposed to be doing and that's what was going on.[41]

However, many mothers got up, got on with their work and did not try to hide it. Betty Smith, practising in Glasgow in the 1940s said, 'The mothers weren't supposed to get up out of their beds till about the tenth day and you very often would go [to visit] and the mother had skipped out for messages.'[42] Midwives accepted the reality that most mothers could not stay in bed for the stated length of time because they had so much to do. Doddie Davidson said:

Keepin the mothers in bed depended on the mother a lot. Some o them wanted tae lie, some o them didna. But they were aye a few days in their bed. Sometimes aboot a wik. Sometimes if they hid ither little anes they wanted tae get up. But some Mams wanted tae lie. It aa dependit on them. Once they got up they were OK.[43]

May Norrie, practising in Froickheim and Carmyllie, Angus, in 1947, was realistic too. She said, 'Oh well, I just left [them] to their own devices. But I knew perfectly well some of them were up and doing things for their family, you know.'[44] Margaret Foggie, in Glasgow in 1934, added another aspect to the postnatal period. She recalled:

The people...were very dispirited somehow. It was very sad. It was a very bad time... I never looked after anyone who had a husband working. You had to try and keep the mothers in bed but it was very difficult. You couldn't really insist on it. But you told the husbands 'Look after these children and remember [she] is not well... Run the messages for her and look after the weans.' They would say, 'Yes,' but...I don't think they did. They used to stand around on the street, talking.[45]

Families' financial difficulties were echoed by Mary McCaskill who explained why she sometimes had to negotiate times of visits:

We visited twice a day for the first four days [postnatally] and thereafter once a day up till the fourteenth day. I know that's been changed but that was what I did. [The mothers] sometimes weren't there. In some parts of Glasgow the mother was in receipt of dole money and they would hop off to sign on. That took precedence over everything else, but usually you just had to work round it. Because you couldn't chain them to the bed...for seven days.[46]

However mothers who would not stay in bed probably did themselves a favour apart from avoiding the muscle-wasting described by Mima Sutherland. A well-known hazard of staying in bed with no exercise was deep venous thrombosis (DVT). Annie Kerr recalled:

> I wid mebbe be there a fortnight. It wis reckoned they shouldna be out o bed till the nine days were up. That wis quite a common thing. Ye had tae wait in yer bed intil a certain time and then get up but ye weren't allowed up because I remember one woman gettin up. The baby began to cry and I took no notice of it. I got on with the bakin, whatever I was doin in the kitchen and when I came in, here she was sittin wi the baby... She had got up...and walked across to the baby, and picked it up. I got sic a shock when I saw her. She was never any the worse of it. They say they liked to get ye up on yer feet. It saved clottin.[47]

Hospitalisation brought other hazards. In the 1950s, with the number of hospital births rising, more mothers were in hospital for postnatal care for varying lengths of time, but with a normal stay of nine to ten days. Cross-infection was more likely to happen in hospital than at home, highlighted by one district midwife in the Outer Hebrides in the 1940s and 1950s who said, 'I don't remember any postnatal infections. You see they were in their own homes.'[48] Another hospital-related issue was episiotomy. More mothers had episiotomies in hospital than at home. With mothers still being kept in bed for about five days (and it was easier to enforce this rule in hospital than at home), an episiotomy nurtured in a warm moist atmosphere was an added potential source of infection. Jan Fenton, working in Dundee Royal Infirmary in the mid-1950s, observed that mothers with infected episiotomies were allowed up earlier than the usual five days in order to have a shower. She had what she thought was a good idea. She said:

> When they [the mothers] were in the wards they would be in for nine days. And ...they were kept in bed for five days... If episiotomies went 'off', they used to let them get up for a shower... And I said to the sister, 'I think it would be much better if we just got them all up for a shower. It would save these episiotomies going off.' And I was told I wasn't paid to think.[49]

Midwives were expected to adhere to hospital policy regardless of changes which would benefit mothers.

Keeping mothers in bed for long periods of time eventually went out of fashion. Successive editions of Margaret Myles' *Textbook for Midwives* demonstrated an unstoppable movement. In the first four editions Myles recommended that 'normal patients' [sic] are allowed out of bed:

> ...on the second day of the puerperium...for [no] longer than three minutes at first, and...encouraged to walk round the bed rather than sit on a chair. The time is gradually increased until the third or fourth day, when she is permitted to go to the 'toilet' and to have a bath-tub.[50]

Myles cited the advantages of this early ambulation as representing better drainage from, and rapid involution of, the uterus; fewer respiratory complications; reduction in thrombotic conditions; more rapid resumption of bowel and bladder function; and stronger, happier mothers with greater experience of handling their babies. A disadvantage was the possibility that, once a mother was out of bed, she would do too much. This would lead to poor establishment of lactation, fatigue and poor recuperation from giving birth, physically and emotionally.[51]

In the sixth edition of *A Textbook for Midwives* (1968), Myles said 'Normal patients are allowed to be out of bed on the first day of the puerperium; they may have a shower (with mobile hand spray) six hours after delivery.'[52] However vulval swabbing by midwives at this time was still *de rigueur*. Myles gave the same directions in her seventh edition in 1971, with the addition of comments on self-vulval swabbing and the use of bidets (with lucid instruction from the midwife and unremitting supervision). However, with the practice of early ambulation now established and apparently with no ill-effects, she stated, possibly to reassure wary midwives (or those who were not allowed to think), 'The practice appears to have no deleterious effect. Primitive women get up early with no harmful effects.'[53] By Myles' 8th edition, early ambulation and self-vulval swabbing were accepted facets of postnatal care.[54]

By 1961, the homebirth rate in Scotland was down to twenty-five percent, with a further decrease to 15.4 percent by 1965.[55] The shortage of maternity beds was exacerbated by the increase in hospital births and the rising birth rate. Corresponding changes in postnatal care developed; mothers took more personal responsibility and, increasingly, were encouraged to tend to their babies themselves. The midwife's role in the postnatal wards changed from one who performed full physical care for mother and baby to one who taught mothers to look after themselves and their babies with support where necessary. The issue of hospital bed numbers, combined with more able and mobile mothers, pointed to the next phase: early discharge home.

Early discharge home
The ten-day postnatal hospital stay gradually decreased to a mean of 5.3 days in 1980. While this suited some mothers, with a few leaving hospital as early as forty-eight hours after delivery, the real reason behind it was the increase in hospital deliveries and subsequent pressure on hospital bed numbers. The corresponding need for antenatal beds exacerbated the problem.[56]

The trend for early discharge, linked to the shortage of hospital maternity beds, is evident in the official reports from 1959. A ten-day stay in hospital after delivery was widely regarded as suitable, although seven or eight days 'or even less' was quite common. However, with the ten-day discharge, it was difficult to obtain enough midwives to fulfil the CMBS's current fourteen days of statutory postnatal visiting. It became even more difficult when mothers were discharged earlier. The RCM argued that mothers who were discharged before ten days were not so happy or confident and had difficulty establishing breastfeeding. In contrast, the Royal College of Obstetricians and Gynaecologists Scottish Standing Committee suggested that, with the prevailing shortage of beds, 'more admissions and shorter stay' might be preferable. Similarly, the British Paediatric Association suggested a pilot 'very early discharge from hospital' scheme, even although they acknowledged that this did not help breastfeeding.[57]

Fourteen years later the Tennent Committee reported on integration in the maternity services. It stated that early discharge was convenient for some mothers but should not be universal and it should not be used solely as a method of increasing bed turnover. Nevertheless, the *Report* conceded that this might happen 'as a temporary expedient in order to provide specialist services for a greater number of patients.'[58]

Midwives' and women's views on the matter were mixed. Betty Smith, midwife, thought that, for some women, a longer stay in hospital was a good thing, declaring:

> [With early discharge] I feel the mothers are getting put out too quickly. When they were in hospital, particularly mothers that had family, after their babies were born they could have the sleep because the staff were there to look after the babies at night. They were having their food brought to them, having their baths – many a patient didn't have a bath to go home to. They were able to have their baths and a rest... Yes, they had an afternoon nap...lying on their tummy. With a pillow maybe under their tummy... They got wakened after that [for tea]. If they get sent home...they don't get that rest... Now some of the patients wanted home but that was up to them. They would request a forty-eight hour confinement. I just feel now they're – because [of] the postnatal blues at about the third and fourth day – that's when they want to cry. They want all the assistance they can get and their bosoms [are sore] – you know.[59]

However, in the 1960s before the trend was established, early discharge was sometimes initiated by maternal request. Fay McLeod observed:

> Sometimes it was within twenty-four hours if they pressed hard enough to get out. I've gone to visit somebody the morning after they've got home and they've been away out somewhere and it's only less than forty-eight hours since the baby was born. Thankfully not too many of them were as silly as that, but you did get the odd one.[60]

Gelda Pryde, in Fife and Angus in the 1970s, commented on differences in postnatal care related to early discharge:

> The whole type of care [changed]. After delivery they were in bed for ten days, swabbed twice a day, three times a day until the tenth day. [Then] when the early discharge came in so many of them [mothers] thought, 'Oh, this is great', but when you went to do their home visit two days later they're...all stressed out and saying, 'Oh I wish I'd listened to you and stayed in hospital for a few days longer'... Quite often, yes, when you would visit them days later, they would wish that they had not been in such a hurry to get home.[61]

Pryde also agreed that the planned early discharge scheme arose mainly because of the shortage of beds brought about by the push for hospital births. This comment confirmed the forecast of the *Tennent Report*, and the recommendation for 'more admissions and shorter stay' of the *Montgomery Report* (see above). She said:

> I can remember this Planned Early Discharge scheme. That was, I think, more governed by the need for beds rather than looking at what the patients' wishes were. It must have been at Forth Park [in the late 1960s] because we were never short of beds in Angus, but I think...it was so that we could do more deliveries in hospital and to get everybody in for delivery then they had to have this planned early discharge. So if they had a normal delivery and everything was fine, they could go home. It was forty-eight hours when it

first came in. It was [official policy]... If it was a first baby they were usually persuaded to stay in or if...it was an unsuitable home for whatever reason, you know their facilities weren't good or there were lots of other children or people sharing their homes or whatever, they were usually kept in. So it was normally uncomplicated para ones, twos.[62]

Although early discharge home developed from the need for maternity beds, it was still strictly controlled.[63] If a mother indicated antenatally that she would like to go home from hospital early, it became policy for the community midwife to inspect the home for suitability. Myles' textbooks gave didactic instructions on how midwives and GPs should negotiate this with a mother. For example, 'an initial visit is paid by the midwife to assess the home conditions and discuss domestic conditions. Overcrowding is not acceptable.' Myles discussed issues such as adequate heating and 'the help of a reliable woman,' before saying, 'about the 36th week an evening visit is paid [by a midwife] to confirm that arrangements have been completed and to gain the husband's co-operation.'[64] These instructions contrast with the situation as late as the 1950s when midwives delivered women in one-roomed over-crowded homes without them necessarily being assessed for suitability while the *Montgomery Report* was trying to promote homebirths.[65]

Transfer not only occurred from hospital to home, but also from hospital to hospital. A mother could be sent to a large specialist maternity unit for the birth because of problems arising ante, or intranatally, and returned to a smaller local unit for postnatal care. Maureen Hamilton, a pupil midwife in Glasgow, then midwife in Campbeltown in 1970, commented:

That was very different [from working in Glasgow] because we dealt with the Air Ambulance from Campbeltown to Glasgow if there were any complications... Often the GPs panicked a bit...[even] when they were cracking on quite well in labour. They sometimes just didn't really give them [the mothers] a chance. They would say, 'Oh I think there are going to be problems. We'll need to get her to Glasgow.' Then she would deliver as soon as she arrived [in Glasgow] which wasn't fair on the patients... [When the mother and baby returned] we had them postnatally... They kept them in the hospital for about seven days then and it was lovely because it was a home from home for them, overlooking the loch. The mothers who came in there loved it.[66]

Ella Clelland also experienced inter-hospital transfer:

I went to the Vert Memorial Hospital [in 1958] just outside Haddington. I was there for about two years as a staff midwife. That was very good. It was GP run. They had no doctors within the hospital, but there were something like thirty-odd GPs within the East Lothian area. Some of them were very old and had been there for quite a long time. Some were quite young with quite new ideas...

We did not do complicated midwifery. Anything complicated was taken into Edinburgh to the Simpson or the Eastern, so we as midwives would know when we needed help. But in the main it was normal midwifery with occasionally a breech delivery or low forceps – no ventouse then – and we called the GP when we felt we had difficulty... Work at the Vert was pretty good experience of the normal side of life and anything that was too abnormal required to be shipped off to Edinburgh and we went in the ambulance with them and took them to hospital there... All being well, we had them for the postnatal period which was ten days. We kept the mothers ten days and with a first baby sometimes fourteen.[67]

Gelda Pryde, practising in Angus in 1973, described postnatal care given in a small general hospital:

The Fyfe Jamieson Hospital [in Forfar] closed and we got a ward in Whitehills which was one of the long-stay units and we did DOMINO deliveries there with the possibility of the mothers staying in for up to twenty-four, [or] forty-eight hours if necessary with the community midwives going in visiting them. The care was by general nurses but [with] the community midwives going in as they would have visited them at home. They visited them in hospital. They really needed minimal care, but it was to have somewhere as an alternative to home for babies with feeding problems where they were getting some support and where home conditions weren't really suitable for the mum to go straight home. This was a sort of respite care almost... The Scottish Office were very interested when we started it.[68]

Contrasts in midwifery practice
High on the agenda of most midwives interviewed was the poverty they encountered, both as pupil midwives and as midwives. This was something which most of them had not previously met. Anne Chapman worked in the dunnies in Glasgow. She said, 'My mother wouldn't believe me when I was telling her that. She would say, "Ye're bletherin lassie."'[69] Margaret Dearnley's 1946 Lennox Castle training involved district midwifery in some areas of Glasgow that left her with some unforgettable memories:

Now, the poverty was dreadful. Very, very bad. I remember going in a house which was all dark, but a great big roaring fire. And there were two or three kids running about... with wee vests on and nothing else and a packed earth floor. And the new mother... was lying on what they call ticking. Now you know the ticking is the bed ticking. She was lying on ticking on a bed, an iron bedstead in a corner. And then the other corner of the room was all the orange boxes with the fruit and everything and her husband was a barrow boy. And these kids played aboot in there and that was where they lived and that's where he stored his fruit.[70]

Margaret Dearnley also recalled seeing huge contrasts in homes, sometimes within a single day's work. She also highlighted how it was normal procedure for midwives to carry tokens with them supplied by the Council to use in gas meters. She remembered particularly one wet Sunday morning:

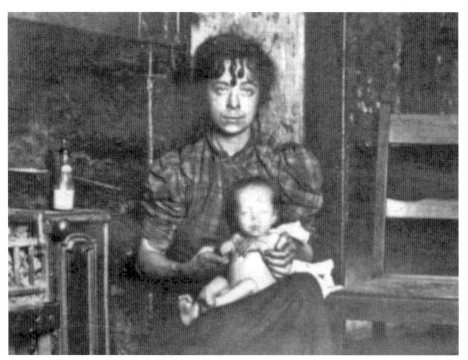

Mother and baby in a very poor home in Glasgow. (Courtesy of Glasgow City Archives, ref: P663.)

Another house I went into...had two apartments...a kitchen with a bed recess and ...what they called their front room...and [an] outside...closet... [It was] a day of torrential rain. I went in to bath the new baby to find the woman...lying there and no fire, nothing, and I said, 'Have you had a cup of tea?' She said, 'No'. And I said to her, 'What's wrong? Why has nobody been in? Where's your husband?' 'Oh, he left when he knew the baby was coming. He left me. He left me three weeks ago and I haven't any money' I went to the lady next door... [which] we'd been instructed to do... She said to me, 'I'm sorry, I can't give you any money. I've given her money before and he's stolen it. He's even tampered with the meter, for the drink...' I said, 'Well, she's lying there and...she's got the baby in beside her for warmth. It's never been washed... She hasn't had a cup of tea; the house is freezing cold. There's nobody there even to light a fire.' So she said, 'Well I'm sorry, I can't do any more.' And shut the door. So I went back to her... and I...[used] tokens given by the Parish for the gas meter...and [lit] the gas heater...boiled the kettle...got her a cup of tea and washed [the baby], got her washed...and I think I lit the fire... I took my uniform off...because I was frightened it would get dirty and it was wet with the rain anyway...

So I left her and went to the next close, two or three doors up. The same kind of house and to be met with the granny of the new baby and the great-granny... all smiling. They said, 'Oh how nice ...' and she says, 'I hope you don't mind but...we just left the baby for you [because] we thought that perhaps you would like to dress the baby for its first outing...to the church.' They were Catholic people. I said, 'That would be nice to do that.' They took my wet clothes from me...into the other room and I was in the front room [with] the new baby and the mother. After I examined [them both] and dressed the baby [in its special clothes] they brought in tea and they had dried my skirts to the best of their ability... They gave me an old umbrella for the worst of the rain... So...the two contrasts in the same style of house...on the one Sunday morning in Glasgow. [One with]...not even the money to put in the gas and [the other], the warmth and happiness and pleasure and everything so nice.[71]

Agnes Morrison also told of contrasts in mid-1940s Leith Walk:

I remember going into one tenement and strangely enough I had delivered two babies within about forty-eight hours of [each other] in the same tenement... [In this family] I think it was about her eighth baby which was being born...and the father had taken time off to be there at home and you know they hadn't all that much and the baby was welcomed; it was just lovely... Two rooms maybe and a kitchen and the little girls in the house were helping. It was just such a happy family... One stair up from there, a first baby being born. It was an immediate atmosphere as soon as you went in, everything immaculate... The baby was eventually born. I asked where the husband was and there wasn't much [letting on]. He came in pretty fou and he had the most terrible scars... His wife had just taken her two hands down his cheeks before he'd gone out. Those awful scratches. Whereas ...those others were so happy [but] hadn't much.[72]

Anne Bayne also encountered extreme poverty in Glasgow in the 1950s. She described a very poor one-roomed home.

We had to do case studies for our Blue Book and [this was one]. I think this woman was para ten [eleventh pregnancy]. She had this one room. She was thrilled because they had actually the sink – the jaw-box in the window. There was a fireplace with a mantlepiece and it was a little open fire, a range, where she did all her cooking. That night the older boy and the father went through into the next room. There was a box bed [with] a sheet over [it] and... five children of varying ages in behind that sheet and... five little peep-holes in the sheet... She had her bed and at the end there was a heap of coal and...a cot and...two in the cot... and Moses basket...at the other side...there was another bath there [with] the last baby...in it and now we were delivering the new one. There wasn't room for the doctor and the midwife and myself to stand on that floor. We took it in turns to sit on the bed. There was a wee paraffin lamp which was all the light we had and we took turns to hold that depending on who was doing what. We had a plate, a soup plate and we had a Higginson's syringe and so we gave the enema out of this plate; she

returned it into the plate. I handed it out of the door and I don't know where
it went, and the plate came back. I took the placenta into that plate and I
bathed the baby in that plate. We would have been finished and away about
four o'clock in the morning and the Green Lady said, 'Now everything is
done. I'll go and phone for your taxi.' By the time the taxi came and I went
down, the mother had told me about how the midwife had been murdered on
the stairs.[73]

In the case of this mother, who would have benefited from postnatal care and support,
Anne Bayne said, 'They went again at ten o'clock to visit her and never got in. Nobody
ever got back to see her postnatally. She didn't open the door.'[74]

Some midwives chose to practise in homes which were materially better-off. Most
midwives spoke about the poverty they saw either during midwifery training, or
practice, yet there were some who practised as private midwives amongst better-off
mothers. These mothers could afford to pay a midwife to attend the birth of the baby,
with or without the GP, and live in the house for some time postnatally. One of these was
Ann Lamb who trained as a midwife in a small training school in Edinburgh in 1927 as
a route to nursing. She joined a nursing association based at the Armstrong Nursing
Home in Aberdeen, enabling her to practise privately both as a nurse and midwife in
many parts of Scotland.

I went from place to place to deliver [babies]. But I delivered them in
hospital too, in Edinburgh, and Aberdeen in the Armstrong Nursing Home,
now St. John's. I have been in Grantown-on-Spey at the hospital...away
down at Montrose, at Carnoustie, in Kirkcaldy. I don't think there is a town
I haven't been in, but not the west coast, Oban and there.[75]

Ann Lamb usually stayed about a month postnatally with mothers. However, she did not
call herself a 'monthly nurse'. This old term, dating from at least the 1500s, applied to
a woman (not a midwife) 'who in a substantial family would be engaged to perform the
more menial tasks during the birth, and to nurse the mother and infant for the following
month.'[76] Later, in the eighteenth century, medical practitioners encouraged monthly
nurses as allies in an effort to consolidate their practice against midwives.[77]

However, Molly Muir, a pupil midwife in the 'old Simpson' in 1934 and private
midwife in the 1930s, used the term 'monthly nurse' to describe what she did.[78] She
described her routine:

When I finished [midwifery training] I went to private nursing. In these days,
if you were a sister in a hospital or anywhere, the salary was eighty pounds
a year whether you had been there two years or twenty years. In private
nursing, if it was a baby case it was four guineas a week. Of course, if you
weren't working you weren't paid. But I did a whole year of baby cases with
no day off because the cases ran into each other. I was acting as a monthly
nurse and you would probably go to the case a week before labour started.
That put you all wrong for your next case. It was very hard work but I loved
it. I loved looking after those babies. I did the postnatal care of the mothers
as well. I used to go to places like Saline and down to North Berwick and

Berwick-on-Tweed – wherever they wanted a midwife. We had our headquarters in Rutland Street. Miss Drummond was our matron and there were about eighty trained nurses and midwives on the staff and they went out to different cases.[79]

Katie Strang also worked privately after two years' midwifery training at Rottenrow (1950-1952). She was one of the few midwives by this time who was not a RGN. To begin with, she obtained private work through her local GP:

So he thought I should do private maternity and he got me my first patient. And he said, 'It's quite an easy one because she's a marvellous mother, she breastfeeds and...it's her fourth baby...' He said, 'She knows far more about it than you will...' So all was well and he came and delivered the baby and everything was fine... That was my first and from then on it became a snowball thing... I never advertised, ever. She [the mother] passed the word on to somebody who was having a baby and so it went on.[80]

To begin with, mothers booked Katie Strang for the birth and postnatal care. However, with the change in place of birth, that began to change too:

[I was booked for the birth] and...when I started off [in 1952] it was usually for four weeks, depending what the mother wanted or how many other children she had. It gradually got less and less [homebirths], and by 1966 they stopped having them at home.[81]

She also said that even when she was employed for the postnatal period only, she did not do much postnatal care. Here she raised a point about visits by other professionals which indicated that even though she, a midwife, was there, the district midwife still visited postnatally:

I was really employed for the baby. [I didn't give] very much [postnatal care] because you see they had this nurse [midwife] coming in and then the health visitor... I used to try and get them to do their exercises... A lot of them weren't keen. I didn't do a great deal really. I had to help them, of course, with breastfeeding and engorged breasts...[82]

Within their own small worlds, private midwives wielded a certain power, protecting the mother from the outside. Katie Strang said:

I always insisted on the mother having a sleep in the afternoon after the two o'clock feed. If anybody came to the door between three o'clock and four, I would say, 'Well I'm terribly sorry but she is sleeping.' Some of them were quite annoyed. I was considered quite a bit of a dragon I think.[83]

One man, in his seventies, agreed with this last point. He remembered Ann Lamb in the house looking after his mother and baby brother when he was boy of seven and said, 'I couldn't stand her. She wouldn't let me in to see Mum.'[84]

Midwives therefore worked with a wide range of people from all backgrounds. Some chose to work privately, which shielded themselves from extremes of poverty that they had probably met during their training. Some, like David Rorie's 'The howdie', went everywhere:

> A' gate she'd traivelled day an nicht,
> A' kin o orra weather
> Had seen her trampin on the road,
> Or trailin through the heather.[85]

Gelda Pryde put it in a nutshell when she said, 'You know, you were talking about bare floorboards one minute – and then two-inch thick pile carpets two hours later.'[86]

Conclusion

The work of midwives postnatally up until the 1980s was regulated by the CMBS and supervised by the LSAs on the Board's behalf. Midwives were required to keep within CMBS *Rules* and other rules imposed by medical opinion, for example, on how long a postnatal mother should stay in bed. This rule changed informally at home over the years as midwives found that they had to be realistic about the conditions in which some mothers were living. Rising numbers of hospital births meant that hospital policies reduced midwives' ability to give individual care to postnatal mothers, and increased medical control of postnatal care even although this came within the midwife's area of responsibility.[87]

Although the basic *Rules* for postnatal examination of the mother and baby remained the same, the pattern, organisation and span of time for midwife attendance changed. The move from fourteen to ten days in 1965 relieved some pressure on over-worked domiciliary midwives alongside the trend in the 1960s towards early discharge and increasing postnatal home visits. The emergence of early discharge home schemes partly aided the hitherto threatened role of community midwives. However, they were restricted mainly to postnatal care and were not fulfilling their full role as midwives. In addition, care for the mother became even more fragmented. In the early decades of the twentieth century, with mostly homebirths, continuity of care was taken for granted. Growing hospitalisation and the tripartite administration of the NHS combined to break up care of women during the child-bearing episode. Early discharge home added another facet of fragmentation: mothers delivered in hospital, by a midwife they did not know, spent one to three days in a postnatal ward looked after by numerous midwives, and then they went home to be visited by more unknown midwives. At the same time, there were not enough community midwives to give adequate care at home. Later in the twentieth century, an attempt was made in Scotland to address some of the issues of fragmentation of care and dissatisfied midwives through initiatives such as the DOMINO scheme and integration of maternity services.

The CMBS undermined midwives' autonomy in 1965 when it allowed nurses and health visitors to care for mothers and babies within the postnatal period. This removed midwives' special place in the field of postnatal care at a stroke. The midwife's status only began to be regained with the gradual implementation of the integration of maternity services in Scotland in the 1970s and 1980s.

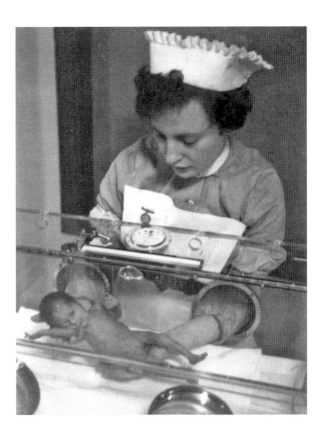

Margaret Nicol (now Ritchie), midwife, attending to baby in incubator, Dunfermline Maternity Hospital 1959. (Courtesy of Margaret Ritchie.)

1.   NAS/CMB 4/2/9, *CMBS Rules*, 26 August 1916, p 9, para 12.
2.   CMBS *Rules*, 31 March 1918, p 20.
3.   M McGuire, *Community Postnatal Care Provision in Scotland: the development and evaluation of a template for the provision of woman-centred community postnatal care*, unpublished PhD thesis, (University of Glasgow: 2001) p 23: The postnatal period differs from the longer puerperium which is defined 'as the period from birth until six weeks after the baby is born....[when] the reproductive organs return to their pregravid state, lactation is established and the woman recovers from pregnancy and childbirth;' the CMBS did not require midwives to visit the mother and baby for the full puerperium.
4.   NAS, CMB, 4/1-5, *CMBS Rules*, 26 August 1916, p 9.
5.   T Murphy-Black, 'Care in the community during the postnatal period', in S Robinson, A Thomson (eds) *Midwives, Research and Childbirth*, Vol 3, (London and Glasgow: Chapman and Hall, 1994), p 121.
6.   NAS, CMB, 1/5, *CMBS Minutes*, 18 March 1937, Vol 22, p 8; 1937 Maternity Services (Scotland) Act, [1 Edw 8 & 1 Geo 6 Ch 30], 1 (1).
7.   *CMBS Rules, 1980, p 10.*
8.   *CMBE&W Handbook and Rules*, (London: William Clowes, 1962), p 40; Murphy-Black, 'Care in the community during the postnatal period', p 121.

9.   LR 117.

10.   Murphy Black, *'Care in the community in the postnatal period'*, p 123.

11.   NAS, CMB 1/8, *CMBS Minutes*, 16 September 1965, p 2.

12.   NAS, CMB 1/8, *CMBS Minutes*, 19 April 1973 p 3.

13.   NAS, CMB 1/8, *CMBS Minutes*, 20 September 1973 p 3.

14.   SHHD, *Maternity Services: integration of maternity work, (Tennent Report)*, (Edinburgh: HMSO, 1973), p 14; NBS, *CMBS Report*, 31 March 1974, p 4.

15.   NAS, CMB 1/8, *CMBS Minutes*, 20 February 1975, Appendix 1, p 1.

16.   Murphy-Black, *'Care in the community in the postnatal period'*, p 124.

17.   NBS, *CMBS Rules*, 31 March 1918, p 23.

18.   Murphy-Black, *'Care in the community in the postnatal period'*, p 120.

19.   NAS, CMB 1/5, *CMBS Minutes*, 26 July 1934, Vol 19, p 24; *CMBS Rules*, 31 March 1939, p 13.

20.   J Raphael-Leff, *Psychological Processes of Childbearing*, (London: Chapman and Hall, 1991), p ix, but see the whole book for insight into maternal and family psychology related to childbearing, and chapter 33 for postnatal psychological complications, pp 477-497; J Watson, *A Complete Handbook of Midwifery for Midwives and Nurses*, (The Scientific Press Limited: London), 1914, pp 319-320. Here, 1 1/2 pages are given to puerperal insanity, mania and melancholia.

21.   V R Bennett, L K Brown, *Myles Textbook for Midwives, (11th ed)*, (Edinburgh: Churchill Livingstone, 1989).

22.   LR 27.

23.   LR 117.

24.   *Ibid*.

25.   *Ibid*.

26.   LR 119.

27.   LR 47; L Reid, 'Midwifery in Scotland 4'.

28.   *Ibid*; LR 101.

29.   LR 110; 'Midwifery in Scotland 4'.

30.   *Ibid; Written testimony*, LR 3.

31.   LR 9; 'Midwifery in Scotland 4'; L Reid, 'Where's your comfort zone?' *The Practising Midwife*, (2010), Vol 13 (3), p 42.

32.   LR 91. 'Slunge' – to souse with water.

33.   LR 9.

34.   LR 27; see chapter 3, endnote 76 for quote, LR 27.

35.   *CMBS Rules*, 1968, p 13; *CMBS Rules Approval Instrument 1980*, did not specify the raised temperature rule as hitherto. However it is implicit in rule 58, p 9.

36.   J Towler, J Bramall, *Midwives in History and Society*, (London: Croom Helm, 1986), p 77.

37.   Watson, *A Complete Handbook of Midwifery for Midwives and Nurses*, p 289.

38.   M Tew, *Safer Childbirth? A critical history of maternity care, (2nd ed)*, London and Glasgow: Chapman and Hall, 1995), p 147; the CMBS *Rules* said nothing about length of stay in bed.

39.   LR 56; Reid, 'Midwifery in Scotland 4'.

40. Z Barnett, 'Yesterday, today and tomorrow in postnatal care', in *Midwives Chronicle*, November 1984, p 360.
41. LR 46; Reid, 'Midwifery in Scotland 4'.
42. *Ibid*; LR 93.
43. LR101; Reid, 'Midwifery in Scotland 4'.
44. *Ibid*; LR 70.
45. LR 50; Reid, 'Midwifery in Scotland 4'.
46. *Ibid*; LR 27.
47. LR 110; Reid L, 'Uncertified midwives in Scotland: the howdies', *The Practising Midwife,* (2009), Vol 12 (5), pp 40-43; Reid, 'Midwifery in Scotland 4'.
48. LR 99.
49. LR 116; Reid, 'Midwifery in Scotland 4'.
50. M Myles, *A Textbook for Midwives, (1st, 2nd, 3rd, 4th eds),* (Edinburgh: E &S Livingstone Ltd., 1955 (reprint), 1956, 1958, 1962), pp 453, 449, 449, 474.
51. *Ibid.*
52. M Myles, *A Textbook for Midwives, (6th ed)*, (Edinburgh: E &S Livingstone Ltd., 1968), p 457.
53. M Myles, *A Textbook for Midwives, (7th ed)*, (Edinburgh: Churchill Livingstone, 1971), p 460.
54. M Myles, *A Textbook for Midwives, (8th ed)*, (Edinburgh: Churchill Livingstone, 1975), p 407.
55. Murphy-Black, *Care in the community in the postnatal period*, p 124.
56. *Ibid*, p 123; Myles, *Textbook for Midwives, (6th ed)*, p 460, *(7th ed)*, p 463; see also Reid, 'Midwifery in Scotland 4'.
57. *Montgomery Report*, p 17.
58. *Tennent Report*, p 14.
59. LR 93.
60. LR 117.
61. LR 69; Reid, 'Midwifery in Scotland 4'.
62. LR 69.
63. Myles, *Textbook for Midwives, (6th ed)*, p 460.
64. Myles *Textbook for Midwives, (8th ed), p 410.*
65. *Montgomery Report*, p 40.
66. LR 112.
67. LR 9.
68. LR 69.
69. LR 11.
70. LR 20. 'Ticking' is a strong cotton fabric, (sometimes striped) which was used sometimes as a mattress cover and sometimes as a layer of material between the mattress and the bed-springs.
71. *Ibid.*
72. LR 35.
73. LR 91.
74. *Ibid.*

75. LR 47.
76. J Donnison, *Midwives and Medical Men*, (New Barnet: Historical Publications, 1988), p 23.
77. *Ibid*, p 40.
78. The situation was confused because it depended on how and with whom a midwife was working: [1] Certified midwives could work by themselves as midwives; [2] Certified midwives could attend a woman in labour under a doctor's supervision when she could be called a maternity/monthly nurse; [3] A RGN could attend a woman in labour under a doctor's supervision but not deliver the baby. Under those circumstances she also could be called a maternity nurse but she was not allowed to act as a midwife. When midwifery training divided into 2 Parts in 1938, after passing Part 1 a woman could practise as a maternity nurse under the supervision of a medical practitioner but not as a midwife unless she had passed Part 2; see Reid, *Scottish Midwives 1916-1983*, p 112-116. 'Monthly nurses' in the twentieth century were usually employed privately and usually worked with a GP.
79. LR 46.
80. LR 89.
81. *Ibid*.
82. *Ibid*.
83. *Ibid*.
84. Personal communication, LR 127.
85. D Rorie, 'The howdie', in D Rorie, *The Lum Hat Wantin the Croon*, (Edinburgh: W & R Chambers, 1935), p 64; David Rorie was a GP in the north-east of Scotland.
86. LR 69.
87. Murphy-Black, 'Care in the community in the postnatal period', p 124.

Chapter 9

On the cusp: midwives and the century

The later years of the twentieth century and the first decade of the twenty-first saw wide changes in maternity care in the UK as a whole and in Scotland in particular. This chapter explores aspects of these changes.

Statutory change came, first with the end of the CMBS in 1983, the beginning of the United Kingdom Central Council (UKCC) with a statutory Midwifery Committee, and its four National Boards, each also with a statutory Midwifery Committee. In 2002, the UKCC was replaced by the Nursing and Midwifery Council (NMC) whose powers are set out within the Nursing and Midwifery Order.[1]

Within its wider aims, the NMC's core function is to establish and improve standards of midwifery and nursing care in order to serve and protect the public.[2]

As previous chapters show, the care of childbearing women in Scotland became increasingly medicalised as the twentieth century progressed. The trend for integration of maternity services marked the beginning of a positive response to consumer criticisms of the 1970s, which challenged the increasing medicalisation of birth and the apparent decreasing level of choice for women.[3]

A breakdown of deference, which began as early as the 1960s, gradually infiltrated into maternity care in general and midwifery in particular. This led to a change in attitude that became particularly visible from the late 1980s.

The move for change

By the 1980s, there was a groundswell of feeling that all was not well in the maternity services and change across the UK was required. In 1986 the new Association of Radical Midwives (ARM) produced *The Vision*,[4] a far-seeing document that recognised these concerns and made proposals for the future of the maternity services. A major player from the consumer point of view was the Association for Improvements in the Maternity Services (AIMS). AIMS was formed in 1960 to improve the quality and provision of maternity services in the UK. AIMS initially fought for *more* hospital maternity beds, the opposite of the objective of their subsequent main campaign in the 1980s.[5]

In 1987 and 1991 there were two significant RCM Reports.[6] Each of these documents, in its own way, indicated a need for change, for more informed choice for women, and for more continuity in the way care is carried out.

The trend continued. In 1991, the Government made a commitment in its *Patient's Charter* that the NHS in Scotland should deliver services responsive to the needs of the user. This document was followed in the same year by *Framework for action* which demonstrated how to put *The Patients' Charter* into effect.[7]

In April 1992, representatives of the Clinical Resource and Audit Group (CRAG) and the Scottish Health Management Efficiency Group (SCOTMEG) came together to form a Framework for Action Working Group on Maternity Services in Scotland. The *Framework for action* identified maternity services as one of the priority groups, with wide variations in clinical care and the provision of services, where watchdog bodies had voiced major concerns, or where the role of the NHS was likely to change significantly.[8]

The CRAG/SCOTMEG group responded by looking at the provision of Scotland's maternity services and how the system could be improved. It involved representatives of both providers and recipients in a wide consultation.[9]

To help with the consultations and dissemination of information, the Working Group held five successful Roadshows across Scotland. This exchange of views and ideas from all sources would stimulate further action at local level. On a national level, Good Practice Days were run in Scotland in 1993 and 1994, demonstrating different aspects of innovative practice and examples of woman-centred care already underway. These days were well attended by midwives, health visitors, GPs and consumer group representatives from across Scotland. At the first one, in October 1993, fifteen examples of Good Practice were presented out of a total of seventy submitted. A key-factor was the need for overall improvement. Positive trends included the use of Parent-Held records; improved Antenatal Contact Communication; the establishment of better midwife-client relationships through increasing home visits, reducing waiting times and anxiety, and introducing team midwifery; and a system of care for women with special problems acknowledging the inappropriateness of the prevailing services to the needs of many women,.[10]

A further Good Practice Day continued the positive trend and confirmation that both professionals and consumers were in the mood for change.[11]

Within the CRAG-SCOTMEG group were sub-groups with varying remits. The consumer sub-group, which asked 'What do women want?', considered the views of consumers about the services at all stages of pregnancy.[12]

This qualitative survey of women from across Scotland revealed a fundamental point: women, all different in their needs, did not all want the same kind of care. Some wanted more control while some wanted more 'management'. There was a clear demand for choice and women repeatedly stated that they wanted to be listened to. They wanted to be acknowledged as individuals with specific and different needs. More specifically, many asked for debriefing and feedback post-birth – something which they felt was not happening sufficiently.[13]

The survey, *What users think*, echoed these findings and demonstrated service shortfalls in information provision, involvement, and individual treatment while poor links between healthcare professionals were identified.[14]

The *Winterton Report*

The UK-wide call for change in maternity services included women, midwives, members of the public *and* politicians. While the CRAG/SCOTMEG Group made progress in Scotland, in 1992 the House of Commons saw the launch of the '*Winterton Report*'.[15]

While the Report did not officially cover maternity services in Scotland, its ramifications were felt across the UK. For the first time, an independent parliamentary committee focussed on what women wanted from maternity services. Significantly, and unusually for a government report, the first third of the *Winterton Report* was devoted to the views of women.[16] Weeping campaigners commented: 'After thirty years of knocking on closed doors...'[17] This Report was the culmination of the Committee's investigation of antenatal, intrapartum, postnatal and neonatal care.

The Report did not represent a victory for midwives, nor was it defeat for any other profession.[18] Of any group, women were the winners. Nevertheless, the Report opened many hitherto closed doors for midwives. For instance, it considered midwives to be the group best placed to provide continuity of care as well as continuity of carers; it made recommendations to improve opportunities for midwives to accommodate women's requests; it suggested the development of midwifery-managed units, midwives' caseloads, and midwives taking full responsibility for care. It spoke out for the right of midwives to admit women to hospital where necessary, without recourse to a doctor; and, the right of midwives to develop and audit their professional standards. It upheld the idea that midwives should have statutory control over their own education. In short, it presented the image of a system for midwives where they could offer continuity of care to a 'defined caseload' in a philosophically acceptable environment within their management.[19]

The report contained over one hundred recommendations, and appeared not only to be pro-mother and baby, but also pro-midwife. Its main conclusion was that maternity services should be geared round the woman and her baby with the mother-infant unit central to care. The maternity services and the care given by the maternity health professionals should become '*woman-centred*'. This sound-bite is still in use even though systems and fashions in maternity care are constantly evolving.

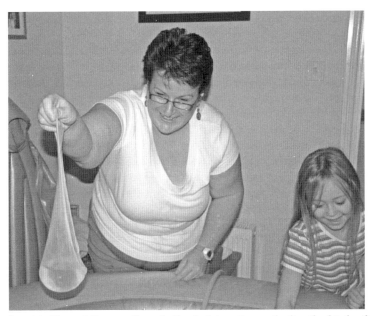

Carrie McIntosh, midwife and Jemma Campbell admiring the caul after the birth of Jemma's sister, Hope. (Courtesy of Carrie McIntosh, midwife, and Alison Campbell, mother.)

Woman-centred care
Woman-centred care could be described as the philosophy at the basis of the care given
to women in the UK at the beginning of the twenty-first century. It recognises that to
achieve the optimum level, the commitment of all concerned is needed. But there was
some confusion and controversy over the meaning when the term first appeared. It is
possible that midwifery hackles were raised as midwives read into the term 'woman-
centred care' an implication that women might not have been the previous focus of care.
Many midwives' fears were voiced.[20]

Even to use the word 'philosophy' presents a dichotomy. On the one hand,
'philosophy' can mean a school of thought, or any system of belief, values or tenets.[21]
This gives a sense of width or multiplicity. 'Philosophy', however, can also mean a
personal outlook or viewpoint, emphasising individuality, but, in so doing, highlighting
the opposite pole. With such wide interpretation of the word 'philosophy' no wonder
there were problems with the meaning of 'woman-centred care'.[22]

Woman-centred care also has two poles, the one placed at the individual care given
by a midwife, and the other, situated at the systems of care offered by maternity services
across the UK and which have many variations. In an effort to help, the RCM stated: 'In
midwifery, woman-centred care has always existed in one form or another, usually
reflecting the personal philosophy of individual midwives.'[23] Midwifery is a woman-
centred caring profession. If a midwife looking after a woman in labour said she were
not giving woman-centred care, even before the sound-bite came into vogue, something
must be wrong. If a midwife said she *were* giving woman-centred care, then her
statement would be accepted, even though she had perhaps never set eyes on the
labouring woman until that day. So, there was some confusion over the meaning of
woman-centred care.

Clarification came from four statements representing the philosophy of woman-
centred care which contrasted with the perceived 'traditional' models of maternity care:
*   Pregnancy, birth and the puerperium are normal life events.
*   Autonomy, self-care and independence are viewed as the right of women.
*   Parents have a right to all information to make informed choices.
*   Social, psychological, physical and spiritual needs of parents should be met
    at all times.[24]

Not every maternity care professional was happy with the *Winterton Report*'s new ideas.
Some obstetricians were 'frankly horrified' at the thought of an increase in non-hospital
births. Some GPs were not happy with the idea that they might be by-passed as
midwives took on the role of referring women where necessary.[25] Grace commented:

> [Looking back], there was a feeling from our [medical] colleagues, 'Don't
> interfere with what they're doing, let the midwives play for a while and then
> they'll come and get us when...it all changes. If we need to sort something
> out we can come in and do it.' I do think [progress has been made from
> that]... There is much closer working together, much closer understanding of
> the priorities which exist in different professional groups... a [greater]
> willingness to be respectful of that.[26]

However, at the time, the *Winterton Report* demonstrated a new concept that created early-1990s waves of intermingled delight, hope, fear, anxiety, thinking, discussion, some progress – and a new feeling of optimism amongst midwives and women.

Tangible progress came in the shape of policy review documents, and with them, another sound-bite: 'changing childbirth'.[27] In Scotland, with approximately one tenth of the population of England, and one-sided media attention, the term 'changing childbirth' became as commonly-used as though this enviably alliterative phrase came from the Scottish *Policy Review*. Although it did not, 'changing childbirth' along with 'woman-centred care' became buzz-words that are still in use. Each country of the UK produced its own policy review document. Each document promoted the same principles and aimed to work towards the same goal: a change for the better in childbirth with woman-centred care at the heart.[28]

Woman-centred care places the emphasis on a woman's own beliefs about her pregnancy, birth and puerperium, her rights, informed choice, maternal autonomy and holistic care. It focuses on women's choices for themselves and their families. This contrasts with the idea of paternalistic, controlling care of women who were expected to do what they were told.[29] It is associated with the concepts of continuity of care and/or carer, where a midwife is able to meet and work with the woman and discover for her and with her the right birth process, whichever form that may take.

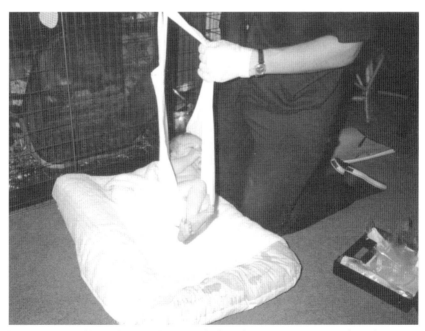

Weighing Lorna Wallace, born at home, Edinburgh 1994. (Courtesy of Linda Bryce, midwife, Mary Wallace, mother, and Lorna Wallace.)

'Continuity' implies fewer midwives involved with any one woman. The aim was for care to be consistent, usually given by midwives well known to the woman, and linked to schemes, for instance team-midwifery, caseload holding and one-to-one midwifery practice.[30] With one or very few midwives involved in a woman's care, supportive woman-midwife relationships could be established, care could be planned in partnership and a standard be set that was appropriate to that woman.[31]

Systems of implementing woman-centred care varied according to geography and demography. The RCM acknowledged: 'Clearly, there is around the country, a huge amount of experimentation with organisational change, and midwives are all at different stages in their thinking and experience of how these can best work. Fashions seem to move quickly in midwifery.'[32] Woman-centred care has the individual woman as the hub and is pertinent to the demographic and geographic requirements of a district, town, country, or people. An important factor is the ability or otherwise of the maternity services and its professionals to provide care following the ideals of the woman-centred philosophy. With the phrase 'choice, continuity and control' becoming very popular in the 1990s, there was a possibility of problems occurring in some NHS maternity services. Sometimes consumer expectations did not always match health boards' abilities to supply what women wanted. Also, some women used to one service might not want to accept a change to midwife-led care. Charlie commented:

> Some mothers want to see their GP early in pregnancy and throughout pregnancy and I think if we have a woman-centred service then that has to be catered for. Many women who have had midwifery-led care... acknowledge that they get a lot more information and support and education through the midwifery-led care that they perhaps wouldn't be afforded through GP-predominant care, but society, I think, still sees a GP as a superior being and therefore they look towards the GP for perceived greater care, and that seeing a midwife doesn't necessarily equate with that until they experience something different.[33]

Midwives and woman-centred care
When the government-led reports and recommendations of the 1990s were issued, many midwives saw this as a chance, not only for women to obtain the kind of maternity care they wanted, but for midwives to regain their lost autonomy. Yet, it did not take long for midwives to feel over-worked, under-paid and insecure, so much so that in 1995 they voted to rescind the RCM's policy of never taking industrial action.[34]

Yet, in the early days, the statement, 'This is the age of the midwife and our time has come,' was greeted to great acclaim.[35] But the concept of woman-centred care presented a challenge to the profession of midwifery and possible difficulties which midwives could encounter. Midwives cited negative feelings as well as positive, particularly when attending homebirths. Any pessimistic feelings about woman-centred care were exacerbated by what some midwives saw as lack of skill in, for example, suturing, resuscitation of the newborn, and siting of intravenous infusions along with inadequacy of midwives' support networks, and unhelpful attitudes by doctors.[36]

However, there were areas where the changes enhanced job satisfaction. An examination of the attitudes of midwives in Glasgow working in the Midwifery Development Unit (MDU) revealed that most MDU midwives felt more positive towards their professional role; there were further positive changes in professional satisfaction, support and development and client interaction; MDU midwives were more certain of their role than hitherto; stress levels amongst MDU midwives were not unduly raised.[37] In England there were also positive reactions, midwives' comments including statements such as: '[My role is] more satisfying as a midwife...[permitting] thinking more freely'; 'working in small groups has meant that we are very supportive towards each other'; and, from a manager, 'I am sure that job satisfaction has increased and areas such as quality of care improved.'[38]

Research, examining midwife satisfaction and continuity of care conducted in a midwife-managed unit in Aberdeen, cited autonomy as the most important predictor of job-satisfaction. Also significant was the length of time a midwife spent with a client along with rapport and trust-building.[39] However, this report was based on findings made in the delivery suite of this Aberdeen unit. Not all midwives could give the commitment required to achieve a possible ideal level of autonomy and continuity of care. The report called for possible modification of new systems of maternity care to give as much job-satisfaction as possible to midwives, while bearing in mind existing differences in hours of work and yet still aspiring to the ideal of woman-centred care. Also, it suggested the need for more research to evaluate the effect of the new systems of care on midwives.

There could be advantages for midwives. They included retention and full use of midwives' skills, increased professional development and accountability, improved recruitment and retention of midwives, and more efficient use of staff leading to a reduction in duplication of work with, hopefully, greater job-satisfaction and increased team-spirit.[40] However, within the practice of woman-centred care, the benefit of the chance for midwives to practise across the child-bearing spectrum could be seen as a problem. Some midwives lacked confidence in their ability to practise in all areas and were therefore unhappy about this opportunity. Some midwives, secure in a niche, lacked confidence or the will to go elsewhere. So, to achieve woman-centred care, it was questioned whether it was really necessary for midwives to be equally competent in all areas of maternity care and if it was desirable or important so long as midwives fulfilled the criteria for woman-centred care.[41] Charlie commented:

> I definitely think that there are midwives who thrive on the challenges of caring for women in a woman-centred, low-risk, midwife-led care unit. There are equally midwives who thrive on the high dependency [unit] dealing with more medically- orientated conditions and working closely with other professionals and using a different repertoire of skills and care to bring about the safe delivery. I think they are different skills...they appeal to different people and they are both midwives.[42]

Regarding woman-centred care and high-dependency needs, while pointing out the woman's right to disagree with professional opinion, Katy said:

> We're working together ensuring the women get the correct care suitable for their needs and whatever they require, so if they have complications [beyond the normal] then a consultant unit is absolutely the place where that woman should be for her labour and birth. There's no disputing these things – unless the woman does. And when she arrives she should get the care that's helpful to her to have the best experience that she could have.[43]

Another possible problem was one of over-protectiveness by some midwives towards mothers. Walsh asked if caseload holding could be attracting midwives who, however subconsciously, enjoyed controlling clients.[44] This would encourage dependency, undermine the woman's autonomy and negate a major part of the principle of woman-centred care. Women's feelings of security were another issue. It was possible that women in the turn-around in maternity services might feel that they were having too much to decide with a consequent loss of security.[45] One woman noted that, when a midwife asked her at booking if she had any questions, she said 'No' because she did not know what questions to ask.[46]

There was a genuine fear that, in the push to give women what it was perceived that they wanted, midwives' 'wants' were being ignored or left behind. Midwives were concerned about Trusts within the NHS, litigation, their changing role, overwork, effects of the big changes in childbirth that were afoot, and working conditions.[47] A research study to try and pin-point how Scottish midwives saw themselves in relation to woman-centred care, their job-satisfaction and impressions of the changes taking place in the maternity services, reported in 1998.[48] The findings of the study had important implications for those concerned with providing and delivering maternity care. The majority of responding midwives were in favour of a change in focus in the maternity services and agreed that they gained job satisfaction from their work. However, there were concerns about the way changes were applied. There was pressure on Trusts to give more for less, concern about workload, skills, responsibilities, and working environment.[49] Similar concerns were voiced elsewhere.[50]

Almost fifty percent of respondents were part-time. This revealed another set of problems centring round feeling undervalued, demonstrated by comments describing a perceived lack of opportunity for professional development and an apparent managerial unwillingness to finance courses and study days:

> Working part-time has affected my chance of becoming a mentor. My manager is not willing to let part-timers attend such study days, which I feel is unfair both professionally and personally.[51]

There was also a feeling of lack of support from their full-time peers. For instance:

> I have much to offer in terms of knowledge and experience, but find that on the whole midwives with families are considered a nuisance.[52]

The study called for consultation of all involved, including consumers, before implementation of new schemes to acknowledge midwives' ownership of their working patterns and provision of care, facilitation of inter-professional working and changes in management-structures of Trusts (still in use in Scotland at the time) so that midwifery matters were handled by midwives rather than by other professionals. Other issues included continuing professional development and education. These aspects of midwifery were falling short and required a co-ordinated approach to improve matters.[53]

Change was in the air throughout the 1990s. Yet, by the end of the decade there was concern that woman-centred care, in spite of media attention and reports, seemed to have made little advance. There were reports of midwife burnout and of schemes of care that had failed, or stopped after their pilot. Midwives were disillusioned, aware of failings in the system yet feeling frustrated and impotent in their efforts to affect change.[54]

Nevertheless, by 1998 further research acknowledged the work that was ongoing to improve maternity services in Scotland. For instance, new evidence suggested that women with normal pregnancies need not have consultant involvement antenatally, as previously recommended.[55] The Scottish Programme for Clinical Effectiveness in Reproductive Health (SPCERH) acknowledged that much work had been done towards improving communication with women, towards enhancing the role of the midwife, towards providing homely settings for births in hospital and fostering continuity of care. However, more was required in terms of collaboration between different professionals sharing care. One aspect was the old question of duplication of care. SPCERH recommended that GPs and midwives should work together to avoid this and develop protocols including clarification of their roles and responsibilities. Women with normal pregnancies would benefit from the choice of community-based antenatal care provided by midwife and/or GP. To address this acknowledgement of the changing needs of late twentieth century maternity services, SPCERH recommended the development of a National Service Framework for the Scottish Maternity Service to be delivered by a managed clinical network cutting across professional, Trust and Health Board boundaries.[56]

Changes in midwifery education

As well as changes towards a more woman-centred and more multi-professional approach to maternity care, midwives began to search for, and universities began to supply, suitable degree courses to develop their education. This became apparent in the 1980s, but escalated in the 1990s and 2000s. Some midwives resisted, but eventually even reluctant scholars were persuaded. Katy recalled:

> Our team leader in 2001 strongly believed in educating midwives so she... pushed for midwives here to do their degrees. It was like educating Rita. All these midwives who had been midwives for a long, long time, including myself, who all said, 'A degree is not going to make me any better. What's a degree going to do? How's that bit of paper going to make me a better midwife?' She really pushed it. The vast majority, a huge number, were enrolled in modules. And, absolutely, it does make you a better midwife. I take back those words where I said, 'I'm as good a midwife as I'm going to be. I don't need this, I don't need that.' It makes you think, it makes you... It re-invigorates you. It motivates. You can never ever learn too much.[57]

The 1990s, in line with the EEC Directives, also heralded new courses for the education of midwives.[58] In response to the EEC Midwifery Directives, the first cohort of 129 single-registered midwives in Scotland qualified in 1995. Since then midwifery curricula in Scottish universities have adapted practice and maternity care philosophy to the current situation when all student midwives in Scotland study a degree course with an Honours option.[59]

When the first batch of 'new' midwives qualified in Scotland in 1995, they were following in the footsteps of their English counterparts who qualified in 1992. A study of these English midwives revealed that they were treated with some suspicion by their previously and differently qualified fellow midwives. In addition, research identified some gaps in their midwifery education.[60]

In Scotland post-1995, anecdotal evidence suggested similar problems. A research study examined newly-qualified single registered midwives' perceptions and experiences of midwifery education and subsequent midwifery practice. Through postal questionnaires, the researchers explored midwives' demography and employment characteristics, their ability to integrate into the midwifery profession, their levels of confidence, their experiences of mentorship and support, their perceptions of education and fitness to practise, and their perceived educational needs.[61]

The study, with a sixty-one percent response rate, revealed some negative aspects which concurred with the English study. There was suspicion and an early lack of support from other midwives although this eased over time. Sore points included difficulty for the 'new' midwives in obtaining a post in Scotland and the poor level of pay. In addition, the first cohort of 'new' midwives in England were paid on a higher grade than the 'new' Scottish midwives.
Written comments included:

> I think it is ridiculous that pre-registration [new] midwives are being offered D-grades for one year – when in England they are promoting a minimum F grade. Because of prejudice in Scotland, we are made to feel second best. It would have been nice to receive support from the Scottish Health Boards when we qualified. Suddenly all adverts stated that positions required 'RGN & RM'...or minimum of 2 years' experience – thereby eliminating direct entry students.[62]

Some midwives said that they lacked confidence in their midwifery ability. This was not helped by other professionals' apparent lack of confidence in them. In addition, many were frustrated by the lack of transfer of evidence to practise. They were not alone: this important point gathered momentum across the UK and, over time, 'evidence-based practice' (EBP) became the watchword. Claire said of her recent personal experience:

> University was good. Our class got on, on the whole. The academic work was obviously hard going sometimes along with everything else that was happening, but I enjoyed it and felt I got a lot out of it and as I progressed through to third year I felt I could actually relate to what I was learning really well. And you wanted to go and read and look at the research through your practice.[63]

However she also commented:

> What happens in practice differs from what you are taught... Guidelines tell us to do spontaneous pushing. At [university] they told us to do spontaneous pushing [in second stage labour] and the vast majority of staff use directed pushing. Change coming in like *KCND* [see below] is all very well, but if the people who are practising won't put it forth, then how are things going to change? This applied even to fairly young, or newly qualified, midwives. My mentor, I think, saw it the same way as I do. There are other things as well,

active or passive third stage, but some people are very resistant to change and I don't understand it. Classroom teaches what the research shows, but it's very different in practice.[64]

The 1998 research also highlighted newly qualified midwives' lack of experience in caring for the 'ill' woman.[65] That is, in the case of midwifery, a woman going through a childbearing episode who has an underlying disease, either pre-pregnancy or contracted during pregnancy or labour. Midwives in the study expressed concerns about their limited knowledge in this field, their lack of practical skills and feelings of being unprepared to practise in some areas. Nevertheless they accepted that, given time and experience, skills that were lacking would develop. A year on from qualification, a substantial majority felt comfortable about their practical skills.

However, concerns remained regarding the care of women who are ill and comments within the research report are still relevant. They include care of pregnant women with underlying illness, and single-registered midwives' lack of a similar depth of knowledge in this field as midwives who are already nurses.[66] This remained an on-going issue in 2010 with more single than dual-registered midwives graduating. In Scotland, in 2010, there were anxieties about maternal ill-health, increasing levels of obesity, diabetes and heart disease which impact on pregnancy and its outcomes. Charlie said:

> We certainly are seeing an increase in pathology in the women, or just poor health in the women, that is compromising how the pregnancy, and certainly the labour, is needing to be managed... [There are] social disorders [in] Scotland across the country and not just in the cities – alcohol, drug misuse, obesity, poor exercise and just a general poor health of the pregnant women. [And] the recent immigrant population, where the health-history of these women is less well-known and has been different in its experience, and their expectations are slightly different. So that too is influencing the care that needs to be provided. So you've got the kind of social dis-ease if you want to call it that.[67]

In the same context of type of care, Charlie also spoke of mature women and pregnancy:

> You also have older women and you have women with pre-existing heart and liver conditions that wouldn't necessarily have had the opportunity of a pregnancy before and [they] now do. It needs a lot more medical management and surveillance, and consequently midwifery management and surveillance, to bring about their safe delivery... [There is a suggestion] that the skills that are required in high dependency care, obstetric-led care, are not gained in the current midwifery education and ...there's a need to have a subsequent training programme in fluid and electrolyte management, understanding of renal /liver function.
>
> ...If you're training to be a midwife and your initial work experience is to be in midwifery-led care then the training programme meets those needs. But if you [move]...into an obstetric-led situation, do you ...have the skills and experience [for that] or should we...acknowledge that we can't put it all

in the basic training and accept that you have to do additional training?[68]

The Scottish Multi-professional Maternity Development Programme (SMMDP) decided to incorporate these problems into a new course. The SMMDP was established in 2004 to address the acquisition of competencies and subsequent updating and retention of skills in maternity care.[69] This was a response to recommendations from the *Report of the Expert Group on Acute Maternity Services* (EGAMS) (see below) which highlighted five main areas where education for health professionals involved in maternity care required to be focussed. They were neonatal resuscitation, maternal emergencies, normality, examination of the newborn, history-taking and assessment.[70] Since then, more courses have been added to their suite. To address some of the problems that Charlie described, the SMMDP began planning and writing a new multi-professional critical care course, *Maternity REACTS*, to be piloted in 2010.

The 1998 research on newly qualified single-registered midwives highlighted attitudes of others to 'direct entry' midwives which were sometimes problematical. Some of the respondents in this study commented on the cynical attitudes displayed towards their midwifery qualification by some managers, midwives and other professionals. They clearly felt a need to champion single registration midwifery. However, comments written by respondents indicated that even as early as one year on from qualification, midwives, for instance, were beginning to review their thinking, direct-entry midwives were more accepted and, as they became more experienced, criticisms and prejudices tended to evaporate. This particular group retained a feeling of optimism which augured well for single-registered midwives in Scotland: of all respondents, only 2.6 % said that they did not want to practise as midwives.[71] Claire showed the developing positive attitude when she said:

> I was told by one sister that you're definitely treated differently in third year because in first year, we're just students, and the same in second year, and in third year we're potential colleagues.[72]

Katy agreed that attitudes regarding direct-entry midwives were improving:

> I think...that there is an acceptance now because a lot of the midwives now are direct entry. [There's not] so much [awareness of it] now as there was years ago... I don't think people consider it now, which is obviously a positive, and I don't think for a minute they ask at any point, were you direct-entry or have you done your nurse training before? ...I think, for the profession [of midwifery], direct-entry is a step forward... It is important that people recognise that we are midwives... Certainly, I think direct-entry is accepted now.[73]

Research in midwifery

Education and research are natural associates. However, up until the 1970s, research was not usually something that midwives 'did'. It is also likely that up until the 1970s the term *training* was frequently used instead of *education* when discussing the route to qualification as a midwife. Research was not contemplated seriously for most midwives whose practice was bound by many CMBS *Rules*, written originally to control the practice of women who wanted to be midwives, but which did not encourage midwives to question what they did. In the first decade of the twenty-first century, the Nursing and Midwifery Council (NMC) says: 'You must deliver care based on the best available evidence or best practice.'[74] Until the 1970s, research in maternity care was a mainly medically-led matter in which midwives might play a secondary role. However, the highlighting and criticism of a distinct lack of scientific rigour in medical decisions and particularly obstetricians' research led to a correction of research methods, systematic reviews of research, and acknowledgement that 'evidence' should inform research: the term 'evidence-based practice'(EBP) came into wide use.[75] Criticism also led to the development of the Cochrane Database in the late 1980s.[76] Through combining results of randomised controlled trials into systematic reviews, this produced convincing outcomes of the effectiveness of various treatments signalling the route to EBP.[77]

Midwives' entry into the research field began in the 1970s and 1980s. Consumers and midwives championed the need for childbirth reforms in the UK at the same time as new nurse-midwives in the US sought recognition for what they did. Any effective systematic evaluation of practice in maternity care occurring in the UK would involve midwifery. Consequently, there was an across-the-spectrum emphasis on basing professional practice on research.[78] This, therefore, particularly from the aspect of midwifery research, improved maternity care and included woman-centred care, expanded knowledge, increased options for women, increased EBP, developed standards, and, expanded a basis and vision for midwifery practice.[79]

The development of research credibility and ability of midwives took time. Would-be researchers responded to the urge to carry out research without a full grasp of research principles and methods. Many initially did not understand that to undertake research they needed also to learn how to do it, either by doing a course in research methods leading to a Master's degree or a PhD, or by supervision from a competent researcher.[80] To begin with, non-researching midwives did not believe the results of their colleagues and turned instead to the work of obstetricians. Subsequently, midwives have embraced the evidence-based research ethos, and question, audit, write, publish, review and listen.[81] Katy commented:

> I think you see yourself evolve throughout your career and, if you were all the midwife you were ever going to be the day that you qualified, then you should really give it up... You will change your opinion [and] there'll be new evidence that will evolve as you carry on throughout your career. Even things that I did that I thought [were correct] last year, I don't necessarily think [are correct] this year.[82]

Ruby thought that midwives should be more pro-active. She said:

> We must get our house in order. We must progress... Research...it's very rarely that it's been done by midwives... The research is medically driven, very medically driven and this means we're still in that kind of vaguely subservient [mode] and, not that you don't value other's work, of course not, but I think we just need...[to] rise out of the depths a wee bit more and continue to rise... [Midwives] are not very good at blowing their own

trumpet. I do [think this stems from history]. You can't just shake that. It's going to take years to overcome.[83]

Yet, still on the subject of subservience, and illustrating how one midwife stood up for herself, Ruby said:

I think midwives today need to be thinking midwives and to have a good analytical profession. You need to have [a degree] level of education realistically. Or equivalent professional development and I think midwives... I think we're seen on that level now... There are still dinosaurs around...not particularly because of time served, it's just the mind-set... The other day, a registrar...was appalled that the midwife didn't do what he told her to do... It's all about the dominance and the subservience. But [here was] a young chap... He'd prescribed a pattern of care. The midwife thought clinically it wasn't a safe option so she thought 'No,' she wasn't going to follow that pattern of care in view of safety. [He was] furious. How dare she not follow his orders? That was exactly what he said... He came off the phone and looked for support from me and I said, 'Absolutely no way. You cannot behave like that.' I was quite shocked that in 2010 we're still [seeing this attitude].[84]

Ruby then conceded, 'But on the whole I would say even my more experienced consultant colleagues, obstetric consultant colleagues certainly wouldn't behave like that.'[85] Katy also commented on the frequency of examining practice:

We do a lot of reflective practice here. We have sessions where we reflect on situations, or on cases, or just something in general that one of us wants to talk about. We talk about what happened. Was there anything that we could do that would change the situation? Are we pleased with what happened? Are we not pleased? How we felt about it and all these different kinds of things. And we discuss it as a team.[86]

Therefore evidence-based practice or care, whether it is done as a result of reading others' research, doing a project or reflecting on practice, is an imperative for professional midwifery. Examples of definitions include 'the conscientious, explicit and judicious use of current best evidence in making decisions about the care of individual patients' and, 'care based on knowledge gained from clinical research.'[87] EBP and the research upon which it is founded have made a notable contribution to the concept of woman-centred care, with increased autonomy for both women and midwives.[88] However, Walsh emphasises the power of qualitative research over quantitative in the field of maternity care when creating an evidence base observing that 'sometimes, what really counts cannot be counted.'[89] This highlights the limitations of quantitative research and the 'profundity of the childbirth experience which, in terms of its effects, cannot be reduced to simple statistics.'[90]

Using research as evidence for practice has become a way of life for midwives. It is also important to be able to articulate and present research findings in a way that managers and politicians will listen to, believe in and act upon.

A Framework for Maternity Services in Scotland and *EGAMS*

The *Framework* was launched on 2 February 2001.[91] The background to the *Framework* with its wide consultation and recommendations may be traced at least to the 1993 *Policy Review* and other progressive reports and documents which succeeded it. Its aim is to deliver consistent, high-quality care that is easily, and preferably, locally accessible. It also recommended a more effective use of resources with joint working between primary, secondary and tertiary services. With this in mind, it set out its philosophy and principles within a template to develop priorities in maternity care, challenging the NHS to meet the needs of women and their partners and empower both professionals and public to rise to that challenge.

Four broad themes are apparent:
- Safety and evidence-based care for mother and baby must remain the foundation of an effective maternity service.
- Pregnancy and childbirth are normal physiological processes in women's lives.
- Maternity services must deliver a woman and family-centred approach to care and support planned in partnership with the woman.
- Maternity services should be essentially community based and midwife managed, wherever possible, with an emphasis on community care.[92]

This philosophical approach, rather than a strategy document or model service specification, outlines a set of broad principles to inform local maternity care strategies. To do this, it covers the main elements of maternity care: preconception, pregnancy, childbirth, postnatal care and parentcraft.

The *Framework* also offers principles for organisation and provision of services and states that service requirements must drive the workforce requirements, areas which provided cause for tension, but which the *Framework* writers agreed could be managed through ongoing workforce planning.[93] In addition, to inform and develop the *Framework*, a new Expert Group on Acute Maternity Services (EGAMS) emerged and reported in 2002.

The *EGAMS Report* comprehensively examined maternity services in Scotland and aimed to provide a mechanism to implement the recommendations of the *Framework*, especially intrapartum care. To do this it set out to consider national, regional and local planning of maternity services and to promote innovative approaches to intrapartum care consistent with the *Framework*'s principles.[94] It concluded that, because of the falling birth rate in Scotland at the end of the twentieth century, the current organisation of maternity services could not be maintained as it was. It suggested the need to organise services so that appropriate care could be provided locally with tertiary services organised on a regional basis.[95] It described levels of intrapartum and childbirth care by location through levels of care ranging from Level I (Ia, homebirth; Ib, stand-alone CMU; Ic, CMU adjacent to non-obstetric hospital; Id, CMU adjacent to maternity unit); Level II, (IIa, consultant-led unit with no neonatal facility; IIb, consultant-led maternity unit with on-site neonatal facility; IIc, consultant-led maternity unit); and Level III, (consultant-led specialist maternity unit). For each of the situations, primary, secondary or tertiary, the *EGAMS Report* describes the lead carer, the clinical situation, the woman's care need and kind of birth that could be catered for.[96]

EGAMS commented on midwives' competencies. One-to-one midwifery care in labour is an important facet of woman-centred care in normal labour. It helps to avoid intervention in low-risk women and has positive outcomes – a key component surrounding spontaneous vaginal birth is the continuous presence of the midwife. But not all midwives are able to provide all elements of midwifery care for low-risk women and one argument claims that many midwives lost core skills and confidence in their ability to do this.[97]

EGAMS included a section on Key Principles to assist NHS Boards to plan, configure and provide acute maternity services in the context of local, regional and national planning. Ten key principles, each broken down into further points, gave a picture of a collective will to improve, modernise, care and inform with the needs of women and their infants at the core. Key principles covered core principles, education, risk, manpower, general principles, planning, the network [according to care levels], transport, information, and change management.[98]

Models of care in pregnancy and childbirth
The word 'model' is used to give an example of a specific philosophy of style or of describing a working practice. A model is usually thought of as the best way of doing things, or best practice. Proponents of a particular model look on it as very nearly ideal and may claim to know through their model how to achieve the best results.[99] The word 'model' has been used in this context for centuries.[100] More recently, within the context of childbirth, different models have been described as the 'obstetric' or 'biomedical' model, and the 'social' or 'midwifery' model.[101] When two models appear directly to oppose each other and the differing philosophies collide, then real conflict may arise between their proponents. There can also be a problem if a model becomes an ideology and taken as an immovable pattern or standard, therefore possibly becoming a deterrent to innovation and progress.[102]

In Scotland, as birth became increasingly medicalised, the biomedical/obstetric model took over the greater part of care for women during pregnancy and childbirth. It remained like that until the later decades of the twentieth century. The inclusion in the medical model of the care of childbearing women is characterised by the use of high-technology equipment, the use of medical and nursing hierarchical systems, and public persuasion to give birth in hospital on the grounds of safety. The social or midwifery model emphasises that the majority of pregnant women have the potential to have a normal, safe pregnancy and birth without medical intervention.[103] Although the characteristics of the models appear to oppose each other, midwives can be found working within both obstetric and social models along different points on a continuum between the two extremes. In an obstetric unit, for instance, working with and under the direction of obstetricians, there are midwives and obstetric nurses. In other settings, for example, at home, in a community maternity unit (CMU) and other midwife-led units, the midwifery/social model prevails and may or may not include GP input.

The broad themes of the *Framework* implemented by the *EGAMS Report* allow for both midwifery/social and biomedical models when necessary or, if a woman wishes it, to be used when giving woman-centred care. Ideally, care is tailored according to the needs and wishes of the individual woman and neither model is ruled out. Midwives may practise at any point within the continuum or range of the two models. Charlie observed:

> Many midwives will practise in the middle. But there are some...who are really leading the field in midwifery-led care in Scotland and they are very proficient at what they are doing, but they could not necessarily work as a midwife further along the continuum where you needed all sorts of additional care or treatments – high tech obstetric-led care. ...I would suggest that...the opposite is [also] true. Midwives who deal with high dependency obstetric-led care are not necessarily comfortable providing midwifery-only care without epidural, without escalation.[104]

Just as models need not be so fixed that they prevent change where necessary, the range within the models will change, grow larger, and the extremities might become closer or further away. Midwives, too, may change their thinking and their position within the midwifery-biomedical spectrum as they gain experience, develop, and gather their own philosophies of midwifery. This could unfold a further strand in thinking. Bryers argues that maternity services require more than just the adoption of a social or midwifery model and cites New Zealand where, although maternity services have been pro-active in adopting a midwife-led and woman-centred approach since the 1990s, there has been no lessening of intervention rates.[105] So, in accordance with the current trend towards partnership between women and all members of the multi-professional maternity care team, an appropriate direction is to advocate a new 'post-modern' holistic partnership model, a woman-centred model of maternity care, based on the practice of promoting woman-centred pregnancy and birth as a normal life event.[106] This would have the added benefit of increasing maternal salutogenesis or feeling of wellbeing with rising long-term benefits in the overall health of the population.[107]

Independent midwifery[108]

While the discussion in this book has focussed on midwifery, and its progress and changes across Scotland, there are midwives in Scotland and the rest of the UK who wish to practise independently along with women who want to employ an independent midwife (IM) to care for her during pregnancy, her labour and birth of her baby and during the postnatal period. IMs become independent usually because they wish to provide continuity of care and this is the main reason women book with an IM. IMs, like any other UK registered midwife, are bound by the NMC code of conduct and NMC rules. They are allocated, or choose, a supervisor of midwives in their main area of work and, like other midwives, have to submit an 'Intention to Practise' form to any LSA where they wish to work. Their practice also adds important further choice to the range of maternity care available.

In 2006, the UK government announced its policy requiring all health care professionals to have professional indemnity/insurance cover (PII). This is scheduled to become mandatory in 2013. Due to the number of independent midwives currently being too small to enable the risk to be pooled and spread in a way that produces an affordable premium, there is no insurance available for independent midwifery services. Inability to access PII would result in the demise of independent midwives in the UK.[109]

In 2007, a campaign for the survival of independent midwifery was launched by Independent Midwives UK (IMUK), and which received significant support. The Department of Health for England proposed a solution: Independent midwives would contract their services to the NHS and thereby access indemnity for these NHS clients. In England this would be through Primary Care Trusts (PCTs) and legislation to enable non-NHS providers to access indemnity from the government scheme run by the NHS Litigation Authority. This was included in the 2008 Health and Social Care Act which applied to England. However by 2010 this clause had still not been implemented as subsequent effects of such legislation on other parts of the NHS in Scotland, Wales and Northern Ireland had not been resolved.[110]

In 2009, the UK government commissioned the *Findlay Scott Review* to look at the feasibility of having indemnity insurance as a condition of every healthcare professional's registration. The review was published in 2010 and recommended that indemnity/insurance should become mandatory and a requirement for registration. However, it also recommended that for those groups (i.e. independent midwives) for whom the market does not provide affordable insurance or indemnity, the relevant Departments of Health in the four countries of the UK should decide if the continued availability of this service is necessary and, if so, should try and find a solution to the problem. At the time of writing (September 2010). their responses to the Review were awaited. Their responses might be an ideal vehicle through which to address this anomaly with solutions coming from the policy-makers.[111]

In 2010, the IMUK was still seeking commercial insurance. This is because the members of the IMUK are in agreement that women in the UK should retain the right to seek midwifery care outside the NHS if that is what they want.[112]

Carrie McIntosh, independent midwife wrote on her website:

> Working independently allows me to work with women on a one-to-one basis which is such a satisfying way to work.
>
> I am registered with the Nursing and Midwifery Council and am bound by the Code of Professional Conduct and the Midwives Rules and Standards. I am a member of the Independent Midwives Association, Association for Improvements in Maternity Services, Royal College of Midwives and am a local representative for the Association of Radical Midwives.
>
> As an Independent midwife I am happy to support women planning a homebirth, on dry land or in water. I can attend as a birth support partner should transfer to hospital be necessary or should you be planning a hospital birth. It is occasionally possible to negotiate an honorary contract to work as a midwife in hospital.[113]

Keeping Childbirth Natural and Dynamic

The *EGAMS Report* provided building materials for the scaffolding of the *Framework*. NHS Boards in Scotland accepted the principles outlined in both the *Framework* and the *EGAMS Report* which endorsed the promotion of pregnancy and childbirth as normal life events and advocated woman-centred care tailored to suit the needs of individual women. Care was planned to be community-focussed and midwife-managed for healthy women, with multidisciplinary maternity team care for complex cases.

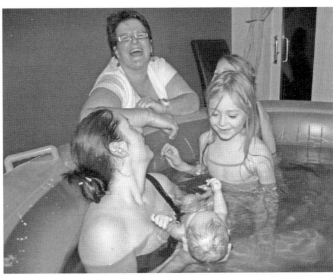

Carrie McIntosh, midwife, with Alison Campbell, mother, and her daughters Jemma, Emily and newborn Hope. (Courtesy of Carrie McIntosh, midwife, and Alison Campbell.)

In 2007, some key aspects of the plans remained outstanding. Two in particular were the position of the midwife as lead professional for the majority of low-risk women and babies, and the need to ensure a normal birth pathway for healthy women regardless of where they planned to give birth. Work on the Scottish Government's *Keeping Childbirth Natural and Dynamic (KCND)* programme started in 2007 to support the multi-professional team to implement the principles of the *Framework* and boost opportunities for healthy women to have as natural a birth experience as possible. For professional guidance, the *KCND* programme has developed the *KCND Pathways*.[114] This focusses on midwifery care, uses an evidence-based midwifery model and reinforces the ideal of woman-centred maternal and infant safety through working within a multi-disciplinary care network. The offer of appropriate information and support enables women to make informed choices about their care options and where they would like to give birth.[115] One intention of the *KCND Pathways* aims to avoid unnecessary intervention. This should be achieved by offering each woman appropriate care from her first early pregnancy consultation. This should also have the benefit of avoiding duplication of care.[116] In 2010, the *KCND Pathways* were evolving across NHS Scotland. Katy commented:

> I think it is progressing... In Perth and Tayside we were fairly far advanced in the *Keeping Childbirth Natural and Dynamic* anyway. I think we had three community maternity units which are still there and now we have an alongside maternity midwife-led unit – that's in Dundee – at Ninewells... That only opened in February [2009] and it's already been a huge success.[117]

KCND assumes the suitability of all healthy women for midwife-managed care with onward referral to the obstetrician, others in the maternity care team and other specialists as required. This is an important philosophical shift in maternity care in Scotland. All women are encouraged, through discussion and information, to make decisions regarding their care and birth preferences, including where they want to give birth. So, although low-risk women are usually happy to have midwife-led care, they can make their own choice, as Katy showed in her comment:

> Low risk women are automatically being streamed through the [midwife-led] unit...unless somebody specifically says, 'I ...don't want to go there because I am having an epidural...' Then they would be directed to labour suite.[118]

KCND also encourages women to document their preferences and keep the document safely in their hand-held records. This is all part of the overall encouragement and support for women to take as active a role as possible. *KCND* also acknowledges that, due to the impact of inequality in health and social exclusion, needs vary in quantity and complexity and procedures are in place to give appropriate information, support and referral based on need.[119]

Risk assessments during pregnancy are part of maternity care and take into account that risk status is dynamic and may change, involving, for example, a move from midwifery to obstetric care. The ideal plan anticipated is that women may move between different care packages or models in both directions depending on clinical recommendation or maternal choice.[120] Katy said:

> Yes, [antenatally] the women [can be] in and out of the medical high risk at some point...then, if everything goes fine, they have a scan or it's fine, then back in the care of the midwife. Together with our obstetric colleagues, I think it is really working very well on Tayside.[121]

The idea of movement fits within the meaning of the word 'dynamic', which it is important to retain when discussing *KCND*. 'Dynamic' is defined as: (1) Vigorous and purposeful, full of energy and enthusiasm... able to get things going and get things done; (2) ... producing or undergoing change and development.[122] This not only concurs with the need for movement within the multi-professional maternity services team in the interests of woman-centred care, but also in an acknowledgement that movement forward in evidence-based practice is also desirable.

The Scottish Government agreed that consultant midwives should be appointed in Scotland with the aim of implementing the programme. Health Boards had appointed sixteen KCND consultant midwives by 2010. Charlie commented:

> I think the KCND consultant midwives are breaking new ground in that they are working within the health system to try and pursue services that would allow midwives to provide more midwifery centred care... In many areas, the arguments are not with obstetricians. I think they've acknowledged that there is a need for that aspect of the service, and some women – that's what they need and want and therefore the KCND consultants are not having that much opposition with obstetricians at all. What they are having difficulty with, and I think it is different in different Health Board areas, but it's prevalent in

more than one Health Board area – they're having a lot of difficulty with GPs particularly over the point of midwife as the first point of contact in the antenatal experience... GPs are seeing that as an infringement into their sphere and, I suppose, control in that field.[123]

However, she also said that some mothers want to see their GP early in pregnancy and throughout pregnancy and commented that, in a woman-centred service, this had to be catered for.[124] Nevertheless, according to comments emerging from the British Medical Association Scotland conference held in Clydebank in 2010, some GPs felt that they were 'being distanced from maternity care. Women are being told by bus-shelter ads, to sidestep us altogether.'[125] However Gillian Smith, Director of the RCM UK Board for Scotland, refuted this when she said:

> It's about trying to get women to refer...early so you can get them in the best health to go forward in their pregnancy. I see the midwives as a sign poster. If a woman has a medical problem, then the most appropriate person she sees is the GP.[126]

The *KCND Pathways*, thoroughly researched and evidence-based, and disseminated across Scotland, give a clear signal promoting woman-centred, midwifery-led maternity care following the ethos that pregnancy and childbirth are normal physiological processes and unnecessary intervention should be avoided.

Refreshing the *Framework*
In April 2010, the Maternity Services Action Group (MSAG) commenced work on a programme to produce *A Refreshed Maternity Services Quality Framework*.[127] This is intended as a refreshment of the *Framework* (2001) in order to provide an up to date perspective on policy and evidence-base for the development of maternity services in Scotland. This is in line with Scottish Government policy whose aim is to ensure that no one is denied opportunity because of race, gender, identity, disability, sexual orientation, religion or belief, or age, in the work towards achieving a just and inclusive Scotland.[128] From the NHS aspect, this is epitomised in *Better Health, Better Care* (BHBC) with its key components: health improvement, tackling health inequalities, and, improving the quality of health care.[129]

Each of the key components is bound up in maternity care. Since the publication of the *Framework*, there is a developing evidence-base linking the experience of pregnancy, early childhood days and poor maternal mental health with inequalities in health, education and socio-economic outcomes for the child. At the same time, care will remain woman-centred and in line with the *KCND* programme. The *Refreshed Framework*, while retaining its original philosophy, will reflect the current situation in maternity services in Scotland including the *KCND Pathways* and includes evidence relating to the critical role of the maternity services in improving health outcomes for women and their children, the overarching principles for maternity services and specific relevant details for each stage from pre-conception to the postnatal period.[130]

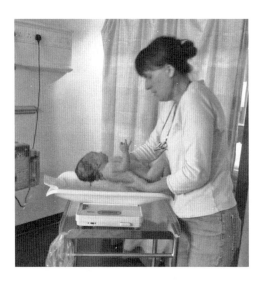

Jenny Patterson, midwife,
weighing baby Katherine Sanders.
(Courtesy of Jenny Patterson,
midwife, and Susan Sanders,
mother.)

Midwifery 2020

In the autumn of 2006, the Department of Health for England launched Modernising
Nursing Careers (MNC) as a joint initiative with the other UK Health Departments.[131] A
number of strands progressed from this including the NMC review of pre-registration
nursing education, preparation of specialist and advanced roles, reviewing career-paths,
and mapping out nursing roles and competencies.

Midwifery 2020 is a UK programme of work regarding midwifery which has
evolved from MNC.[132] In response to changes in society, population, politics and the
environment, the UK Chief Nursing Officers (CNO) recognised the need for the
midwifery profession to anticipate, be ready for change, and respond to the question:
'What kind of midwifery services do we want to see by the year 2020?' In line with
similar programmes already underway in healthcare settings, they commissioned a paper
in February 2007 to reflect on the requirement of a programme to describe the future
contribution of midwifery to maternity care in the UK. The paper recognised that
midwives have a unique and specialist contribution to the health and wellbeing of
women and their babies. It proposed the establishment of a programme of work designed
to enable midwives to lead and deliver care in the current rapidly evolving healthcare
environment. The programme is intended to offer a route for midwifery through the
changes. It would also identify possible changes to the way midwives work, their role,
responsibilities and any appropriate changes required in training and professional
development needs.[133]

Improved care of, and outcomes for, mothers and babies and their families must
always be of primary consideration and the Project Initiation Document (PID) of
Midwifery 2020 included the need for the midwifery profession to meet the future health
and social needs of women and their families as its aim. The objectives included: review
the current role of midwives in the UK; gather evidence and use for future direction of
midwifery services; examine ongoing midwifery service models; consider midwifery
education and any required changes; examine midwifery career pathways and create

situations for midwives to enlarge on their abilities to develop and deliver research-based practice; explore how the support roles of maternity care assistants can best be used; and, consider how midwives can be supported and encouraged to remain in practice.[134]

Each of the four countries of the UK had a project to support the infrastructure. England undertook *Education and career progression and quality*. This entailed scoping current midwifery education and its fitness for purpose, and development of clinical academic careers. Scotland lead the work in *workforce and workload*. This included the collation of UK-wide data on workforce (age profiles, Agenda for Change (AfC) banding, whole-time equivalent numbers of midwives by health board or regional authority and attrition rates).[135] Wales examined the core role of the midwife. Northern Ireland and Scotland reviewed the public health aspects of midwifery.

The project had a wide vision of where the midwifery profession in the UK wanted to be in 2020 and how it was going to get there.[136] This came together in the Midwifery 2020 Report, *Delivering Expectations*, which was launched on 9 September 2010. In a pre-launch article, Bradshaw and Bagness stressed the key requirement that education presented to fuel the drive and ambition required to meet the demands of twenty-first century midwifery care.[137] The *2020 Report* also identified education, research and development in its key messages highlighting the vision of how midwives can lead and give care in a changing environment. The other key messages included: the scope of the midwife role; the need to strengthen evidence-based and quality-based practice; midwifery care and contribution to the challenges of inequality and improving public health; midwives' potential in leadership and strategic roles; and, the need to present midwifery as an attractive career choice.[138]

These key messages presented challenges to midwives across the UK. At the time of writing (September 2010), further review of these messages and any resulting action remain to be seen, but it is evident that nothing will stand still.

Conclusion

In the twenty years surrounding the cusp of the twenty-first century, midwifery in Scotland has moved from what was a glimmer of hope for progress to real positive change. Evidence of the upsurge of public opinion, work from groups like CRAG-SCOTMEG and activity amongst the ranks of midwives, all combined to propel movement in the maternity services in Scotland forward. The *Winterton Report* spurred on the early 1990s maternity services reports from the four countries of the UK, and woman-centred care with its highs and lows, new systems and drive for change.

Change came too in the development of midwifery education from its early twentieth-century rule-ridden philosophy to an analytical research-based form of learning which allows midwives to think, reflect, and use initiative in the pursuance of evidence-based practice. This attitude matched the ethos of the *Framework for Maternity Services in Scotland,* the recommendations of the *EGAMS Report* and the courses for multi-professional development which the SMMDP continues to promote and present across Scotland.

Not everyone can agree on how care should be given. The old word 'model' suddenly leapt on to a maternity care continuum as different approaches were compared, contrasted and contested. These differences came together in a diplomatic way with the *KCND programme* which emphasised the need to keep childbirth as normal as possible for healthy women. At the same time, *KCND* with its 'traffic-light' system offered suitable routes for woman-centred care which incorporated different models and made it possible for women to move between models where necessary and if that was what they wanted. In its own way, *KCND* has also confirmed the concept of improved communication between health professionals and improved midwifery career-paths through offering wider horizons.

1. *Nursing and Midwifery Order* (SI2002/253), (London: NMC, 2001); C McKenzie, 'Midwifery Regulation in the United Kingdom', in D Fraser, M Cooper, *Myles Textbook for Midwives (15th ed)*, (Edinburgh: Churchill Livingstone, 2009), pp 81-100.
2. *Ibid*.
3. Hall, MacIntyre, Porter, *Antenatal Care Assessed*, pp 2, 8, 23; *Tennent Report*.
4. Association of Radical Midwives (ARM), *The Vision*, (Droitwich: Spa Printing and Copying, 1986).
5. Christie D, Tansey E, (eds), *Wellcome witnesses to twentieth century medicine: Maternal care*, Witness seminar transcript, Vol 12, (London: The Wellcome Trust Centre for the History of Medicine at UCL, 2001), p 70, (Alison MacFarlane); see also Christie, Tansey, *Maternal Care*, endnote 186.
6. RCM, *The role and education of the future midwife in the United Kingdom*, RCM, (London: RCM 1987); RCM, *Towards a healthy nation*, (London: RCM, 1991).
7. Scottish Office Home and Health Department (SOHHD) 1991, *The patient's charter: a charter for health*, London: HMSO, 1991); SOHHD, *Framework for action*, London: HMSO, 1991).
8. *Ibid*.
9. SOHHD, CRAG/SCOTMEG Working Group on Maternity Services, *Antenatal care*, (Edinburgh: HMSO, 1995), p 1.
10. SOHHD, CRAG/SCOTMEG Working Group on Maternity Services, *Innovations in practice: abstracts of presentations*, (Edinburgh: HMSO, 1993).
11. SOHHD, CRAG/SCOTMEG Working Group on Maternity Services, *Innovations in practice: abstracts and presentations*, (Edinburgh: HMSO, 1994).
12. Bostock Y, Reid M, *Pregnancy, childbirth and coping with motherhood: what women want from maternity services*. (Edinburgh: SOHHD, 1993), p 9.
13. Bostock , Reid, pp 14, 44.
14. SOHHD, *The patients' charter: what users think*, (Edinburgh: HMSO, 1994).
15. House of Commons Health Committee, *Second Report: Maternity Services, (Winterton Report)*, (London: HMSO, 1992).
16. Christie, Tansey, *Maternal care*, p 78 (Luke Zander).
17. J Lawson, *'Power to mothers and midwives'*, *MIDIRS Midwifery Digest*, (1992), Vol 2 (2), pp 127-130.
18. Lawson, *'Power to mothers and midwives'*.
19. *Ibid*; 'caseload' refers to a personal caseload where named midwives care for

individual women, Fraser, Cooper, *Myles textbook for midwives, (15th ed)*, p 1073.

20. B Dimond, 'Fears for the future', *Modern Midwife*, (1995), Vol 5 (4), pp 32-33.
21. *Collins Dictionary and Thesaurus* (Glasgow: Collins, 1989).
22. L Reid, 'Woman-centred care – midwives in Scotland', *Nursing Times*, (1997) July 2-8, pp 52-53.
23. RCM Supplement, *Woman-centred Care*, (January, 1996), p 1.
24. G Skinner, S Roch, 'Creating confidence by building on experience', *British Journal of Midwifery* (1995), Vol 3 (4) pp 284-287.
25. Lawson, *'Power to mothers and midwives'*.
26. LR 130.
27. Welsh Office, *Maternal and Early Child Health*, (Cardiff: HMSO, 1991); Northern Ireland Maternity Unit Study Group, *Delivering Choice: Midwife and GP-led Maternity Units*, (Belfast: HMSO, 1994); DH, *Changing Childbirth. Part 1: Report of the Expert Maternity Group*, (London: HMSO, August 1993); SHHD, *Provision of Maternity Services in Scotland – A Policy Review*, (Edinburgh: HMSO, July 1993).
28. *Ibid*.
29. Skinner, Roch, *'Creating confidence by building on experience'*.
30. A Fleissig, D Kroll, 'Achieving continuity of care and carer', *Modern Midwife*, (1997), Vol 7 (8), pp15-19.
31. L Page, B Jones, P Bentley, et al, 'One-to-one midwifery', *British Journal of Midwifery* (1994), Vol 2 (9), pp 444-447.
32. RCM Supplement, *Woman-centred Care*, No 2, (April, 1996), p 2.
33. LR 129.
34. L Reid, E Hillan, M McGuire, 'The challenge of negotiating the maze of woman-centred care in Scotland', *British Journal of Midwifery*, (1997), Vol 5 (10), pp 602-606.
35. C Flint, 'Inaugural address', *RCM Midwives Chronicle*, (1994), 107, pp 335-339.
36. L Floyd, 'Community midwives' views and experience of homebirth', *Midwifery*, (1995), (11), pp 3-10.
37. D Turnbull, M Reid, M McGinley, Shields N, 'Changes in midwives' attitudes to their professional role following the implementation of the midwifery development unit', *Midwifery*, (1995), (11), pp 110-119.
38. N Leap, 'Caseload practice within the NHS', *Midwives Chronicle*, (1994), 107, pp 130-135.
39. V Hundley, F Cruikshank, J Milne et al, 'Satisfaction and continuity of care: staff views of care in a midwife-managed delivery unit', *Midwifery*, (1995) (11), pp 163-173.
40. T Murphy Black, 'Systems of midwifery care in use in Scotland', *Midwifery*, (1992), (8), pp 113-124.
41. Skinner, Roch, 'Creating confidence by building on experience'; L Reid, E Hillan, M McGuire, 'The challenge of negotiating the maze'.
42. LR 129.
43. LR 131.

44. D Walsh, 'Is woman-centred care becoming a pious platitude?' *British Journal of Midwifery*, (1996), Vol 4 (4), pp 173-174.
45. Reid, Hillan, McGuire, 'The challenge of negotiating the maze'.
46. Personal communication.
47. B Dimond, 'Fears for the future'.
48. E Hillan, M McGuire, L Reid, *Midwives and woman-centred care*, University of Glasgow and RCM Scottish Board, (Edinburgh: RCM Scottish Board, 1997); L Reid, E Hillan, M McGuire, 'Woman-centred care: midwives' need to be heard', *The Practising Midwife*, (1998) Vol 1 (12), pp 22-25.
49. L Reid, 'Organisation of Health Services in the UK', in D Fraser, M Cooper, *Myles Textbook for Midwives (15th ed)*, (Edinburgh: Elsevier, 2009), pp 1027-1038; Trusts in the NHS in Scotland ceased in 2000.
50. Audit Commission, *First class delivery: improving maternity services in England and Wales*, (Oxford: Audit Commission publications, 1997); E Hillan, M McGuire, L Reid, P Purton , 'Woman-centred care: a midwifery perspective', *RCM Midwives Journal*, (2000), Vol 3 (12), pp 376-379.
51. L Reid, E Hillan,, M McGuire, 'Woman centred care: part-time midwives – are they getting a fair deal?' *The Practising Midwife*, (1999), Vol 2 (1), pp 27-29.
52. *Ibid*.
53. Hillan, McGuire, Reid, *Midwives and woman centred care*, pp 18-19.
54. J Sandall, 'Midwives, burnout and continuity of care', *British Journal of Midwifery*, (1997), Vol 5 (2) pp 105-111; Hillan, McGuire, Reid, Purton, 'Woman-centred care: a midwifery perspective'.
55. J Tucker, M Hall, P Howie et al, 'Should obstetricians see women with normal pregnancies? A multicentre randomised controlled trial of routine antenatal care by general practitioners and midwives compared to shared care', *British Medical Journal*, (1996), Vol 312, pp 554-559; Scottish programme for clinical effectiveness in reproductive health (SPCERH) and the Dugald Baird Centre for Research on Women's Health, *Maternity Care Matters: an audit of maternity services in Scotland 1998*, (SPCERH Publication Number 9, SPCERH, Aberdeen, 1999), p 7.
56. Scottish Executive (SE), 2001, *A Framework for Maternity Services in Scotland*, SE; SPCERH, Maternity care matters, pp 8-9.
57. LR 131. The voices of five contemporary midwives are introduced by pseudonyms: Charlie, Claire, Grace, Katy and Ruby.
58. Council Directives of 21 January, (80/154/EEC), *Official Journal of the European Communities*, No L 33/1, (1980) and (80/155/EEC), *Official Journal of the European Communities*, No L 33/8 (1980).
59. The term 'direct-entry' midwives is sometimes used instead of single-registered . midwives.
60. M McGuire, L Reid, E Hillan, *The perceptions and experiences of newly qualified single registered midwives in Scotland*, (Glasgow: University of Glasgow, 1998) p 3; C Maggs, 'Direct but different: midwifery education since 1989', *British Journal of Midwifery*, (1996), Vol 2 (2), pp 612-616.
61. McGuire, Reid, Hillan, *Perceptions and experiences*, p 4.

62. *Ibid*, p 7.
63. LR 132.
64. LR 134.
65. McGuire, Reid, Hillan, *Perceptions and experiences*, p 15.
66. *Ibid*, pp 11, 17.
67. LR 129.
68. *Ibid*.
69. www.scottishmaternity.org
70. SEHD, *Report on the Expert Group on Maternity Services (EGAMS Report)*, (Edinburgh: Scottish Executive, 2002), pp 67-68.
71. *Ibid*, p 17.
72. LR 132.
73. LR 131.
74. NMC, *The code: standards of conduct, performance and ethics for nurses and midwives*, (London: NMC, 2008).
75. A Cochrane, *Effectiveness and efficiency*, (London: Nuffield Provincial Hospitals Trust, 1972).
76. R Mander, 'Evidence-based practice', in D Fraser, M Cooper, *Myles' Textbook for Midwives (15th ed)*, (Edinburgh: Elsevier, 2009), pp 67-79.
77. D Walsh, *Evidence-based care for normal labour and birth*, (London: Routledge, 2007), p 2.
78. A Luyben, 'The midwife as a researcher', in Mander R, Fleming V, (eds), *Becoming a midwife*, (Abingdon: Routledge, 2009), pp 115-126.
79. Luyben, 'Midwife as a researcher'.
80. A Thomson, 'Is there evidence for the medicalisation of maternity care?' *MIDIRS Midwifery Digest*, (2000), Vol 10 (4), pp 416-420.
81. L Reid, 'Best practice: aims and realities', in L Reid, *Midwifery: freedom to practise?* (Edinburgh: Elsevier, 2007), pp 9-29.
82. LR 131.
83. LR 133.
84. *Ibid*.
85. *Ibid*.
86. LR 131.
87. D Sackett, W Rosenburg, J A Gray, et al, 'Evidence based medicine: what it is and what it isn't.' *British Medical Journal* (1996) Vol 312 (7023), pp 71-72, quoted in Mander, R, Evidence-based practice; L Albers, 'Evidence' and midwifery practice, *Journal of midwifery and women's health*, (2001) Vol 46 (3), pp 130-135.
88. Reid L, 'Best practice: aims and realities', p 14.
89. Walsh, *Evidence-based care*, p 4; I Chalmers, M Kierse, J Neilson, *A guide to effective care in pregnancy and childbirth*, (Oxford: Oxford University Press, 1989), quoted in Walsh D, *Evidence-based care*, p 4.
90. Walsh, *Evidence-based care*, p 4.
91. SE, *A Framework for Maternity Services in Scotland*, (Edinburgh: SE, 2 February 2001); 2 February is the day after St Bride's Day and, whether by

accident or by design, was an appropriate day for the launch of the *Framework*.
St Bride is the Celtic saint of midwives. Legend says that she helped Mary give
birth to the infant Jesus. Bride's flower is the snowdrop; midwives and
snowdrops have long been associated.

92. *Framework*, p 22.
93. *Ibid*, pp 22-23.
94. *EGAMS Report*, 2002, p 3.
95. L Reid, 'Normal birth in Scotland' in L Reid, *Midwifery: Freedom to practise*, pp
     240-260.
96. *EGAMS Report*, p 5.
97. *Ibid*, p 57.
98. *Ibid*, pp 77-83.
99. E Van Teijlingen, *A social or medical model of childbirth? Comparing the
     arguments in Grampian (Scotland) and the Netherlands*, unpublished PhD thesis,
     (University of Aberdeen, 1994), pp 323-327; L Reid, 'Best practice: aims and
     realities' in L Reid, *Midwifery: freedom to practise?* pp 9-29.
100. Oliver Cromwell's 'New Model Army' was formed in 1645, and Bryers uses
     'model' to describe the working pattern in the provision of district nursing,
     community midwifery and health visiting in the *Gàidhealtachd* and subsequently
     across Scotland in the early twentieth century: H Bryers, *Midwifery and
     Maternity Services in the Gàidhealtachd and the North of Scotland, 1914-2005*,
     unpublished PhD thesis, University of Aberdeen, 2010, Chapter 1.
101. Walsh, *Evidence-based care*, pp 7-11; Reid, *'Best practice: aims and realities'*,
     pp 16-20; L Stephens, 'Midwifery-led care', in L Reid, *Midwifery: freedom to
     practise?* pp 146-149; Bryers, *Midwifery and Maternity Services*, pp 90-107.
102. Bryers, *Midwifery and Maternity Services*, p 91; Reid, *'Best practice: aims and
     realities'*, p 17.
103. Van Teijlingen, *A social or medical model of childbirth?* p 299; L Reid, *'Best
     practice: aims and realities'*, pp 9-29.
104. LR 129.
105. Bryers, *Midwives and Maternity Services*, p 105; Skinner J, 'Risk, let's look at
     the bigger picture', *Women and Birth* (2008), (21), pp 53-54.
106. Bryers, *Midwives and Maternity Services*, p 105; D Walsh, *Improving maternity
     services* (Oxford: Radcliffe Publishing, 2007) p 94.
107. Walsh, *Improving Maternity Services,* pp 88-89; S Downe, C McCourt, 'From
     being to becoming: reconstructing childbirth knowledge', in S Downe, (ed)
     Normal Childbirth: Evidence and debate (London: Churchill Livingstone, 2004)
     p 4; L Durkin, T Palmer, 'Towards a woman-centred model of care', *The
     Practising Midwife*, (2010), Vol 13 (3), p 21.
108. Many thanks to Carrie McIntosh and her independent midwife colleagues for
     their help with this section.
109. www.independentmidwives.org.uk
110. *Ibid*.
111. *Ibid*.
112. *Ibid*.

113. Carrie McIntosh: www.mcmidwives.co.uk/Carrie.html
114. NHS Quality Improvement Scotland (QIS), *KCND Programme, Pathways for Maternity Care*, (Edinburgh: QIS, 2009).
115. H MacGregor, G Butcher, L Powis, 'Scotland's pathway says 'no' to intervention', *Midwives*, June/July (2009), p 29. The *KCND Pathways* use a 'traffic light format': 'green' indicates midwife-led care, 'amber' demonstrates the need for further assessment and 'red' indicates the clear recommendation that the maternity care team is required.
116. *Ibid*.
117. LR 131.
118. *Ibid*.
119. *KCND Pathways*, p 2.
120. *Ibid*, p 3.
121. LR 131.
122. *Encarta World English Dictionary*, (London: Bloomsbury, 1999), p 587.
123. LR 129.
124. *Ibid*.
125. L Moss, 'Doctors: We're being cut out by empire-building midwives', *The Scotsman*, 12 March 2010, p 17.
126. *Ibid*.
127. Maternity Services Action Group ((MSAG), *A Refreshed Maternity Services Quality Framework* (Draft), (Edinburgh: MSAG, Jan 2010).
128. *Refreshed Framework* (draft), pp 3, 4.
129. Scottish Government Health Department, *Better Health, Better Care*, (Edinburgh: Scottish Government, 2006).
130. *Refreshed Framework* (draft).
131. Department of Health (DH), *Modernising Nursing Careers: setting the direction*, (London: HMSO, 2006). The DH did not include the profession of midwifery in its publication title. Midwives across the UK will be disappointed that the DH has not acknowledged the distinction of midwifery as a profession in its own right.
132. DH, *Modernising Nursing Careers: setting the direction*, (London: HMSO, 2006).
133. UK CNOs, *Midwifery 2020, Project Initiation Document V6, 2007*.
134. *Ibid*.
135. In 2004, under the title, *Agenda for Change*, the NHS initiated pay re-structuring along with the requirement for most NHS staff to undergo annual development reviews. L Reid, 'Organisation of the health services in the UK', in Fraser, Cooper, *Myles Textbook for Midwives*, p 1035.
136. www.midwifery2020.org
137. G Bradshaw, C Bagness, 'Midwifery 2020 (1): education and career progression', *The Practising Midwife*, (2010), Vol 13 (8), pp 4-5.
138. N Kent, 'The road ahead', *Midwives*, (September 2010) pp 24-25; NHS, Midwifery 2020, England, Northern Ireland, Scotland, Wales, Midwifery 2020, *Delivering Expectations*, Final Report, (launched Edinburgh, September 2010).

Chapter 10

'I feel very positive about midwifery today...'

Scotland is a country of geographic and demographic contrasts. Its population of almost 5.2 million is distributed unevenly across four distinct regions: the Highlands and Islands, the lowland Central Belt, the South West, and the upland Scottish Borders.[1] The population density contrasts sharply between the remote areas of, for instance the Highlands and Islands and the easily accessible Central Belt. The Highlands cover more than fifty percent of mainland Scotland, but most of the population lives in the Central Belt covering only ten percent of the land area. Overall, this translates into the uneven distribution of eighty percent of the population of Scotland living in twenty percent of the land area.[2]

An uneven distribution of population leads to an uneven distribution of midwives and maternity services, and requires different ways of working. The *Framework* and the *EGAMS Report* succeeded in highlighting problems arising, particularly in maternity care, within this uneven mix of demography and geography and in suggested practical, realistic ways of managing the problems.[3] These documents also demonstrated a desire to continue the move towards offering a more normal way of birth to more women, with a lessening of the medical or obstetric model of childbirth and the development of the midwife-led or social model. From this thinking, the *KCND Programme* emerged with its aims of increasing normal birthing opportunities for healthy women through an evidence-based midwifery model within a multidisciplinary care network.

Within the principles and standards of the *Framework*, the *EGAMS Report* and the *KCND Programme*, there are wide issues not least of which is that midwives are practising in this country of geographic and demographic contrasts. This gives rise to different thinking, ways of practice, career paths. With the help of the voices of five contemporary midwives, this chapter explores aspects of, and creates a snapshot of, issues surrounding midwifery and childbirth in twenty-first century Scotland. To give grounding to the discussion, it will offer a brief résumé of what has gone before. This brings the past into focus before the voices of five midwives from the first decade of the twenty-first century have their say and bring the book to a conclusion.[4]

Spotlighting the past

With the implementation of the 1915 Midwives (Scotland) Act, midwifery in Scotland changed from being alegal, unlicensed and unregulated, to a profession which eventually covered the care of women during normal pregnancy, labour and the postnatal period.[5] However, in the early decades of the twentieth century, midwives had little input into the care of pregnant women. Their main remit lay in the care of mothers during labour and the postnatal period, along with the newly-born infant. By 1983, midwives still held a subordinate role in antenatal care, with management of women in labour controlled by members of the medical profession, and postnatal care, particularly in hospital, subject to hospital policies.[6]

Opinions of midwifery practice varied. Many midwives practising across the UK on the district in the post-war years did so autonomously.[7] Oral testimonies also depict midwives working very hard, especially intranatally and postnatally, some in extreme circumstances but making autonomous decisions while still under the control of their LSA. In contrast, Ann Oakley, historian and sociologist, has emphasised the restrictions on midwives.[8] Evidence suggests that both points of view are right. These views highlight contrasts in midwifery practice which varied from place to place within the UK and across Continental Europe. Within Scotland, these contrasts existed in all areas of midwifery practice. Student midwives' Blue Books demonstrated contrasts in antenatal care from town to town, varying from care in municipal clinics to none at all. In rural areas, disparity also existed. Sometimes GPs and midwives appeared to work together, as Ella Clelland demonstrated in Callander. However, other oral testimonies revealed tensions where some GPs did not like working with certified midwives and some did not believe what the midwife had to say. Sometimes there was no certified midwife and howdies looked after mothers in childbirth.

History also reflects contrasts in what midwives were trained and officially permitted to do, and what they were allowed to do in practice. Oakley comments that midwives were 'in danger of becoming mere handmaidens to obstetricians,' a fair point, especially as hospitalisation of childbirth increased.[9] Yet oral evidence from midwives on the district revealed an initiative and confidence which diverges from the handmaiden theory. Nevertheless, the continuing issues of where and how women, having a normal labour, should give birth affected midwifery practice and the role of the midwife. Her role as a decision-making professional diminished and became blurred with the change in place of birth from home to the hospital labour ward, medical assumption of responsibility, the development of new technologies, hospital policies and protocols.[10]

Midwives in hospitals found themselves in an uncomfortable situation. They were pulled between obeying hospital policy and meeting mothers' primary needs.[11] Midwives practising on the district had more freedom. They could take account of the individuality of mothers and their situations, and make their own decisions. But as the place of birth changed from home to hospital, the care for mothers over the whole childbearing episode became increasingly fragmented. The role of the community midwife, restricted for a time to postnatal care, became progressively more threatened and denigrated. Early discharge home of many postnatal mothers exacerbated the problem. This dictated the way community midwives practised. In the time available to them, postnatal care was rushed and they finished up giving less care to more mothers.[12]

This apparent loss of autonomy was the price midwives in Scotland paid for a legal identity, acquired initially through the implementation of the 1915 Midwives (Scotland) Act. Although their autonomy was contained within the Act, it was, in practice, nebulous and affected by the provisions of the Act. The paradox of legal autonomy of midwives and legal entitlement of women to choose their maternity care on the one hand, and overall control by the medical profession on the other, existed throughout the time of the CMBS between 1916 and 1983, and led to tensions between obstetricians, GPs, midwives and women.[13] The CMBS, while endeavouring to create a safer environment for mothers in Scotland by placing strict *Rules* on midwifery and eliminating the howdies for the sake of mothers and the livelihood of certified midwives, still insisted that doctors should have overall control of maternity care. The 1937 Maternity Services (Scotland) Act attempted to co-ordinate maternity services. It advocated more partnership-working between maternity care professionals. This short-lived hope for something nearer to parity than midwives were enjoying at the time was dashed after the changes occurring during World War Two, the implementation of the NHS and its tripartite administration, the rise of the GP as first contact for pregnant women, the increasing trend for hospital births, and corresponding medicalisation of maternity care.

Examination of aspects of the history of midwives in Scotland has brought to light fluctuations in midwifery autonomy between 1916 and 1983, when the CMBS oversaw midwifery training and practice in Scotland. These fluctuations can be attributed to changes in legislation and practice in the care of pregnant and childbearing women, the input and opinions of those in other professions, the change in the geographic location of practice, and the actions and attitudes of midwives themselves.

Improved education eventually helped to create greater confidence among midwives although this took time. Midwives' power remained limited. The CMBS itself was answerable to the DHS (latterly the SHHD). Furthermore, within the Board, even as the number of midwives on the Board grew, they remained subordinate to the medical members for many years. Margaret Kitson, a midwife with a long career in midwifery practice and education, recalled: 'When I first joined the Central Midwives Board [in 1973] it was very, very medically dominated. It was necessary, to begin with, ...just to sit down and be quiet and listen.'[14] In clinical practice, the erosion of midwives' responsibilities and skills became increasingly obvious after the coming of the NHS.

In spite of variations in midwives' autonomy and freedom to make decisions about their practice, and the continuing obstacle of medicalisation of childbirth and midwifery, there were signs by the last decade of the CMBS's existence that midwives' confidence in their professional abilities was developing.[15] Firstly, the improved education of midwives and midwife teachers helped midwives to feel more able to stand beside their medical colleagues. This led to a lessening of medical domination. Secondly, the generations changed. Older obstetricians gradually retired and a more equal partnership between midwives and obstetricians developed.[16] Confidence grew in the CMBS, on the UKCC, and was revealed in practice by midwives' actions, attitudes and initiative.[17] Nevertheless, what these midwives also showed was that they still required the blessing of the doctors with whom they worked. So, the 1980s reveals the developing confidence of the midwife, along with increasing autonomy by 1983, but suggests that to capitalise on this, midwives required the goodwill and confidence of themselves and colleagues, other professionals and the women with whom they worked.

Normality in childbirth
The concept of woman-centred care brought with it a different thinking towards pregnancy and childbirth. An important part of the philosophy is that pregnancy, birth and the puerperium are normal life events. In principle, within the notion of normality in childbirth, there is the idea that all women can give birth normally unless or until circumstances say otherwise.[18] The *EGAMS Report* states: 'The promotion of normality in childbirth is integral to a quality maternity service, but it is essential that recognition of the ill mother and infant is paramount.'[19]

The concept of normality in childbirth is a difficult one: the words 'normal', 'natural', 'usual' become mixed together in a melting-pot of definitions.[20] Answers to the question, 'What is normal?' have ranged from, 'a vaginal delivery' to, 'anything that is not a caesarean section.'[21] Similarly, formal definitions all add a different dimension to the idea of normal. For example, normality is, 'the way things are under normal circumstances'; and 'usual, conforming to the usual standard, type or custom; healthy, physically, mentally and emotionally; occurring naturally, maintained or occurring in a natural state.'[22] These definitions, while all correct, are not specific enough to stand alone in the pregnancy and childbirth situation.

The World Health Organisation (WHO) defines normal labour as: 'low risk throughout, spontaneous in onset with the fetus presenting at the vertex, culminating with the mother and infant in good condition.'[23] This definition stresses the physiological with little emphasis on the psychological well-being. Increasingly, the holistic attitude to labour and childbirth is taken into account and an acknowledgement that the experience represents a major *rite de passage* in a woman's life.[24] Over the two decades straddling the millennium differing definitions of normal pregnancy and childbirth have developed. Most have similar philosophies around the words 'normal' and 'natural' and agree on the requirement for positive reductions in unnecessary intervention in, and medicalisation of, childbirth and the requirement for a calm non-threatening environment, the accent on holism, and the use of alternative methods of pain relief with encouragement of mobility.[25] In 2007, the Information Centre for the Maternity Care Working Party (MCWP) adopted a working definition for normal labour and birth and described it as a measurement of the process of labour and not [its] outcomes. The 'normal delivery' group should include women whose labour starts and progresses spontaneously without drugs, and who give birth spontaneously. It should also include women, provided they do not meet the exclusion criteria below, who experience augmentation of labour, artificial rupture of membranes (ARM), entonox inhalational analgesia, opiods, electronic fetal monitoring, managed third stage of labour, antenatal, delivery or postnatal complications including, for example, postpartum haemorrhage, perineal tear, repair of perineal trauma, admission to Special Care Baby Unit (SCBU), or Neonatal Intensive Care Unit (NICU). Exclusion criteria from the 'normal delivery' group include women who experience induction of labour with prostaglandins, oxytocics or ARM, epidural or spinal analgesia, forceps or ventouse delivery, caesarean section and episiotomy.[26]

There are differing opinions therefore of what constitutes normal childbirth. Sandall suggests that it is 'straightforward birth that is as natural as possible, and in which any interventions that are used are evidence-based and do more good than harm.'[27] The concept may also be influenced by further factors, for example culture, geography and obstetric policy.[28] In addition, in the pursuit of woman-centred care, what the woman wants must be taken into account and, while many embrace the 'normal experience', some will opt for a more medicalised approach.

Choice: what the woman wants
At the beginning of the twentieth century, as the social model of maternity care prevailed, most women in Scotland had no alternative about how or where they were cared for in childbirth.[29] Now, women are encouraged to have 'choice in childbirth'. But

for a woman to have choice she needs to know what she is choosing and why. In short, choice had to become 'informed'. This conforms to the concept of woman-centred care. Women in becoming informed became partners in their care rather than merely recipients of care. A woman and her midwife and if necessary, the rest of the maternity care team, through working, discussion and using evidence-based information and care will discover together the appropriate pathway for her.[30] However, there are other factors which might influence a woman's choice. These include geography, risk factors and a woman's acceptance or otherwise of what is the optimum pathway.

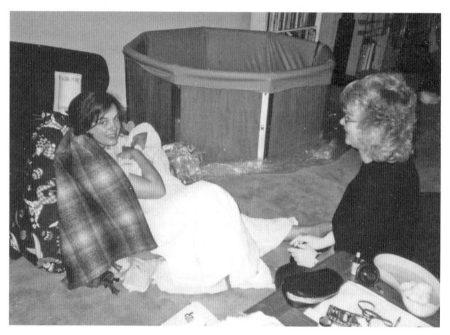

Linda Bryce, midwife, with Catherine Murray John, mother, and baby Alexander. (Courtesy of Linda Bryce and Catherine Murray John.)

Geography
The physical geography of Scotland presents challenges to the maternity services. Bryers argues that remote and rural issues have a direct bearing on the management of maternity services and affect both women and the maternity care team.[31] Women are exposed to the problems of distance and weather, which put limitations on their access to specialist care if necessary. Women who need, or want, to give birth in an obstetric-led unit may have to leave home before the expected date of delivery in order to stay in hospital accommodation and be sure of being there on the day. This then has the added trauma of separation from partners and other children. If a woman goes into labour before her planned move to the 'central' unit, she might face a long, possibly hazardous journey in labour, and the increased risk of a birth en route or unplanned homebirth.[32] Issues surrounding the maternity care team highlight differences in attitudes between those working centrally and locally. Sometimes differing interpretations of evidence-based care challenge maternity

care professionals working in different situations.[33] Other related issues surround the importance and challenge of team-working as well as the development and maintenance of skills, competencies and confidence for staff working in remote and sparsely populated areas. Another challenge is social: to live and work in a small community means building up relationships and this, for the professional, can create social risk.[34] There is no city anonymity in the rural spaces. However, the social space is there for improved partnership-working for further development of remote and rural-friendly maternity services.

It is also necessary to provide urban-friendly maternity services using woman-centred care. Tertiary and many secondary units in Scotland are inevitably in centres of high urban population, and they are sometimes the only local maternity unit for an area. In the years following the turn of the twenty-first century, there was concern over a perceived assumption that tertiary units were all about interventions and consultant control.[35] Latterly, with the emphasis on individualised care, these centres were seen to provide care for women at all levels from high to low risk, for women who present with very complex medical and obstetric histories, to those who need midwifery-only care to give birth safely and normally.[36] Perception nonetheless lingers as Ruby explained:

> I would have a client coming in from the ...peripheral [rural] unit with huge anxiety... I think they're scared they're going to be medicalised. And then they get here and they think, 'Ooh,' [and give] a big sigh of relief. They've got it built up in their head. That's an aspect that...needs addressing.[37]

However, when a woman is transferred to a consultant-led unit from a CMU, or from a planned home labour, then the very fact that all is not going to plan will create anxiety even if, in the end, she gives birth normally. Many of these units have adjacent midwife-led units or 'normality rooms' which seem to engender less anxiety. Claire described them: 'They are just a little bit nicer than the other rooms ...with the bed out of the way with a throw over it, a rocking chair, a bean bag, and a mat, all those kind of things.'[38]

Ruby commented:

> the city women [as opposed to those transferred from rural areas] who come to the midwife-managed unit [within the tertiary unit]...they are ready for that. That's in their head. That's what they're going to do. They're having a baby. That's what their choice is.'[39]

Risk

For a long time, the concept of risk has been the driver of how maternity services were run in Scotland. The Encarta Dictionary simply and primarily defines risk as, '[The] chance of something going wrong; the danger that injury, damage, or loss will occur.'[40] Parliamentary agreement to the passing of the 1915 Midwives (Scotland) Act was based on the perceived risk posed to women in Scotland when many members of the medical profession were on World War One military service and when most midwives were unqualified and unregulated. The strict provisions of the 1915 Act, and subsequent *Rules* of the CMBS, were premised on the concept of risk. Of particular concern to the CMBS was the risk posed by previously uncertified midwives, the *bona fides* who could, at the time, become certified without examination.

Bryers examines the concept of risk and how risk concepts and theories have influenced maternity services.[41] She associates Pickstone's three phases, equating to the changes in health services over the twentieth century, with stages of risk development: 'productionist', 'communitarian' and 'consumerist'.[42] The productionist agenda is associated with the early growth of a risk society.[43] This was made more urgent by the poor physical health of the population and high early twentieth-century maternal and infant mortality rates. While it could be said that measures to improve health in general, and maternal and infant health in particular, were for the sake of the beneficiaries, they could also be seen as governmental means of societal management and control.[44]

The communitarian phase can be seen as a progress towards a state of social solidarity by means of either charity or through the development of public services like the Highlands and Islands Medical Service (HIMS) and the NHS.[45] The young NHS, created during this phase, was class-ridden, paralleling post-World War Two British society, and doctor-driven.[46] In maternity services, midwives could only come a poor second to the perceived expertise of socially highly-ranking consultant obstetricians and the 'doctor knows best' culture of the day.[47]

The consumerist phase illustrates the population from the 1960s tending to take good health for granted.[48] Attitudes changed and medicine became a commodity. This also marked the beginning of a public watchfulness and an emerging dissatisfaction and eventual challenging of the medicalised approach to childbirth.[49]

Bryers suggests that perceptions of risk vary depending on the viewpoint of the society or profession or individual.[50] From this, as far as childbirth is concerned, there seems to be a natural division of thinking between obstetricians and midwives when it comes to attitudes to, and models of, care in pregnancy and childbirth. Nevertheless, within each profession there are some individuals who embrace the philosophy of the opposing model and who prefer to work within it.

Risk assessment depends in some measure on human judgement, decision making and subjective and objective opinions.[51] As already shown by midwives' testimonies, sometimes members of the medical profession did not agree with midwives' assessment.[52] The coming of the NHS in 1948 handed much maternity care impetus to obstetricians and GPs, and removed strength from midwives. Mortality and morbidity statistics were used to extrapolate results which treated many childbearing women as unnecessarily high-risk. Their individuality was lost and birth moved into hospital.[53] Intuition, experience, environmental influence, and social factors were subsumed as irrelevant in the face of quantitative statistics denoting a perceived risk and which played a significant role in the medicalisation of childbirth.[54] Birth was no longer seen as a normal physiological episode in a woman's life. It was only normal in retrospect.

Education and research have been empowering for midwives. So too has been the developing respect for midwifery, as midwives became accepted for their abilities to assess risk. Charlie commented:

> The process of clinical risk – incident reporting and the need for risk discussions, [and] management... That, I think, has improved professional respect and intra-professional working... It's been a challenge. But most of the people leading the clinical risk incident reporting have been midwives so

I think they have had a challenge to make sure that this isn't just a process within midwifery – that this is across the professions, but I think they're getting there. They're building lots of bridges.[55]

A woman's choice: the optimum pathway

The *KCND Pathways* set out a recommended route for care of women in pregnancy and childbirth. Its woman-centred service promotes ongoing risk assessment and uses evidence-based care which makes sure women have the appropriate professional support at all times during their maternity care. To be truly woman-centred can sometimes present a difficult challenge. This intensifies with Scotland's geographical diversities, allowance for risk factors, sometimes high maternal expectations, and the possibility that a woman might not want what the professional thinks she will want. Charlie observed:

> ...I don't think that you can assume that [all] women want the same. There has been...an assumption that women want midwifery-only care without intervention, without the benefits of mechanical or pharmaceutical drug therapy... In reality many women want that from the outset. [They] don't think that they should suffer in labour, so they want the epidural early, not just when someone thinks that it is indicated. They want their baby induced when it's convenient for the family to have that baby... You can put forward all the arguments, but they're not necessarily going to be persuaded... [It is] the same as the women who want an elective section. The...'too posh to push' argument – should we deny their choice?
>
> I think all you can do, if you're going to promote a woman-led service where there's choice, is put forward the evidence for and against what they're choosing. If you can satisfy yourself that they have considered that information and understand the consequences, then I think...you have to give them the service that they want. Who are we as professionals to stand in superior judgement of them?[56]

Ruby, discussing homebirth, agreed that women should have the service that they want:

> I am [happy with the idea of homebirth]. And if they want a home[birth], you say, 'that's fine' and you go through the process. [Then] if you came across a stumbling block you [might say], 'Perhaps that's not the best, given your history, whatever.' They would hear you out...and at the end of the day they either take your advice or they don't. You would just advise them of the professional [opinion] or under the circumstance, 'I think it's great, we'll just plan for that, that's super,' or you say, ' Well, I'm sorry, my professional opinion would be that I don't think this is a good option for you because of X, Y and Z.' They do what they will with your information. And I think you just have to... remind yourself that you can't afford to be judgemental. You have to maintain a good relationship with her...no matter what [decision she makes]. You might not like it...I've had [to be] in situations I wouldn't have chosen to be in. But who does? At the end of the day, it's all part of it isn't it?[57]

Ruby added:

> I think patients can say what they want, [and] should be offered [the information] to make that choice. I don't really see any barriers to that across Grampian. I feel in the Highlands and Islands you might have a different situation.[58]

Bryers echoed this important point when she referred to possible difficulties of maternity service provision in different remote situations.[59]

Acknowledgement of a woman's right to choose, is part of acknowledging women's (and in the wider Health Service, patients') part in the care of their own person, and their responsibility for themselves. Grace commented:

> ...Women are responsible as well [as] the one who is guiding the care, because even within somebody with the worst and most complex history...who might say I don't want A or B, how can you ever make her do things which she doesn't want to do? So we are guidance here.[60]

So, maternity care in the new millennium seems to be changing because of what women want, and professional acknowledgement that women, as long as they have and understand all the relevant information, have a right to choose what they want. In addition, maternity care is changing according to changes in the clientèle and their needs. Charlie said:

> [As well as] social dis-ease ... you also have older women and women with pre-existing heart and liver conditions who wouldn't necessarily have had the opportunity of a pregnancy before and now do, but it needs a lot more medical, and consequently midwifery, management and surveillance ...to bring about their safe delivery. I think the continuum is getting longer...diverging, and therefore the midwifery profession has to diverge or extend.[61]

Working together in the first decade – with women

The current attitude of guidance rather than overbearance, individualised woman-centred care rather than the same routine for all, seems to be in the ascendancy. This attitude is a far cry from the days when professionals and their protocols had to be obeyed. Now the accent is on partnership, not only between maternity care professionals, but between the members of the multi-professional team, whether singularly or collectively, with the women in their care: a woman-centred model.

Midwives have always worked with women. That has not changed, just as the physiological mechanism of normal birth has not changed. The place where a woman gives birth in Scotland has changed from an estimated ninety-five percent homebirths in the first decade of the twentieth century to approximately 1.46 percent homebirths in 2008 with pockets of increased incidence in different areas.[62] However, the incidence of births in CMUs and other midwifery-led units is rising, helped by the changing culture towards midwife-led and woman-centred care. However, most births in Scotland still take place in a maternity unit but, as Grace said, that does not mean that a normal birth should be any less normal:

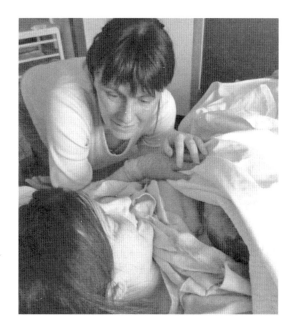

Jenny Patterson, midwife, with Susan Sanders, mother, and baby Katherine. (Courtesy of Jenny Patterson and Susan Sanders.)

The majority of women in Scotland...have their babies in hospital. If we believe that there is a physiology of normal labour and birth...then that experience should be the same whether in hospital or at home. [Coming] into hospital should not alter what nature has put together. So [a woman] should be able to have her baby in the same way with the same principles and ethos of care, support and attention that we associate with a home setting. The natural process should be exactly the same whether in hospital or at home, and whether it's delivered by a midwife or an obstetrician. Normal physiology is normal physiology. As professionals within the service, we should be working with that... Any action to change or intervene should come only if it's required.[63]

However, Grace pointed out that a hospital may present a problem which could alter the course of labour:

It is an abnormal environment. Taking someone from a known comfortable, environment... and bringing her into [one] with unknown people, smells, sights and sounds... could potentially hamper the body's natural responses to the onset of labour. We see that... [often] when someone comes in, the contractions have stopped. But our job...is to acknowledge this, ...build relation-ship and trust, create a safe, pleasant environment, even if it's not her living-room, show kind, caring and interested practice and then, hopefully, the process can start again and continue normally... Our challenge is, [with] the right ethos and principles of care, to make the labouring and birthing environment better within a hospital... I believe you can... We need to make sure that care in hospital is as good as at home.[64]

The ethos of the *KCND* programme rests on the desire to acknowledge and maintain normality in pregnancy and childbirth if possible, to acknowledge where this is not possible and, in the interests of dynamism in woman-centred care, to be able to offer relevant multi-professional care. Health, social, and population changes as well as women's choices, acting together or separately, demonstrate clearly the need to acknowledge that woman-centred care requires the use of obstetric as well as midwife-led units and the expertise of those who work in them. Not all midwives are happy working in 'high-tech' units, just as some midwives who work in an obstetric-led unit would be uncomfortable attending a homebirth. Ella Clelland, who worked in Callander in the 1980s, epitomised this feeling when she had to take a labouring woman from the security of home to hospital. She said:

> Modern labour rooms are quite different from what I remember and when Sister came on she was saying, 'Well this is the room, here is this machine, here is the oxygen, here is this, here is that, here is the thing for checking the bilirubin, blood gases and all.' My eyes were like organ stops and I said, 'I've just discovered I don't know how to work the bed-pan machine let alone all this. There's no way you are leaving me with that lot.' However, put me on top of Ben Ledi with somebody having twins and I would be able to cope.[65]

When the term 'woman-centred' care first became used, the drive for continuity, change and new schemes of care seemed to pursue the idea that to be complete, midwives should be competent in all areas of midwifery. The hope and excitement of the notion of woman-centred care became partially subsumed for many midwives in the stress and burnout which followed.[66] Now, the *KCND Pathways* have the ability to allow women to move between midwifery-led and multi-professional (which also includes midwives) team care depending on need. From this follows the possible conclusion and acknowledgement that midwives have preferences about not only where, but also how, they work. Charlie commented:

> If we have a hub and spoke organisation of delivery units – a 'hub' [giving] multi-professional care because of pathology or need – ...through a process of risk assessment and triage, the women who do not need ...multi-professional care can be safely cared for by midwives in a 'spoke' of CMUs or midwife-led birth units. With that framework, the women who should be coming in to the...hub are...the high-dependency case list or potential risk cases. That would be the theory if that system [were] working fully. So you then have to consider...'What is a midwife?'[67]

The World Health Organisation (WHO) and the International Confederation of Midwives (ICM) have agreed definitions on the role and responsibilities of a midwife.[68] Yet one of the sub-groups of *Midwifery 2020* has discussed the re-definition of a midwife. Charlie commented:

> Look at the midwives [who] care for women in a collaborative manner with obstetricians and anaesthetists and deal with all their pathologies. Is that midwife the same midwife that we need to care for the low risk women? This midwife is working much more autonomously. Are the skills, the knowledge

and the experience the same? ...The knowledge and the skills [to be a midwife] start out the same, but if you have these centres of intervention as tertiary units are becoming, then these midwives need something different. They don't need the social, the psychological support to support a woman through a long and difficult labour without epidural or opiate. They need knowledge and skills of high-dependency care and that's not what we're predominantly teaching in midwifery.[69]

Charlie pointed out that the skills required for each area of midwifery are different and said that some skills may appeal to some midwives but not to others. Nevertheless, they are all midwives.[70]

This returns the discussion to the diversities between the obstetric/medical model and the social/midwifery model. There is a growing body of opinion agreeing the need for maternity care to be provided along the range of care, from a social to a medical model.[71] If this were to be followed, woman-centred care in Scotland would provide a variety of maternity care between low and high risk, would enable women to have local access to Level I maternity care, the spoke (low risk); and access to Level II or III , the hub (high risk) services when necessary.

Although the *KCND Pathways* and their principles of care are in use across Scotland, the system is not the same in all health board areas. For example, Grampian's 'hub' in Aberdeen has 'spokes' radiating from it as far as Elgin sixty-six miles away on the mainland, and Lerwick 217 miles away by sea or air. Lothian, however, has two well-supplied units, one Level III in Edinburgh with some midwife-led rooms, one Level IIc maternity unit but currently no CMU. Charlie commented, 'This [hub and spoke] is a growing organisation of services but it is not predominant in Scotland yet.'[72] However, Grace demonstrated her desire to promote normal birth within her level IIc unit when she said:

We have nine labouring rooms and two pools. All our rooms are normal birth rooms. So, that's what I'm saying, in theory if you are in labour and all is well it doesn't matter what room you're in.[73]

Ruby agreed that different thinking appears in different areas of Scotland. She said:
It fits with KCND. Just equitable care...trying to spread out... [Given the geography] I don't think realistically we'll ever provide equitable care across Scotland... We have to accept that homebirths in one of the remote islands on the north coast is a difficult care-pattern to provide because it means flying midwives on and off the island every 24 hours, ...but [even though] there are geographical complications, we've now got a universal set of notes for women to use [known as hand-held notes]. That's a standardised package... [It contains] care aspects which include the pattern that's laid out across Scotland so...it sets out the standard of care. I think that's really positive.[74]

Charlie also thought positively and highlighted the standard:
If you look at the pathway and [are] shown [the woman's] notes – they're based on the assumption that you're assessing risk at every contact with the

woman and making sure that the care is appropriate and provided by the best person for the job.[75]

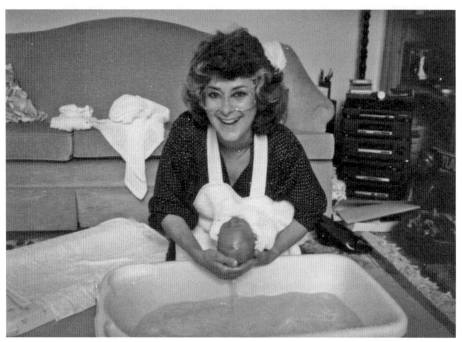

Cara with midwife Linda Bryce. (Courtesy of Linda Bryce and Claire Burnet, mother).

Working together in the first decade – with other professionals

Working within the *KCND Pathways* involves the use, when necessary, of referral from one member of the team to another. It also involves working together with mutual respect and partnership. Up until the later decades of the twentieth century, a midwife could neither refer a woman directly to hospital nor call out a flying squad. Anne Bayne, working in Tullibody in the 1950s, commented that 'it was shocking then that you couldn't, on your own, call out a flying squad and a doctor couldn't phone from home... [He] had to say, 'Yes I've been to see her. Yes, we need the flying squad.'[76]

The situation has moved on from that time. Increasingly, midwives are the lead professionals within the multi-professional team for healthy women with uncomplicated pregnancies. They work within a shared philosophy of practice that supports, protects and maintains normality. Although pregnant women may choose to see their GP and obstetrician if they wish, *KCND* aims for most to use midwives as the first point of contact.[77] Midwives then have the responsibility of providing a woman with current evidence-based information and involving her from the beginning with decisions regarding the care of herself and her baby. In theory, members of the multi-professional team are complementary and work together with mutual respect and trust. Charlie commented:

I think services have evolved. There's much more use of clinical risk assessment, referring on, if risk factors are identified... The last Confidential Enquiry [highlighted the need to] make sure that the right professional with the right skills was in attendance, that you referred early, that you didn't wait until there were complications and you were out of your depth before referring on to the right person.[78]

Given the reported reactions of some members of the medical profession when the *Winterton Report* was published, some midwives still appear to feel hesitant about seeking advice of their medical colleagues or making a referral on what would be hoped was an equitable professional footing.[79] However, Grace commented:

> If an obstetrician looking after a woman with a high risk pregnancy had an issue with her that he couldn't deal with by himself, he wouldn't hesitate in making a referral, say, to a cardiologist... It's not really that different [with] a woman who starts off with midwifery-led care [and needs]...input from an obstetrician – that referral is the same. [It's not saying] that the [midwife] can't do their job... I think we need an acknowledgement nationally that professions need to work together in order to deliver a service – there's maybe a difference in interpretation of what working together actually means.[80]

Ruby was positive about referral. She said:

> [I have no problems referring]...and I think this is throughout Grampian. I think it's born out of healthy relationships. Certainly, as a community midwife myself, I never hesitated. I'd pick up the phone, 'Hi, it's me. I've got this lady here, can I...?' – 'Yes no problem.' My colleagues were the same when I was on the community and I can't see that things have changed.[81]

Grace brings the discussion back to guidance at team level with the comment that 'if the guidance [offered to a woman] needs to be assumed [through referral] by different people through the course of a pregnancy, it shouldn't diminish that team at all.'[82] Yet, it still takes time to break down old stereotypes. Ruby commented:

> I think, historically, we were very subservient... We did ourselves no favours... We went about with these silly caps on our heads. Well, that's subservient for a start. It was a very strange set up. So, visually, we looked like maids...subservient to our professional colleagues... That just set the stall out really.[83]

Ruby also commented on the improvement in relationships achieved as midwives have gained a higher level of education, although she added that not everyone would agree with this view. 'There are still dinosaurs around.'[84]

Kirkham suggests that any problems that midwives might have with obstetrics is not medical but social and organisational. She asserts that society in general is very medicalised, not just to do with the medical profession, but as a result of bureaucracy and an industrial model of organisation. This is akin to the productionist and constructivist periods discussed above.[85] In addition, midwives mostly working within the hierarchical settings of a hospital frequently experience problems obeying the protocols of the hierarchy while endeavouring to be 'with woman' in its fullest sense. Kirkham suggests 'striving to see midwifery and medical models as complementary, not as alternatives.'[86] This concurs with Charlie's opinion when discussing the continuum with extremes of models, but within the range, the size of which will fluctuate, differing models could function where necessary in harmony.[87] Given time, willingness and mutual respect, inter-professional working between all members of the multi-professional team should be an accepted reality. Charlie said:

> There is good progress... There have always been tensions between parts of that team – midwifery/obstetrics, midwifery/ general practice and so on... They probably still are there at some level, but I think, if we really want a service which provides truly world-class maternity care for women and their families, then [the team] has to work together with an acknowledgement [and] a respect for each discipline.[88]

Grace agreed:

> I do think [progress has been made from that]. I think there is much closer working together, much closer understanding of the priorities which exist in different professional groups. You can't see the world always through other people's eyes. If you have one world view, it's hard to see another person's, but I think what you have now is a much more willingness to be respectful of that.[89]

Working together in the first decade – leadership and respect
The first decade of the twenty-first century has seen an acknowledgement of the need for strong midwifery leadership in Scotland. This has overtly manifested itself in the appointment of, firstly, midwife consultants and, secondly, sixteen *KCND* midwife consultants who were selected to implement the *KCND Pathways*. With less publicity, but nonetheless valuable, have been the midwives taking on leadership roles in various guises in their place of work. Midwifery leaders have been present since the 1915 Midwives (Scotland) Act in the shape of the Local Supervising Authorities (LSA) and their Inspectors of Midwives (IOM). However, the CMBS considered that midwives were not adequate for the role of IOM and these posts were the province of MOHs and health visitors. Even after the term Supervisor of Midwives (SOM) had taken over from IOM, Mary McCaskill's quote on how she handled a pending inspection indicates a respect for the power that the SOM held, the *Rules* that went with it, and their powers of suspension if she did not obey. But this did not indicate respect for the person of the SOM.[90]

With respect goes trust. Lack of trust in midwives is also historical, shown, for example in strict CMBS *Rules* and a top-down approach to practice which did not begin to disappear until the late twentieth century. Even in the CMBS, for many years midwife members had to sit down, be quiet, and listen.[91] Midwives came from the bottom of the social pile, the Sarah Gamps of the world. Leaders of the nursing profession in the late nineteenth century used every journalistic outlet they could to denigrate and pull them down. A member of the Edinburgh Obstetrical Society thought midwives were 'rather an accident' and was 'waiting for them to die a natural death.'[92] Some of this lack of respect and trust may have been born of jealousy. By the late nineteenth century it was obvious that midwives in England and Wales were going to achieve legal registration well before the nursing profession. Some lack of respect and trust may have been because of fear of loss of earnings as members of the medical profession saw their 'cases' slipping through their fingers into the less expensive hands of the midwifery profession. Some lack of respect and trust may also have been born of gender bias. It was Dr Elsie Inglis (1864-1917) who, when volunteering her services as a surgeon in World War One to the Royal Army Medical Corps (RAMC), received the response, 'My good lady, go home and sit still.'[93]

Whatever the reason for lack of respect or trust from others, midwives also need to respect themselves and each other. Charlie commented:

> The midwives' profession hasn't really been good to itself has it? ...I've always said that, if we had professional respect within our profession, we would be so much stronger and be able to overcome the challenges.[94]

This is an important point which in itself is a challenge. Katy said:

> I think we have to challenge people. [Sometimes things are said]... It's unacceptable to speak to somebody in that manner. There is a way to speak to somebody... We could start with, from the head of midwifery down, treating each other with respect and [foster] respect and dignity in the workplace. They're trying to do these things. Everybody has to do it... Starting off, [by] treat[ing] our students well.[95]

Katy made the last comment because she had had to deal with a traumatised student midwife with memories of a bad previous experience. There are plenty of anecdotes relating treatment meted out to students, but there is another side too. Claire commented:

> Even when it got to third year and I had my own views about certain things for delivery... I think it's the way we [those in my set] managed to do it. Not be arrogant or rude and just put it across to her [midwife in charge] in a nice way. If we'd been looking after the women for the majority of the shift and someone was coming in [to supervise]... It's about how you put it.[96]

Ruby saw working with students and others as an important part of the senior midwife's remit and said, 'Our consultant midwife... She would come and work as in 'work', hands on, with the woman and with a student, guiding other midwives.'[97] She also remarked on the importance of good leadership:

> I think now, more than ever... good positive leadership is an imperative. Leadership takes many guises – [some are] not the kind of leader you want. But in our setting we need positive, forward thinking, really gutsy people, not to go off on one, but really open-minded and aware of the broader picture... Leadership in the past has been very much experiential. To work for ten years and get a promoted position wasn't really thoughtful. I think that was...to our detriment... Any position needs to be well thought out... I think

that is happening...now. This is about having...the desired attributes to lead.[98]

Ruby then made the link between leadership and respect:

> Back in 1981, ward sisters, as they were called then, were very visible. Visibility led to credibility because that's how people function... That's still very much the case. It's about the visibility factor. [You need to be] visible in a clinical area. I read this quote: 'Delegation works if the person who is delegating works'... That's so true. You gain respect, that person gains credibility. The ward sister was incredibly visible, she was very much a leader and teacher... You'd high regard and the utmost respect for these people. They are now becoming visible again.[99]

Good leadership can also lead by example at all levels across the multi-professional team. Grace advocated diplomacy:

> You never change anything by being aggressive in your approach. Being more diplomatic may take longer, but it possibly will [be more successful]... I think we've become better at doing that. We need to be direct but take account of other people's feelings and thoughts. ...be prepared to work together and I...see this happening... I do see the intent to hear everybody's viewpoint. If there is a change in practice, or a new idea, we discuss it first. It is about inclusion, talking together, getting the best, being more cohesive.
>
> I see the desire...to work together for the benefit of women. You need to be respectful of people's egos, but what I see now in midwives is, particularly if they have good leadership, much more of a willingness to put forward their ideas, to articulate their thoughts on a better service for women. They're bringing ideas forward in a non-aggressive way. There's much more awareness of the potential of midwifery and...much more confidence in the potential values of good midwifery. Midwives are still realising that potential, but there's real confidence there at all levels. It fits with the ethos of the KCND programme. [It] acknowledges midwifery's place within maternity care and encourages good dialogue between professional groups for the better provision of care for women and their families. It has been a very beneficial programme from a midwifery point of view. Just acknowledging the need for [KCND] consultant midwives says something about midwifery practice in Scotland and offers another resource to the maternity service. It has also given midwifery a very good career pathway. All round, I think it's wonderful for women.[100]

Working together in the first decade – the teaching role, mentors and role models
From the beginning of their student days midwives are taught that they are also teachers: of women, students of any kind, other midwives and doctors. The Scottish Multi-professional Maternity Development Programme (SMMDP) runs an Instructors' Training Course that has helped many midwives teach on further courses and in their daily work. Charlie described the benefits:

Their confidence grew and professional respect was shared... Two midwives from a CMU said that being trainers had brought a whole new aspect to their professional life [and] place of work... They found that their confidence, working inter-professionally, was much better... [This happened] in different ways. They had used the techniques they had learned as instructors back in their work place and found it worked and people were coming to them asking them to do a session on that in the work place or apply it to something else.

A midwife who became an instructor for the 'Examination of the Newborn Course' was now acknowledged by paediatricians as experts in examination of the newborn and [was] asked to train the junior medical staff. [She was] being consulted upon, for instance, if they were examining a baby. That's been very empowering for some of them... That's been another vehicle for inter-professional training and working.[101]

All student midwives in Scotland, as well as many midwives in new posts, have a named mentor who has passed a mentorship course to guide their progress. Claire had two in the course of her training:

To begin with, we followed our mentors in all areas. My first placement was just to be with her... I helped at about five hands-on births before the first Christmas. She was very good – she said I was like a scared rabbit. For the first year I think I probably was, but she was very good at helping me. We observed deliveries first, then she did some, with her hands over mine, and then, we were on nightshift the first time and she said, 'Right, we're not going to call another midwife, you deliver and I'll conduct the delivery.' I still remember that... Then I was given another mentor who then stayed with me right the way through. She also was lovely. I was lucky.[102]]

Claire's next quote demonstrates how a mentor can be a role model and how easily a different procedure could have been followed depending upon the midwife in charge:

[The woman] had a lovely [birth] on all fours leaning over on the beanbag and I put the baby through her legs and she had skin to skin [contact] immediately. [I] didn't touch the cord...because – there was no need and [the mother had mentioned a natural third stage]. The baby went to the breast and fed immediately. Everything was set for natural third stage... She was happy, the baby was feeding, she was comfortable... [My mentor] agreed with me and said that everything was fine and just to leave the cord attached. Baby was feeding well and then, after about half an hour, she said, 'Oh, I think, I feel a fullness,' and she just kneeled up and the placenta came out. We really hadn't done anything. So then we cut the cord and it was wonderful for that girl because I think the first time round everything had been so 'done to her'. I was pleased because I felt that we had executed her birth plan well and she felt happy... My mentor was really excited for us... A natural third stage is such a rarity in most places and I was so pleased. It was just wonderful and really what she wanted.

I feel if I'd had a mentor with a different opinion who believed in active third stage...[the woman] would have had an active third stage when she didn't need or want it. With much credit to the midwife, I think that she was fine with it, she didn't try and overrule. It could have been very different.[103]

'We're getting stronger as a profession...'

I feel very positive about midwifery today [2010]. I think we are coming out of what I consider was a bit of a professional dip in midwifery with a very slow recovery. Then the *Framework*, the *EGAMS Report* and *KCND* all evolved to push that whole mechanism forward and I think that's been hugely positive and a huge boost not only to midwifery. I think our medical and other professional colleagues now have a different approach to us as midwives.[104]

Midwives have seen many challenges since the 1915 Midwives (Scotland) Act and, while it is satisfying to hear good and happy accounts of what is happening in midwifery at the beginning of the twenty-first century, and the *KCND* programme with its *Pathways* has shown every sign of being a success, it is important to remember that there are still challenges to be faced.

One challenge is for midwives, newly-qualified in Scotland, to obtain a post in Scotland. There appear to be more midwives qualifying from Scottish universities than there are posts available. Some new midwives travel to maternity units in England to obtain posts, but this is unsatisfactory when their homes are in Scotland.[105] Claire, who did not have a post when she qualified in 2009, and who sees her career pathway to be in midwife-led care, emailed recently:

I have managed to get a job. I shall be working...full time. I'm not sure when I start yet, or how long the contract is initially for (four or twelve months?) but am *very* relieved. It was getting a bit scary. They were able to give some, I'm not sure how many, new midwives' jobs under the Job Guarantee Scheme, as I believe the normal funding is insufficient at the moment in most places... [I'm] so happy the scheme is in place in Scotland or I wouldn't have a post yet, or perhaps ever.[106]

It follows, therefore, that midwives are only too happy to get a job, to the extent that they will accept what is offered as long as it is as a midwife. This raises a question regarding the possible effect that this could have on midwives' dreams or aspirations about where and how they work. Charlie discussed midwives and where they worked on the range of models and how they reached that point:

Most hospitals have core staff who don't...rotate round departments. Or, in a team organisation there will be some core staff and the other team members will rotate between community and in-hospital care. So, some people aspire to a core post where they are experienced, consolidating, doing the type of midwifery that they wish to and that may be in an obstetric-led labour ward or midwives-led unit... So they are different people... and the requirements of those two people are different... I don't know at what point they become different ... When they're newly qualified...do they feel able to work right across that spectrum? And, as they work through their post-registration experience, do they devolve along that continuum because of their experience and their job opportunities? Or, do they actually pursue their career differently?[107]

The challenge of the continuum is an important one. Should midwives be able to find and settle to work where they feel most comfortable, at either end, or at some point in the middle? It does not happen like that as Charlie explained:

They may just evolve into that role [in an obstetric-led department]... In some units, the staffing in the midwife-led units can be quite a strong core and it can be some time before vacancies occur. Therefore it's difficult for midwives, who see that as their ideal role, to get into a midwife-led unit and...it may be easier for them to get into another rotational post, rather than to be a core midwife.[108]

Another challenge, linked to the range and models of care, belongs to the use of peripheral midwife-led units and CMUs: the hub and spoke analogy. Using this system, *KCND* pathways, with the two-way referral process in use if necessary during pregnancy are employed. If all is well, labour is expected to be normal and plans go ahead for normal birth in as local a situation as possible. However, there may be differences in attitudes between midwives giving midwifery-led care locally and those in the maternity care team in the central unit with a possible clash of interpretation of evidence-based care. This can lead to confusion and lack of confidence. Charlie commented that she wondered if midwives are at risk of 'moving into a two-tone midwifery'. This point was made in relation to the diverging of midwives on the continuum, which is increasingly evident. However, she added:

There's not a hierarchy. One is not better than or superior to the other. The demands are different... They [midwives in obstetric-led care] work more in collaboration with the others...rather than in the more autonomous sphere that we have around midwifery...and may need to do an additional [skills] training... It's no different from the midwife [who] wants to do midwifery-led care   then she may well do [an] additional course in aromatherapy or waterbirth or hypno-birthing... I would be ...concerned that those in control and power and influence...may see it as a hierarchy. I would like to consider that those midwives who are leading the field in midwifery-led care are acknowledged as experts.[109]

Those 'in control and power and influence' over midwifery, and the varied care that midwives give should be ideally, midwives, who understand what it is that a midwife is and does. However, this does not always happen. In the 1960s, midwives in Scotland found themselves losing administrative autonomy which filtered from management into education of midwives as well. That anxiety continued to exist fifty years later. No philosophy of care, and those who choose to work within it, is necessarily better than the other or whatever lies in between. As Katy said, 'It's not a competition.

It's not consultant units versus [CMUs]. We're working together, ensuring the women get the correct care suitable for their needs.'[110] Yet, the difficulty lies in persuading others, especially in difficult financial times. Charlie commented:

> [We need more funding] because it is a woman-to-woman service or a midwife-to-woman service and so you need the midwives on the floor to be able to provide that care. [Low staffing levels] are because of lack of funding and I think there is lack of understanding of how intensive it is... to provide midwifery care. A health service manager who applies a non-midwifery work tool to calculate staff sees this big number of staff – midwives, in comparison with nurses providing another aspect of the health service that they're responsible for and they don't necessarily understand the need. There's been a lot of work done on midwifery workforce tools to try and get a more robust workforce tool (across the UK). But...that tool itself was devised for a more hospital-orientated service and so much of the care now is community-led. Added to that, the community can be far-flung...the rurality aspect of midwifery community care wasn't catered for... That had to be factored in and the workforce tool adjusted. So now...it's been applied again to ... calculate the needs of the service. But health service managers are commissioned to find a cut in services. And it's very difficult for the health economies to do that.[111]

This highlights, firstly, the challenge for midwives faced with management from other professionals who do not understand the needs of the service nor midwifery practice. The 2010 plans for the Refreshment of the *Framework* would be an appropriate opportunity to make a further case for midwifery leaders to have a higher profile within management so that a midwifery voice can be heard at the highest level. The second challenge is the tension between acute maternity services and the drive to make financial savings. Here again, midwife leaders need to be heard at the top table. For instance, CMUs are highly regarded but are seen to have high staffing costs, especially if only the birth numbers and not their total caseload are considered. Katy agreed that the service provided by a CMU is quite expensive but argued:

> A CMU gives a really good service and I think it's worth it. The money's now, but if you think of the health benefits... [It's keeping] the costs neutral... It balances out. I think women's self-esteem is boosted. Generally...there is much less likelihood of maternal morbidity, long-term.[112]

Consequently, the development of midwifery as a strong profession, supported by midwifery leadership at national and health board levels, will impact on improving health and well-being of individual women and families; and at a population level, of Scotland as a whole, and the future generation.[113] However, a senior midwife arguing for the continuing existence of a CMU, or for more midwives in any maternity unit, has a real fight on her hands to be heard at health board level. This contrasts with the clout of a doctor or a general manager. This is about recognised leadership and respect for what midwives are actually doing.

Another challenge is to do with education of midwives and the link between university and the clinical areas. Claire acknowledged that an attempt was made:

> Our midwife skills facilitator...was a teacher either in the skills part of the 'uni' or in the hospital. [Also] some of the midwives came up to the university to teach us from the hospital... There was a little bit of coming and going. I think I would have preferred more...to maybe align things a bit. Yes, I think we need more...communication between them.[114]

Ruby felt that there was a lack of togetherness between the midwives of the university staff and those of the clinical areas, and that university staff should be more visible in the clinical areas. She said, 'My perception is it's about the visibility factor. So, if you're not visible in a clinical area, you lose credibility.'[115]

A big difficulty seems to be matching what is taught in the classroom with what is taught in the clinical area. Claire said, 'We realised that a lot of the things that we were taught in the university weren't carried out in practice.' However she added, 'But we tried to think in a positive way, how can we go in and help these things change?'[116] To effect change was also the way to go for Katy:

> We'd get student midwives saying, 'I'm really disillusioned with midwifery because none of what we've been taught in the class...all these fantastic things... And we go into reality and it's not like that.' So we [decided to] have a study day once a year for students, no mentors, purely students...with the midwives who work here... [The students come from] different hospitals all over Scotland. We'll have fifty places on it. It's about what midwifery's about, about working together...about how people perceive midwifery... It's been amazing. Every year – this is the third or the fourth year – as soon as you mention it we've got all the places booked.[117]

Katy also was positive about the progress of students:

> Students are now much more vocal. I remember going to a conference in England and thinking, 'their students are really confident.' But I noticed ours are changing. The students are becoming more vocal and appear to be happier... I think things are improving... They seem to be much more normality-focussed and happier and more confident than previously.[118]

Last words – for the moment...

Midwives have proved themselves very able to speak up for themselves. This book has followed the changes in midwifery in Scotland, to a great extent through their voices, opinions and narratives of their experiences. The last words here are left for midwives to comment on changes and improvements that they see in maternity care in Scotland, and their hopes for, and importance of, midwifery as a profession.

Claire commented on changes in the three years that she was a student midwife:

> Midwifery became even more special for me when I realised how much satisfaction I got from it... I feel like putting a sticker on the wall that says, 'Remember how excited and wonderful you thought this was. Don't lose that.' You look back to first year and think, 'Oh, I can really see how I've

grown...' In third year, I started to get real satisfaction out of what I was doing and I felt that I was working positively for the woman...'

I also felt more able in third year to speak up for women. It was a turning point, the day when I was brave enough to say, 'This is what this lady wants,' and she was able to have it. To begin with, every woman I delivered was in the semi-recumbent position. Then I helped women birth in left lateral, on knees, leaning over the bed, standing, all sorts of different positions... I think it was because I was able to assert more. We should be able to work round what the woman feels she wants. Things certainly changed [with *KCND*], but it depends on the midwife [and her attitude]. I think *KCND* is only as good as the people who are going to take it on, and some midwives in Scotland are more accepting of *KCND* than others. I can see it moving forward, but slowly... I would like to be one of the strong midwives like my community midwife.[119]

Lack of integration of maternity services was historically a problem which fragmented care. Charlie commented on how this has improved:

There is greater integration between hospital and primary care through the conduit of the midwife. Midwives are moving in and around both environments. You'll still get midwives predominantly community-based, or hospital-based but do a bit of community. But, although it'll be different in different geographical areas, I think there is better information, communication and more symmetry of care between one and the other.[120]

Ruby commented on how positive and optimistic she felt for midwifery in Scotland, adding:

My big hope is for the body of midwives to continue to get stronger mentally and as a profession... Midwives have to take responsibility, look at their practice and evaluate it properly – not just do it because we've always done it... We're evolving, but I think there's a lot to be done yet. As a body of professionals, we very much need to have strong leaders and enthusiastic motivators, individuals to take us forward without being threatening... Everybody has a contribution and it's about getting the right dynamics. We must get our house in order and approach any changes and their politics in a positive manner. We must progress, do more midwifery driven research... Blow our own trumpet... Keep going.[121]

Katy commenting on midwifery and maternity care across Scotland, said:

I don't think it needs to be the same throughout Scotland. There are all sorts of different models to use within women's choice and woman-centred care. I'm the eternal optimist... Yes, we're in uncharted water financially...but if you think of the public health benefits of a normal birth...I think it balances out. Women's self-esteem is boosted generally and, if you've had a normal birth, there is much less likelihood of long term maternal morbidity... You can't overestimate how important it is that a woman has good self esteem and feels happy about her birth.... There's all sorts of good midwifery practice going on throughout Scotland, but we need to bang our own drum. The tall poppy syndrome has to go. Midwives must see that [the] benefit of the service we are giving is positive, life affirming and immense from both the midwife's and the woman's point of view.[122]

The importance of midwifery also has a wider public health importance and Grace summed this up in her comments:

Part of *Midwifery 2020* deals with the midwife's role in public health... But, just the birth experience is a massive public health issue on its own and women can be profoundly affected by it. No-one ...should have a traumatic birth experience... Even if it's complex, they should not be traumatised by this to the 'nth' degree... That's where midwifery can have a huge impact on public health. Women's health, their long-term health, their relationships... We have a massive role and responsibility there. Perhaps we have not always actually acknowledged the impact of what we do.[123]

Grace also demonstrated how far midwifery in Scotland has come from the early twentieth century until 2010:

Any new guideline needs to reflect sensitive, appropriate care... Things are now not just done because it's 'aye been that way'. I feel quite positive about that. Midwives are much more confident to raise points...in a reasonable, sensitive, diplomatic way... It's not perfect. Nothing is. But the desire is there to work together for the benefit of women. We also have a career pathway that identifies the importance of midwifery to the health of the population. We are growing midwives who are critical articulate thinkers and able to initiate and evaluate change, but in a very positive, proactive way.[124]

Looking at the past is sometimes uncomfortable. Nevertheless, to cherish and appreciate the past with all its varying features, brings knowledge which enables confident progress within the present, and aids positive strong construction and planning for the future. *Midwifery in Scotland: A History* has offered an exploration of aspects of midwifery's history in Scotland since the early twentieth century through archival papers, documents and books, and through the voices of midwives.

This exploration of midwifery history has demonstrated that midwives practise within different models and varying strands of the profession. However, through being with, and caring for and about women around the time of their babies' births, midwives are, through their history, a part of the hope and inspiration for the future.

1.   GRO for Scotland, Mid-2008 Population Estimates Scotland, National Statistics publication for Scotland, (28 April 2009), p 1.
2.   SEHD *A framework for maternity services in Scotland*, (Edinburgh: SEHD 2001), p 25.
3.   Framework, 2001; SEHD, *Report of the Expert Group on Maternity Services in Scotland*, (Edinburgh: SE, 2002).

4.   The voices of five contemporary midwives are introduced by pseudonyms:
     Charlie, Claire, Grace, Katy and Ruby.
5.   The word 'alegal' means neither illegal nor legal.
6.   Scottish Health Service Planning Council, *Shared Care in Obstetrics: A Report
     by the National Medical Consultative Committee*, (Edinburgh: SHHD, 1983),
     para 1.6.
7.   J Allison, *Delivered at Home*, (London: Chapman and Hall, 1996).
8.   Oakley, *Captured Womb*.
9.   *Ibid*, p 76.
10. R Mander, 'Autonomy in midwifery and maternity care', in *Midwives Chronicle*,
     (October, 1993), pp 369-374.
11. S Hunt, A Symonds, *The Social Meaning of Midwifery*, (Basingstoke: McMillan
     Press, 1995), p 141; T Murphy-Black, 'Care in the community in the postnatal
     period', in S Robinson, A Thomson (eds), *Midwives, Research and Childbirth,
     Vol 3*, (London: Chapman and Hall, 1994), pp 120-146.
12. Murphy-Black, *'Care in the community in the postnatal period'*, pp 120-146; M
     McGuire, *Community postnatal care provision in Scotland: the development and
     evaluation of a template for the provision of woman-centred community
     postnatal care*, unpublished PhD thesis, (University of Glasgow: 2001), p 28.
13. J Garcia, R Kilpatrick, M Richards, (eds), *The Politics of Maternity Care*,
     (Oxford: Clarendon Press, 1990), p 2; Mander, *'Autonomy in midwifery and
     maternity care'*, pp 369-374.
14. LR 120.
15. E van Teijlingen, G Lowis, P McCaffery, M Porter, *Midwifery and the
     Medicalization of Childbirth: Comparative Perspectives*, (New York: Nova
     Science Publishers, 2000), p 1, defines medicalisation of childbirth and
     midwifery as: 'the increasing tendency of women to prefer a hospital delivery to
     a home delivery, the increasing trend toward the use of technology and clinical
     intervention in childbirth, and the determination of medical practitioners to
     confine the role played by midwives in pregnancy and childbirth, if any, to a
     purely subordinate one.'
16. LR 120.
17. For example, Chapter 4, endnote 97, LR 116; chapter 4, endnote 102, LR 9;
     chapter 7, endnote 46, LR 116.
18. L Reid, *Keeping childbirth natural and dynamic: a resource*, (Edinburgh:
     Scottish Multi-professional Development Programme (SMMDP), 2008) p 11.
19. *EGAMS Report*, Core Principle 7, p 77.
20. Reid, *Keeping childbirth natural and dynamic*.
21. Reid, 'Best practice: aims and realities' in Reid, *Freedom to practise*, p 22.
22. *Encarta World English Dictionary*, (London: Bloomsbury, 1999) p 1290.
23. WHO Department of Reproductive Health and Research, *Care in Normal labour.
     A practical guide*, (WHO Geneva, 1997), quoted in, C McCormick, 'The first
     stage of labour: physiology and early care', in, D Fraser, M Cooper, *Myles
     textbook for midwives (15th ed)* (Edinburgh: Elsevier, 2009), pp 457-475.
24. Cassidy, *Myles Textbook*, 1993, p 149.

25. B Beech, B Phipps, 'Normal births: women's stories', in S Downe (ed) *Normal Childbirth: evidence and debate*, (London: Elsevier, 2004), pp 59-70; RCM, *Vision 2000*, (London: RCM, 2000).
26. Maternity care working party, (MCWP) *Making normal birth a reality, Consensus statement from the MCWP*, (London: National Childbirth Trust, RCM and Royal College of Obstetricians and Gynaecologists, 2007); Reid, *Keeping Childbirth Natural and Dynamic*.
27. J Sandall, 'Promoting normal birth: weighing the evidence', in S Downe (ed), *Normal Childbirth*, pp 161-171.
28. R Mander, 'The midwife and the medical practitioner', in R Mander, V Fleming (eds), *Failure to Progress: the contraction of the midwifery profession*, (London: Routledge, 2002), pp 170-188.
29. Bryers, *Midwifery and Maternity Services*, p 362.
30. *KCND Pathways*, p 2.
31. Bryers, *Midwifery and Maternity Services*, p 360.
32. L Reid, 'Normal birth in Scotland', in L Reid (ed) *Midwifery: Freedom to Practise*, (Edinburgh: Elsevier, 2007), p 254.
33. LR 131; Bryers, *Midwifery and Maternity care*, p 360.
34. *Ibid*; J Tucker, J Farmer, H Bryers, A Kiger, E van Teijlingen, M Ryan, E Pitchforth, *Sustainable maternity service provision in remote and rural Scotland: implementing and evaluating maternity care models for remote and rural Scotland*, (RARARI, Dumfries, 2006), pp 47-49.
35. L Reid, *Scottish normal labour and birth course manual*, (Edinburgh, SMMDP, 2005), p 17.
36. *Ibid*, p 10.
37. LR 133.
38. LR 132.
39. LR 133.
40. *Encarta*, p 1619.
41. Bryers, *Midwives and Maternity Services*, p 86.
42. *Ibid*; J Pickstone, R Cooter, *Medicine in the twentieth century*, (Singapore, Harwood Academic Publishers, 2000) p xiii.
43. P Godin, *Risk and Nursing Practice*, p 7.
44. Bryers, *Midwives and Maternity Services*, p 87.
45. *Ibid*; Pickstone, Cooter, *Medicine in the twentieth century*, pp 3, 13.
46. Bryers, *Midwives and Maternity Services*, p 87.
47. *Ibid*; V Navarro, 'The mode of state intervention in the health sector', in, N Black, D Boswell, A Gray, S Murphy, J Popay, (eds), *Health and disease, a reader* (Milton Keynes, Open University Press, 1984) pp 163-169; Pickstone, Cooter, *Medicine in the twentieth century*, pp 3, 14; A Oakley, 'Doctor knows best', in Black, Boswell, Gray, et al, (eds), *Health and Disease*, pp 170-175; L Chertok, *Motherhood and personality* (London: Tavistock, 1969); *Maternity care in Great Britain: a survey of social and economic aspects of pregnancy and childbirth*, Joint Committee Royal College of Obstetricians and Gynaecologists and the population investigation committee, (London: Oxford University Press,

1948) pp 54, 69.
48. Bryers, *Midwives and Maternity Services*, p 88.
49. J Carter, T Duriez, *With child: Birth through the ages*, (Edinburgh: Mainsteam Publishing, 1986), p 181; Bryers, *Midwives and Maternity Services*, p 88.
50. Bryers, *Midwives and Maternity Services*, p 89.
51. *Ibid*, p 84.
52. See Chapter 4, endnotes 70, 71 and 72; each of these quotes illustrates that the midwife correctly noted the level of risk and the GP dismissed it.
53. Bryers, *Midwives and Maternity Services*, p 89; S Downe, C McCourt, 'From being to becoming: reconstructing childbirth knowledges', in Downe S, (ed) *Normal Childbirth: Evidence and debate*. (London: Churchill Livingstone, 2004), pp 8-9.
54. Bryers, *Midwives and Maternity Services*, p 89.
55. LR 129.
56. *Ibid*.
57. LR 133.
58. *Ibid*.
59. Bryers, *Midwives and Maternity Services*, p 88.
60. LR 130.
61. LR 129.
62. L Reid, *Scottish Midwives 1916-1983*, p 4; www.birthchoiceuk.com/AllReferences.htm#88
63. LR 130.
64. *Ibid*.
65. LR 9.
66. Hillan, McGuire, Reid, *Midwives and Woman-centred care*.
67. LR 129; maternity triage: a process of sorting, through risk assessment and a woman's choice, how she is to be cared for in pregnancy and labour; S Kennedy, 'Telephone triage in maternity care', *Midwives*, (2007), Vol 10 (10), pp 478-480.
68. ICM *Definition of the midwife*, (London: ICM, 2005); WHO, *Definition of the midwife*, (Geneva: WHO 1992).
69. LR 129.
70. *Ibid*.
71. Bryers, *Midwives and Maternity Services*, p 364; D Walsh, M Newburn, 'Towards a social model of childbirth: Part one', *British Journal of Midwifery* (2002), Vol 10 (8), pp 476-481; E van Teijlingen, 'A critical analysis of the medical model as used in the study of pregnancy and childbirth', *Sociological research online*, (2005), http://www.socresonline.org.uk/10/2/teijlingen.html
72. LR 129.
73. LR 130.
74. LR 133.
75. LR 129.
76. LR 91.
77. *KCND Pathways*, pp 2-3.
78. LR 129; Centre for Maternal and Child Enquiries (CMACE), *Saving Mothers'*

Lives 2003-2007, (London: CMACE, 2007).

79. LR 130, see Chapter 9, endnote 26.
80. LR 130.
81. LR 133.
82. LR 130.
83. LR 133.
84. *Ibid.*
85. M Kirkham, 'Midwifery and medical models: do they have to be opposites?' *The Practising Midwife*, (2010) Vol 13 (3), p 14.
86. Kirkham, *'Midwifery and medical models'*.
87. LR 129.
88. LR 129.
89. LR 130.
90. See chapter 3, endnote 76; IOMs were later called Supervisors of Midwives.
91. See this chapter, endnote 14.
92. See chapter 2, endnote 9.
93. A F Cahill (ed), *Between the Lines*, (Durham: Pentland Press, 1999), p 1.
94. LR 129.
95. LR 131.
96. LR 134.
97. LR 133.
98. *Ibid.*
99. *Ibid.*
100. LR 130.
101. LR 129.
102. LR 132.
103. LR 132; active management of the third stage includes the use of uterotonic drugs, clamping and cutting of the cord soon after birth and removal of the placenta within a given time.
104. LR 133.
105. L Moss, 'Midwives struggle to find work as Scots posts dry up', *The Scotsman*, 23 November 2009, p 18.
106. LR 132, by email 4 March 2010; *One year job guarantee for nurses and midwives: guidance for 2009-2010*, www.scotland.gov.uk/Resource/Doc/280040/0084326.pdf. Since then, Claire has heard that her contract is for one year.
107. LR 129.
108. *Ibid.*
109. *Ibid.*
110. LR 131.
111. LR 129.
112. LR 131.
113. Personal communication, Helen Bryers.
114. LR 132.
115. LR 133.

116. LR 132.
117. LR 131; see also www.brithinangus.org.uk.
118. LR 131.
119. LR 132.
120. LR 129.
121. LR 133.
122. LR 131; tall poppy syndrome: a tendency to denigrate high-achievers.
123. LR 130.
124. *Ibid.*

Appendix 1

Members of the Central Midwives Board for Scotland 1916-1983 showing years of service as a Board member, the appointing body and status.

Name of CMB member	Year appointed	Year demitted	Appointing person or body	Doctor, Midwife or lay
Lady Balfour	1916	1919	Lord Pres of PC	Lay
Sir Archibald Buchan-Hepburn	1916	1930	Assoc of CC for Scotland	Lay
Sir Robert Kirk Inches	1916	1918 (died)	Con RB in Scotland	Lay
Lady Susan Gordon Gilmour	1916	1921	QVJIN	Lay
Archibald Campbell Munro	1916	1923 (died)	SMOHS	Doctor
Sir J Halliday Croom	1916	1921	UC Edin and St And	Doctor
Murdoch Cameron	1916	1921	UC Glas and Abd	Doctor
James Haig Ferguson	1916	1934 (died)	RCOP Edin, RCOS Edin, RCOPS Glas; 1921 QVJIN; 1926 RCOP Edin, RCOS Edin, RCOPS Glas	Doctor
Michael Dewar	1916	1926 (died)	BMA (Scot Com)	Doctor
John Wishart Kerr	1916	1921	BMA (Scot Com)	Doctor
Alice Helen Turnbull	1916 (July)	1933	Lord Pres of PC (1919 SBH)	Midwife
Isabella Lewis Scrimgeour	1916 (July) Re-appointed 1927	1926 1928 (died)	Lord Pres of PC (1919 SBH); SBH	Midwife
Sir John Lorne MacLeod	1918	1921	Con RB in Scot	Lay
Lady Helen Hermione Munro-Ferguson	1919	1921	Lord Pres of PC	Lay
Kate Leslie Scott	1921	1926	SBH	Midwife
Sir Robert Cranston	1921	1924	Con RB in Sco	Lay
J A C Kynoch	1921	1926	UC Edin and St And	Doctor
Robert Gordon McKerron	1921 Re-appointed 1931	1926 1936	UC Glas and Abd UC Glas and Abd	Doctor

246

Name	Year		Body	Role
Robert Jardine	1921		RCOP Edin, RCOS Edin, RCOPS Glas	Doctor
E H L Oliphant	1921		BMA (Scot Com)	Doctor
Archibald Kerr Chalmers	1923		SMOHS	Doctor
Sir Malcolm Smith	1924		Con RB in Scot	Lay
Mary E Cairns	1926		SBH, later DHS	Midwife
Ella M Millar	1926		Con RB in Scot	Lay
Margaret M White	1926		QVJIN	Midwife
B P Watson	1926		UC Edin and St And	Doctor
John M Munro Kerr	1926		UC Glas and Abd	Doctor
Robert C Buist	1925	1939 (died)	BMA (Scot Com)	Doctor
James B Miller	1926		BMA (Scot Com)	Doctor
Robert W Johnstone	1926	Re-appointed 1936	UC Edin and St And / UC Edin	Doctor
Lillias Ann D Wishart	1929	1953	SBH	Midwife
Rt Hon Lord Polwarth	1930	1939	Assoc of CC for Scotland	Lay
Isabella Cromarty Dewar	1931	1936	QVJIN / QIDNS	Midwife
John McGibbon	1931	1946	UC Edin and St And	Doctor
George Wallace	1933	1941	DHS	Lay
Douglas Alexander Miller	1934	1936	RCOP Edin, RCOS Edin, RFOPS Glas	Doctor
Peter Taylor	1936	Re-appointed 1942	DHS	Lay
		1939 1943		
James Hendry	1936	1945	UC Glas	Doctor
R J Thomson	1936	1939	Assoc of CC for Scot	Lay
James Cook	1936	1939	BMA (Scot Com)	Doctor
Donald McIntyre	1936	1941	RCOP Edin, RCOS Edin, RFOPS Glas	Doctor
Margaret Rachel Gouk	1937	1946	DHS	Midwife
Margaret Wilson Risk	1937	1946	DHS	Midwife
George Henry Kimpton	1937	1939	DHS	Lay

Name				Role
Dugald Baird	1937 Re-appointed 1961	1951 1962	UC Abd; 1961, SOS for UC Abd, Edin, Glas, St And	Doctor
Robert Howat	1939	1941	DHS	Lay
Frances Ann Wilkinson Allan	1939	1948	DHS	Midwife
J D Tod	1939	1941	Assoc CC for Scot	Lay
David Dale Logan	1939	1953	BMA (Scot Com)	Doctor
William Leslie Cuthbert	1939	1953	BMA (Scot Com)	Doctor
Mary McGhie	1940	1952	DHS	Midwife
Clarice M M Shaw	1941	1946	Assoc CC Scot	Lay
David Robertson	1941	1949	Con RB in Scotland	Lay
Sir Alexander Stuart Murray MacGregor	1941	1948	SMOHS	Doctor
Margaret Fairlie	1941	1953	UC St And	Doctor
William Francis Theodore Haultain	1941 Re-appointed 1953	1951 1958	RCOP Ed, RCOS Edin, RFOPS Glas RCOG	Doctor
J Y Sutherland	1943	1944	DHS	Lay
T A Grieg	1944	1947	DHS	Lay
Isa Hamilton	1946	1952	QIDNS	Midwife
Jean P Ferlie	1946	1963	SOS ; 1953, Cert mids prac in Scotland	Midwife
J A Fisher	1946	1958	Assoc C C Scot; later, SOS for Assoc C C Scot, Con RB, Scot C of C Assoc	Lay
Robert Aim Lennie	1946	1960	UC Glas; later SOS for UC Abd, Edin, Glas, St And	Doctor
N D Walker	1947	1948	SOS	Lay
A S McDermid	1948	1951	SOS	Midwife
J Cochrane	1948	1953	SOS	Lay
Janet Love	1948	1953	SOS	Midwife
William Leslie Burgess	1948	1949	SMOHS	Doctor
Nora Wattie	1949	1968	SMOHS	Doctor

Name				
C McGregor	1951	1953	SOS	Midwife
J Gibson	1951	1953	Con RB in Scotland	Lay
George Panton Milne	1951 Re-appointed 1973	1954 1978	UC Abd SOS	Doctor
David MacKay Hart	1951	1973	RCOP Edin, RCOS Edin, RFOPS Glas (1954 SOS for these bodies), 1959, RCOG	Doctor
J Bruce Dewar	1953	1968 (died)	SOS	Doctor
J H Beckett	1953	1961	Cert mids prac in Scot (In 1961, appointed Education Officer to the Board) Retired 1973	Midwife
Phyllis Bennett	1953	1960	Cert mids prac in Scot	Midwife
Elsie Renwick	1953	1968	Cert mids prac in Scot	Midwife
J Wolrige Gordon	1954	1968	SOS	Lay
J M Steel	1954	1959	SOS	Midwife
J Stenhouse	1954	1959	SOS	Midwife
M J A Urquhart	1954	1959	SOS	Midwife
Mary McAllister	1954	1959	SOS for Assoc CC Scot, Con RB, Scot C of C Assoc	Lay
Catherine Harrower	1954	1961	BMA (Scot Com)	Doctor
Sheelagh P O Bramley	1959 Re-appointed 1968	1963 1978	SOS SOS	Midwife
Mary Fraser	1959	1966	SOS	Midwife
Katie Watt	1959	1963	SOS	Midwife
E Chalmers Fahmy	1959	1963	SOS for RCOP Edin, RCOS Edin, RFOPS Glas	Doctor
R Burnside	1959	1962 (died)	SOS for Assoc CC Scot, Con RB, Scot C of C Assoc	Lay
Charles W Norman	1959	1963	SOS for Assoc CC Scot, Con RB, Scot C of C Assoc	Lay

E M H Burrows	1960	1973	Cert mids prac in Scot	Midwife
Hugh B Muir	1961	1968	BMA (Scot Com)	Doctor
Margaret M Grieve	1961	1963	Cert mids prac in Scot	Midwife
G Douglas Matthew	1963	1978	SOS for UC Abd, Edin, Glas, St And 1963, SOS for SUC	Doctor
Margaret J W Taylor	1963	1968	SOS	Midwife
Ellen Hodge	1963	1973	SOS	Midwife
T N MacGregor	1963	1973	SOS for Medical Corporations	Doctor
J Kelly	1963	1968	SOS for LA Assoc	Lay
M B A Ross	1963	1966	SOS for LA Assoc	Lay
H H Conner	1963	1968	Cert mids prac in Scot	Midwife
J M Lamont	1963	1973	Cert mids prac in Scot, 1968, SOS	Midwife
W E Donaldson	1966	1978	SOS for LA Assoc	Lay
R Gatt	1966	1973	SOS	Midwife
R M Bernard	1968	1973	SOS	Doctor
C J Tudhope	1968	1978	SOS	Lay
Ena Logie	1968	1970	SOS for LA Assoc	Lay
Margaret C Barron	1968	1978	SBMOH later, Scottish Affairs Committee of the Faculty of Community Medicine	Doctor
Joseph McGlone	1968	1973	SCBMA	Doctor
Annie S Grant	1968	1973	App Education Officer to the Board 1 Aug 1973, ret Aug 1982	Midwife
N J Stephen	1968	1973	Cert mids prac in Scot	Midwife
A J Gardner	1970	1971	SOS for LA Assoc	Lay
Mary McCue	1971	1974 (died)	SOS for LA Assoc	Midwife
V M Bremner	1973	1976	SOS	Midwife
Maureen M Baird	1973	1976	SOS	Midwife

Name	Date	Detail	Date	Role
John D O Loudon	1973	SOS for Medical Corporations	1978	Doctor
John M Crawford	1973	RCOG	1976	Doctor
W A Ross	1973	SCBMA	1975	Doctor
Margaret G Auld	1973	Cert mids prac in Scot	1977	Midwife
Lena Margaret Kitson	1973	Cert mids prac in Scot	1983	Midwife
Mary M Turner	1973	Cert mids prac in Scot	1983	Midwife
M M Bicker	1973	CMB app for Cert mids prac in Scot, 1978, SOS	1983	Midwife
C R Playfair	1975	SOS for LA Assoc and 1978, for Health Boards	1983	Midwife
John MacKay	1976	SCBMA	1983	Doctor
Marjorie E Marr	1976	SOS, 1978, Cert mids prac in Scot	1983	Midwife
Anne D Dewing	1977	SOS	1980	Midwife
M Mackay	1977	CMB app for Cert mids prac in Scot	1978	Midwife
John W Crawford	1977	RCOG	1981	Doctor
George Gordon	1978	SOS	1983	Doctor
E T Gourlay	1978	SOS	1983	Midwife
M D Wardle	1978	SOS	1983	Midwife
James Willocks	1978	SOS for RMC	1981	Doctor
H T Falconer	1978	SOS for Health Boards	1983	Midwife
Hamish W Sutherland	1978	SOS for SUC	1983	Doctor
Murdoch Murchison	1978	Scottish Affairs Committee of the Faculty of Community Medicine	1983	Doctor
M L Brown	1978	Cert mids prac in Scotland	1983	Midwife
Mary L Taylor	1980	SOS	1983	Midwife
P R Myerscough	1981	SOS for RMC	1983	Doctor
N B Patel	1981	RCOG	1983	Doctor

Appendix 1 Key:

Assoc of CC for Scotland	Association of County Councils for Scotland
BMA (Scot Com)	British Medical Association, Scottish Committee
Cert mids prac in Scot	Certified midwives practising in Scotland
Con R B in Scotland	Convention of Royal Burghs in Scotland
DHS	Department of Health for Scotland
LA Assoc	Local Authority Associations
Lord Pres of P C	Lord President of the Privy Council
SMOHS	Society of Medical Officers of Health for Scotland
QIDNS	Queen's Institute of District Nursing (Scottish Branch)
QVJIN:	Queen Victoria Jubilee Institute of Nurses (Scottish Branch)
RCOP Edin	Royal College of Physicians of Edinburgh
RCOS Edin	Royal College of Surgeons of Edinburgh
RCOPS Glas	Royal College of Physicians and Surgeons of Glasgow
RFOPS Glas	Royal Faculty of Physicians and Surgeons of Glasgow
RMC	Royal Medical Colleges
SBMOH	Scottish Branch of Medical Officers of Health
SCBMA	Scottish Council of the British Medical Association
Scot C of C Assoc	Scottish Counties of Cities Association
SOS	Secretary of State for Scotland
SOS for e.g. Health Boards etc	Secretary of State for Scotland on behalf of, for example, Health Boards, etc.
SUC	Scottish University Courts
UC Edin and St And	University Courts of the Universities of Edinburgh and St Andrews
UC Glas and Abd	University Courts of the Universities of Glasgow and Aberdeen

Appendix 2

The changing place of birth in Scotland 1900-2010: percentage of births at home

Year	Percentage of Births at home	Year	Percentage of Births at home
Early 20th century	95	1965[12]	15.4
c1918-1930[1]	75	1968[13]	7
1935[2]	67	1969[14]	6.4
1946[3]	48	1970[15]	4.7
1948[4]	44	1971[16]	3.36
1949[5]	39	1975[17]	1.0
1950[6]	36	1980[18]	0.5
1951[7]	33	1981[19]	0.5
1952	32	1985	0.6
1953	31	1990	0.6
1954[8]	30.6	1995	0.8
1955[9]	30	1998	0.9
1957	29	1999	0.9
1960[10]	26.5	2000	0.9
1961[11]	25	2008[20]	1.46

Appendix 2 Fig 1   Homebirths in Scotland 1900-2010

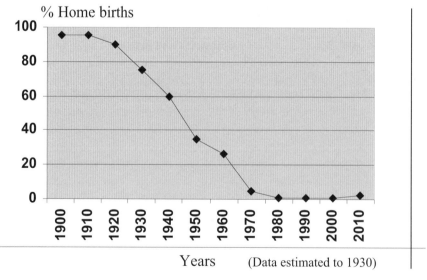

Years   (Data estimated to 1930)

1. T Murphy-Black, 'Care in the community during the postnatal period', in S Robinson, A M Thomson, (eds), *Midwives, Research and Childbirth*, Vol 3, (London, Glasgow: Chapman and Hall, 1994), p 121.
2. H P Tait, *Vital Statistics*, from I Duguid, MTD, Teaching Notes, 1955.
3. G Cumberlege, *Maternity in Great Britain*, (London: Oxford University Press 1948), p 53.
4. H Tait, 'Maternity and Child Welfare', in G McLachlan, (ed), *Improving the Common Weal*, p 420.
5. *Statistical information extracted from the Montgomery Report*, Appendix III, p 56.
6. T Murphy-Black, 'Care in the community during the postnatal period', in Robinson, Thomson, (eds), *Midwives, Research and Childbirth*, vol.3, p 123.
7. *Montgomery Report*, Appendix III.
8. Tait, Vital Statistics, from Duguid, *Teaching Notes, 1955*.
9. *Montgomery Report*, Appendix III.
10. SHHD, *Shared Care in Obstetrics*, (Edinburgh: HMSO, 1983).
11. SHHD, *Report on an Enquiry into Maternal Deaths in Scotland 1965-1971*, (Edinburgh: HMSO, 1974), p 14.
12. SHHD, *Provision of Maternity Services in Scotland: A Policy Review* (Edinburgh: HMSO 1993), p 11.
13. A Grant, 'Intranatal care in hospital', *Nursing Mirror*, 1 August, 1969, pp 18-19.
14. *GRO (Scotland)*.
15. *Policy Review*, p 11.
16. *GRO (Scotland)*.
17. Tait, 'Maternity and Child Welfare', in McLachlan, (ed), *Improving the Common Weal*, p 420.
18. T Murphy-Black, *'Care in the community during the postnatal period'*, p 123.
19. *GRO (Scotland)*.
20. Although this overall statistic seems very low, there are pockets of increased incidence of homebirth in different areas of Scotland.

Appendix 3

Document transcripts

1. Parchment awarded to Mrs Jane Downes in 1881 (see Page 8).
(Courtesy of Edna Walker)

EDINBURGH ROYAL MATERNITY AND SIMPSON MEMORIAL HOSPITAL

*I hereby certify that Mrs. Jane Downes
acted as a Nurse in this Institution from 1st May 1881
to 31st July 1881 and that during the period she performed her
duties in a most exemplary manner. She was most kind and considerate to those
entrusted to her care and gave entire satisfaction.
She was present at the Delivery in ....68 Cases*

*She delivered under the superintendence
of the House Surgeon in ..... Cases*

*She delivered and had the entire management in ....20 Cases
She nursed during the Puerperal period.... 68 Cases*

*Alex Steiner (Signed)
Medical Officer.*

*Geo. W. W. Ashdown. Alexander Bowie. (Signed)
House Surgeons.*

2. An Advertisement for a Course in Midwifery, Mr Joseph Gibson, 1723
(see Page 11). (Courtesy of Keith Adam of Blairadam)

An

ACCOUNT

Of what Mr GIBSON proposes to do in a

Course of MIDWIFERY

To discourse of the Semen *Masculinum* , and in it to demonstrate the *Animalcula*.
To make some Observations on the *Pelvis*, of great Use in Midwifery, and by the By to give the difference between a Male and a Female *Skelet*.
To examine the Parts subservient to Generation in Women.
To talk of the *Menstrua Mulierum*.
To discourse of Generation; to illustrate which we shall give so much of the History of *Incubation* and of *Vegetation*, as is necessary.
To account for the *Growth* and *Nutrition* of the *Foetus*.
To talk of its *Placenta Uterina, funis umbilicalis* and *membranes*.
To discourse of Extra-Uterine Foetus's.
To give the Signs of Conception.
To enumerate the Causes of Sterility.
To discourse of Superfetation and Moles.
To offer something concerning the Management of Pregnant Women.
To observe the Situation of the *Foetus in Utero*, Term and Manner of Delivery.
To give the Signs which precede and accompany a Natural Delivery.
To propose what ought to be done before, in the time of, and after the Operation.
To condescend upon the Circumstances which prognosticate a difficult Labour, and the means by which it may be render'd happy.
To discourse of difficult Labours, whether from the Fault of Mother or Infant, or of Both.
And to propose the best ways of being assisting in such labours.
To talk of Monsters and their Extraction.
To discourse of the Caesarian Section, and the Use of Instruments in the practice of Midwifery.
To give the Regimen of a *Puerpera* and her infant.
To recapitulate the most material Parts of what has been deliver'd.

Mr Gibson begins this Course at Edinburgh on Wednesday the Sixth of November Next, and may be Spoke with at his house in Leith.

3. Certificate awarded to Margaret Reid, midwife, in 1768 (see Page 12). From M Myles, *A textbook for Midwives* (6th edition) (E & S Livingstone, 1968). The image on the certificate represents the French obstetrician, François Mauriceau (1637-1709).

These are to certifie

That Margaret Reid, Midwife, Attended three Courfes of my Lectures upon the Theory and Practice of Midwifery as also the Lying-in Ward in the Royal Infirmary for the Space of   Months by which means She had an Opportunity of Operating in all the different sorts of Births.
Edinburgh 11 Day of June 1768

Thomas Young MD

Profefsor of Midwifery in the University of Edinr.

Bibliography

Primary Sources
CMB Papers
Central Midwives Board for Scotland, *Annual Reports from 1916-1983*:
1917-1923 NAS, CMB 1/1-3.
1925-1930 NAS, CMB 2/10-14: National Archives for Scotland (NAS), West Search Room, Charlotte Square, Edinburgh.
1931-1935: NLS, GHB6, National Library for Scotland, Edinburgh.
1963-65
1967-1983: Royal College of Midwives (RCM) UK Board for Scotland, 37 Frederick Street, Edinburgh.
Central Midwives Board for Scotland, *Minutes of Meetings 16 February 1916 – 30 June 1983:* NAS, CMB 1/1-9: NAS, West Search Room, Charlotte Square, Edinburgh.
Central Midwives Board for Scotland, Schedule, *Rules framed under Section 5 (1) of the Midwives (Scotland) Act, 1915 (5 and 6 Geo. V. c.91), 17 April 1916 and 26 August 1916, NAS, CMB 4/1-5, NAS, West Search Room, Charlotte Square, Edinburgh.*
Central Midwives' Board for Scotland, *Rules Framed by the Central Midwives' Board for Scotland*, 1918, 1922, 1926, 1928, 1930, 1931, 1939, 1944, 1947, 1948, 1949, 1950, 1951, 1954, 1956, 1958, 1959, 1960, 1962, 1964, 1965, 1968, 1980, (Edinburgh: George Robb & Co, 1918-1944; Oliver and Boyd, 1947-1968; SHHD, 1980). RCM UK Board for Scotland, 37 Frederick Street, Edinburgh.
Central Midwives Board for Scotland *Rules 1980 Approval Instrument 1980.*
Central Midwives Board for England and Wales, *Handbook and Rules*, (London: William Clowes and Sons, 1962).
CMBS, CMBE&W, NICNM, an Bord Altranais, *The Role of the Midwife*, (London: Hymns Ancient and Modern, 1983).
Memorial of the Medical Faculties of the Universities, The Royal Medical Corporations, and the Medical Officers of the Maternity Hospitals in Scotland to The Right Honourable H M Secretary for Scotland and the Right Honourable The Lord President of H M Privy Council Anent a *Midwives Bill for Scotland*, 19 August, 1915, NAS, CMB 4/2/6, NAS, West Search Room, Charlotte Square, Edinburgh.

Other archival papers
Colville Papers, Box CC, paper 9/26, 1723. Blairadam Archives, Blairadam, Maryburgh, by Kelty, Fife.
CMBS Blue Case Books, currently (2010) held at RCM UK Board for Scotland, 37 Frederick Street, Edinburgh).
A Lamb, *Memories, handwritten and tape-recorded*, Northern College, Aberdeen, 1994-1995.

Government Publications

Acts of Parliament

Midwives (Scotland) Act, 1915, [5 & 6 Geo.5 Ch 91].
Midwives and Maternity Homes (Scotland) Act, 1927, [17 & 18 Geo 5. Ch 17].
Maternity Services (Scotland) Act, 1937, [1 Edw 8 & 1 Geo 6], 1 (1).
Midwives (Scotland) Act, 1951, 14 & 15 Geo 6 Ch 54.
Nurses, Midwives and Health Visitors Act, 1979, Ch 36.

Parliamentary Debates

House of Lords Fifth Series, 1914, Vol 15; 1915, Vol 20;
House of Commons Fifth Series, 1912, Vol 37; 1915, Vol 25, 26, 27; 1927 Vol 203, 207; 1936, Vol 317; 1937, Vol 319.

Census

Census of Scotland 1911, *Report on the Twelfth Decennial Census of Scotland, Vol 2 Occupations,* (London: HMSO, 1913).

Reports

Department of Health (DH), *Changing Childbirth, Part 1: Report of the Expert Maternity Group,* (London, August 1993).

DH, *Report of the standing maternity and midwifery advisory committee, (Peel Report),* (London: HMSO, 1970).

DH, *Modernising Nursing Careers: setting the direction,* (London: HMSO, 2006).

Department of Health and Social Services (DHSS), Committee of Enquiry into the *Cost of the National Health Service, (Guillebaud Report)* Cmnd. 9663, (London, HMSO, 1956).

DHS Circular no 84/1951, *Dressings for confinement and lying-in period,* (8 August 1951), notes belonging to Isobel Duguid, RGN, SCM, MTD.

DHS, *Report of the Committee on Scottish Health Services,* Cmnd 5204, *(Cathcart Report),* (Edinburgh: DHS, 1936); Chapter XIV, .Maternity and Child Welfare', pp 170-182.

DHS, Scientific Advisory Committee: Clinical Sub-Committee, *Maternal Morbidity and Mortality in Scotland,* (Douglas and McKinley Report), (Edinburgh: HMSO, 1935).

DHS and Scottish Health Services Council, *Maternity Services in Scotland, (Montgomery Report),* (Edinburgh: HMSO, 1959).

DHSS, SHHD, Welsh Office, *Report of the Committee on Nursing,* Cmnd 5115, *(Briggs Report),* (London: HMSO 1972).

House of Commons Health Committee, *Second Report: Maternity Services, (Winterton Report),* (London: HMSO, 1992).

Information Services Division, Common Services Agency for the Scottish Health Service, *Scottish Health Statistics 1983,* (Edinburgh: HMSO, 1984).

Ministry of Health, (MH) *Maternal Mortality,* (Campbell J M) Reports on public health and medical subjects No 48, (London: HMSO, 1924).

MH, *Report of the Maternity Services Committee, (Cranbrook Report), London: HMSO, 1959.*

MH, DHSS, Ministry of Labour and National Service, *Report of the Working Party on Midwives,* (London: HMSO, 1949).

MH and SHHD, *Report of the Committee on Senior Nursing Staff Structure, (Salmon Report)*, (London: HMSO 1966).

NHS, Midwifery 2020, England, Northern Ireland, Scotland, Wales, Midwifery 2020, *Delivering Expectations, Final Report*, (launched Edinburgh, September 2010). www.midwifery2020.org

NHS Quality Improvement Scotland (NHS QIS), *KCND Programme, Pathways for Maternity Care*, (Edinburgh: NHS QIS, 2009).

Northern Ireland Maternity Unit Study Group, *Delivering Choice: Midwife and GP-led Maternity Units*, (Belfast: HMSO, 1994).

SBH, Departmental Committee's *Report on Puerperal Morbidity and Mortality*, (*Salvesen Report*), (Edinburgh: HMSO, 1924).

Scottish Executive Health Department, (SEHD) *A Framework for Maternity Services in Scotland*, (Edinburgh: Scottish Executive, 2001).

SEHD, *Report on the Expert Group on Maternity Services (EGAMS Report)*, (Edinburgh: Scottish Executive, 2002).

Scottish Government Health Department, *Better Health, Better Care*, (Edinburgh: Scottish Government, 2006).

SHHD, *Maternity Services: Integration of Maternity Work*, (*Tennent Report*), (Edinburgh: HMSO, 1973).

SHHD, *Provision of Maternity Services in Scotland: a Policy Review,* (Edinburgh: HMSO, 1993).

SHHD, *Report on an Enquiry into Maternal Deaths in Scotland 1965-1971*, (Edinburgh: HMSO, 1974).

SHHD*, Report on an Enquiry into Maternal Deaths in Scotland 1976-1980*, (Edinburgh: HMSO, 1987).

SHHD, *Shared Care in Obstetrics: A Report by the National Medical Consultative Committee, (Edinburgh: HMSO, 1983).*

SOHHD, CRAG/SCOTMEG Working Group on Maternity Services, *Antenatal Care*, (Edinburgh: HMSO, 1995).

SOHHD, CRAG/SCOTMEG Working Group on Maternity Services, *Innovations in practice, Abstracts of presentations*, (Edinburgh: HMSO, 1993).

SOHHD, CRAG/SCOTMEG Working Group on Maternity Services, *Innovations in practice: abstracts and presentations*, (Edinburgh: HMSO, 1994).

SOHHD, *Framework for action*, London: HMSO, 1991).

SOHHD, *The patient's charter: a charter for health*, (London: HMSO, 1991).

SOHHD, *The patients' charter: what users think*, (Edinburgh: HMSO, 1994).

Welsh Office, *Maternal and Early Child Health*, (Cardiff: HMSO, 1991).

Reports (non-governmental)

Boddy K, Parboosingh I J T, Shepherd W C, *A Schematic Approach to Prenatal Care*, (Edinburgh: 1976).

Chamberlain G, Gunn P, *Birthplace, Report of the Confidential Enquiry into Facilities Available at the Place of Birth,* (Chichester: John Wiley, 1987).

Chamberlain G, Wraight A, Crowley P, (eds), *Home Births*: The *Report of the 1994 Confidential Enquiry by the National Birthday Trust Fund*, (London: Parthenon, 1996).

Corporation of Glasgow, *Report of the Medical Officer of Health, City of Glasgow,*
(1934).
Council Directives of 21 January, 1980: (80/154/EEC), *Official Journal of the*
European Communities, No L 33/1; (80/155/EEC), *Official Journal of the European*
Communities, No L 33/8, (1980).
Cumberlege G, *Maternity in Great Britain*, A Survey of Social and Economic Aspects
of Pregnancy and Childbirth undertaken by a Joint Committee of the Royal College of
Obstetricians and Gynaecologists and the Population Investigation Committee,
(London: Oxford University Press, 1948).
Hillan E, McGuire M, Reid L, *Midwives and Woman Centred Care*, (Edinburgh: RCM
Scottish Board, and University of Glasgow, 1997).
McGuire M, Reid L, Hillan E, *The perceptions and experiences of newly qualified*
single registered midwives in Scotland, (Glasgow: University of Glasgow, 1998).
MacKenzie W L, *Report on the Physical Welfare of Mothers and Children, Vol 3,*
Scotland, (Dunfermline: The Carnegie United Kingdom Trust, 1917).
Maternity Services Action Group (MSAG), *A Refreshed Maternity Services Quality*
Framework, (Draft), (Edinburgh: MSAG, 2010, Jan).
UK CNOs, *Midwifery 2020, Project Initiation Document V6*, (2007).

Secondary Sources
Abel-Smith B, *A History of the Nursing Profession*, (London: William Heinemann,
1960).
Albers L, 'Evidence' and midwifery practice', *Journal of midwifery and women's*
health, (2001), Vol 46 (3), pp 130-135.
Allison J, *Delivered at Home*, (London: Chapman and Hall, 1996).
Askham J, Barbour R, 'The negotiated role of the midwife in Scotland', Robinson,
Thomson,(eds), in *Midwives, Research and Childbirth*, Vol 4, pp 33-59.
Askham J, Barbour R, 'The role and responsibilities of the midwife in Scotland', in
van Teijlingen E, Lowis G, McCaffery P, Porter M, (eds) *Midwifery and the*
Medicalization of Childbirth: Comparative Perspectives, (New York: Nova Science
Publishers, 2000), pp 173-178.
Association of Radical Midwives (ARM), *The Vision*, (Droitwich: Spa Printing and
Copying, 1986).
Audit Commission, *First class delivery: improving maternity services in England and*
Wales, (Oxford: Audit Commission publications, 1997).
Barnett Z, 'Yesterday, today and tomorrow in postnatal care', *Midwives Chronicle*,
(November 1984), pp 358-364.
Beech B, Phipps B, 'Normal births: women's stories', in Downe (ed), *Normal*
Childbirth pp 59-70.
Bennett V R, Brown L K, (eds), *Myles Textbook for Midwives*, (*11th ed*), (London and
Edinburgh: Churchill Livingstone, 1989).
Berghahn M, *Continental Britons*, (Oxford: Berg Publishers, 1988).
Bisset-Smith G, *Vital Registration*, (*2nd ed*), (Edinburgh: William Green, 1907).
Black N, Boswell D, Gray A, Murphy S, Popay J, (eds), *Health and disease, a reader*
(Milton Keynes, Open University Press, 1984).

Bostock Y, Reid M, *Pregnancy, childbirth and coping with motherhood: what women want from maternity services*, (Edinburgh: SOHHD, 1993).

Botanic Treatment of Disease, (Glasgow: The Botanic Medical Hall, 1912).

Bradshaw G, Bagness C, 'Midwifery 2020 (1): education and career progression', *The Practising Midwife,* (2010), Vol 13 (8), pp 4-5.

Bramley S, Turner M, 'Obituary: Mrs Margaret Fraser Myles 1892-1988', *Midwifery*, (1988), (4), pp 93-94.

Brotherston J, 'The National Health Service in Scotland: 1948-1984', in McLachlan , (ed) *Improving the Common Weal,* pp 105-159.

Brotherston J, Brims J, 'The Development of Public Medical Care: 1900-1948', in McLachlan, (ed), *Improving the Common Weal,* pp 35-102.

Bryers H, *Midwifery and Maternity Services in the Gàidhealtachd and the North of Scotland, 1914-2005*, Unpublished PhD thesis, (University of Aberdeen, 2010).

Cameron A, 'Licensed to practise within their bounds: the Faculty of Physicians and Surgeons and the regulation of midwives in eighteenth century Glasgow', presented at *History of Nursing Research Colloquium*, Oxford Brookes University, 18 March, 2000.

Campbell R, Macfarlane, A, *Where to be Born? The Debate and the Evidence*, (*2nd ed*), (Oxford: National Perinatal Epidemiology Unit, 1994).

Campbell R, Macfarlane A, 'Recent debate on the place of birth', in Garcia , Kilpatrick , Richards , (eds) *Politics of Maternity Care,* pp 217-237.

Catford E F, *The Royal Infirmary of Edinburgh 1929-1979, Edinburgh: Scottish Academic Press, 1984).*

Chalmers A K, 'On the need for a midwives act in Scotland', *The Journal of Midwifery, The Nursing Times*, Feb 21 (1914), pp 251-254.

Chalmers A K, *The Health of Glasgow 1818-1925*, (Glasgow: Corporation of Glasgow 1930).

Chalmers I, Kierse M, Neilson J, *A guide to effective care in pregnancy and childbirth*, (Oxford, Oxford University Press, 1989).

Chertok L, *Motherhood and personality*, (London: Tavistock, 1969).

Christie D, Tansey E, (eds), Wellcome witnesses to twentieth century medicine: Maternal care, *Witness* seminar transcript, Vol 12, (London: The Wellcome Trust Centre for the History of Medicine at UCL, 2001).

Clark, M, 'Changing clinical practice in nursing', in Duncan, McLachlan, *Hospital Medicine and Nursing in the 1980s,* pp 41-52.

Cochrane A, *Effectiveness and efficiency*, (London: Nuffield Provincial Hospitals Trust, 1972).

Collacott R, 'Neonatal tetanus; a major disease of the Scottish islands', in Cule J, Turner T, (eds) *Childcare through the centuries,* (British Society for the History of Medicine: Cardiff, 1986), pp 136-151.

Collins Dictionary and Thesaurus, (Glasgow: Collins, 1989).

Coombs A, 'Finding Herring Gutters', *Women's History Notebooks*, (2001), Vol 8 (1), pp 13-20.

Cooter R, Pickstone J, *Medicine in the Twentieth Century*, (Amsterdam: Harwood Academic Publishers, 2000).

Corporation of Glasgow Public Health Department, *Scheme for Maternity and Child*

Welfare, (Glasgow: Committee on Health, 1926).

Cowell B, Wainwright D, *Behind the Blue Door: The History of the Royal College of Midwives 1881-1981, (London: Baillière Tindall, 1981).*

Cronk, M, 'Midwifery: a practitioner's view from within the National Health Service', *Midwife, Health Visitor and Community Nurse*, (1990), Vol 26 (3), pp 58-63.

Croom J H, 'The Midwives (Scotland) Act: its Object and Method', read before the *Maternity and Child Welfare Conference*, (Glasgow, March 1917).

Daiches D, *Scotland and the Union*, (London: John Murray, 1977).

Davies C, Beach A, I*nterpreting Professional Self-Regulation: A History of the United Kingdom Central Council for Nursing, Midwifery and Health Visiting*, (London: Routledge, 2000).

Death certificate, *Record of Corrected Entries*, p 68, 20 August 1891, following Report of Result of Precognition, cited in Hutchison I, *Elizabeth Sanderson, née Rae, 1854-1907.* Unpublished paper, (2009).

Dimond B, Fears for the future. *Modern Midwife*, (1995), Vol 5 (4), pp 32-33.

Dingwall R, Rafferty A M, Webster C, *An Introduction to the Social History of Nursing*, (London: Routledge, 1988).

Donnison, J, *Midwives and Medical Men*, (New Barnet: Historical Publications, 1988).

Dow A D, *The Rottenrow: The History of the Glasgow Royal Maternity Hospital 1834-1984*, (Carnforth: The Parthenon Press, 1984).

Downe S, McCourt C, 'From being to becoming: reconstructing childbirth knowledges', in Downe, *Normal Childbirth*, pp 3-24.

Downe S, (ed) *Normal Childbirth*: *Evidence and debate* (London: Churchill Livingstone, 2004).

Duncan A, McLachlan G, (eds), *Hospital Medicine and Nursing in the 1980s*, (London: The Nuffield Provincial Hospitals Trust, 1984).

Dupree M, Crowther A, 'A Profile of the Medical Profession in the Early Twentieth Century: *The Medical Directory* as a Historical Source', in *Bulletin of the History of Medicine*, (1991) (65), pp 209-233.

Durkin L, Palmer T, 'Towards a woman-centred model of care', *The Practising Midwife*, (2010), Vol 13 (3), p 21.

Educational Advisory Group, Scottish Board of the RCM, *Social and Statistical Facts for Student Midwives*, (London: Pitman Books Limited, 1982).

Encarta World English Dictionary, (London: Bloomsbury, 1999).

Ewan E, Innes S, Reynolds S, Pipes R, *Scottish Biographical Dictionary of Women*, (Edinburgh: Edinburgh University Press, 2006), p 24.

Ferguson T, *Scottish Social Welfare 1864–1914*, (Edinburgh: E&S Livingstone, 1958).

Fleissig A, Kroll D, 'Achieving continuity of care and carer', *Modern Midwife*, (1997),Vol 7 (8), pp 15-19.

Fleming, V, 'Autonomous or Automatons? An Exploration Through History of the Concept of Autonomy in Midwifery in Scotland and New Zealand', *Nursing Ethics*, (1998), Vol 5 (1), pp 43-51.

Flint C, 'Inaugural address', *RCM Midwives Chronicle*, (1994) Vol 107 pp 335-339.

Flint C, *'Sensitive Midwifery'*, (London: Heinmann Midwifery, 1986).

Fraser D, Cooper, M (eds), *Myles Textbook for Midwives* (*15th ed*), (Edinburgh:

Churchill Livingstone, 2009).

Fraser W H, Morris R J, (eds) *People and Society in Scotland Vol II, 1830-1914,* (Edinburgh: John Donald, 1990).

Galt J, (1779-1839), 'The howdie: an autobiography', in *The Howdie and Other Tales,* (Edinburgh: T N Foulis, 1923), pp 3-28. Reproduced from the original manuscript.

Garcia J, Kilpatrick R, Richards M, (eds), *The Politics of Maternity Care,* (Oxford: Clarendon Press, 1990).

Gordon E, 'Women's spheres' in Fraser, Morris, (eds) *People and Society in Scotland Vol II,* pp 206-235.

Grampian TV, *St Kilda, Thursday 8 September (2005)*; www.grampiantv.co.uk/content

Hall M, MacIntyre S, Porter M, *Antenatal Care Assessed,* (Aberdeen: Aberdeen University Press, 1985).

Hillan E, McGuire M, Reid L, *Midwives and Woman-centred care,* University of Glasgow and RCM Scottish Board, (Edinburgh: RCM Scottish Board, 1997).

Hillan E, McGuire M, Reid L, Purton P, 'Woman-centred care: a midwifery perspective', *RCM Midwives Journal,* (2000), Vol 3 (12), pp 376-379.

Hogarth J, 'General Practice', in McLachlan, (ed) *Improving the Common Weal,* pp 163-212.

Hundley V, Cruikshank F, Milne J et al, Satisfaction and continuity of care: staff views of care in a midwife-managed delivery unit, *Midwifery,* (1995), (11), pp 163-173.

Hunt S, Symonds A, *The Social Meaning of Midwifery,* (MacMillan Press: Basingstoke, 1995).

Hunter B, 'Oral History and Research, Part 1: Uses and Implications', *British Journal of Midwifery,* July (1999), Vol 7 (7), pp 426-429.

Hunter D, 'The re-organised Health Service', in Clarke M G, Drucker H M, (eds), *Our Changing Scotland: A Yearbook of Scottish Government, 1976-77,* (Edinburgh: EUSPB, 1976), pp 26-37.

Hutchison I, *Elizabeth Sanderson, née Rae, 1854-1907,* Unpublished paper, 2009.

Hutchinson R, *Calum's Road,* (Edinburgh: Birlinn, 2006).

Jenkinson J, *Scottish Medical Societies, 1731-1939,* (Edinburgh: Edinburgh University Press, 1993).

Johnstone R, 'Chairman's Review of the Board's Progress since 1915', NAS, CMB 1/7, *CMB Minutes,* 26 February, (1953), pp 2-3.

Johnstone R, 'Scotland's contribution to the progress of midwifery in the early eighteenth and nineteenth centuries', *The Journal of Obstetrics and Gynaecology of the British Empire,* (1950),Vol 57, pp 583-594.

Kennedy L, *In Bed with an Elephant,* (London: Bantam Press, 1995).

Kent N, The road ahead, *Midwives,* (September 2010), pp 24-25.

Kinnaird J, 'The hospitals', in McLachlan, (ed) *Improving the Common Weal,* pp 213-275.

Kirkham M, 'Midwifery and medical models: do they have to be opposites?' *The Practising Midwife,* (2010), Vol 13 (3), pp 14.

Kitzinger, S, *Birth at Home,* (Oxford: Oxford University Press, 1979).

Lamb A, 'Life at Larryvarry', in Roberts A, *Tales of the Braes of Glenlivet,* (Edinburgh: Birlinn, 1999), pp 118-129.

Lawson J, Power to mothers and midwives, *MIDIRS Midwifery Digest*, (1992), Vol 2 (2), 127-130.

Leap N, 'Caseload practice within the NHS', *Midwives Chronicle*, (1994),Vol 107, pp 130-135.

van Lieburg M, Marland H, 'Midwifery regulation, education and practice in the Netherlands during the nineteenth century', *Medical history*; (1989), Vol 33, 296-317.

Loudon I, *Death in Childbirth*, (Oxford: Clarendon Press, 1992).

Loudon, I, 'Midwives and the quality of maternal care', in Marland, Rafferty, (eds) *Midwives, Society and Childbirth*, pp 180-200.

Luyben A, 'The midwife as a researcher', in Mander, Fleming, (eds), *Becoming a midwife*, pp 115-126.

McBryde B, *A Nurse's War*, (London: Hogarth Press, 1986).

MacDonald S, 'Dirty knives sealed fate of St Kilda people', *The Sunday Times*, 25 Jan (2009).

MacGregor, A, *Public Health in Glasgow 1905-1946*, (Edinburgh and London: E and S Livingstone Ltd, 1967).

MacGregor H, Butcher G, Powis L, 'Scotland's pathway says 'no' to intervention', *Midwives*, June/July (2009), p 29.

McGuire M, *Community Postnatal Care Provision in Scotland: the development and evaluation of a template for the provision of woman-centred community postnatal care*, unpublished PhD thesis, (University of Glasgow: 2001).

McKenzie C, 'Midwifery Regulation in the United Kingdom', in Fraser, Cooper, (eds), *Myles Textbook for Midwives (15th ed)*, pp 81-100.

MacKenzie L, 'Notification of Puerperal Fever', *The Transactions of the Edinburgh Obstetrical Society*, Session LXXXVII, 1927-28, pp 38-44. (Reproduced in the *Edinburgh Medical Journal*, New Series, (1928), Vol XXXV, (3).

McLachlan G, (ed), *Improving the Common Weal: Aspects of Scottish Health Services 1900-1984*, (Edinburgh: Edinburgh University Press, 1987).

MacLeod J, *Notes on Maternal Mortality and Morbidity with Special Reference to Maternity Work in General Practice*, unpublished MD Thesis, (University of Aberdeen, 1935).

MacNaughton M, Mabel Liddiard Memorial Lecture: 'Perinatal Mortality in Scotland', *Midwives Chronicle and Nursing Notes*, March (1992), pp 46-50.

Maggs C, 'Direct but different: midwifery education since 1989', *British Journal of Midwifery*, (1996), Vol 2 (12), pp 612-616.

Main J, 'Nursing: nursing, midwifery and health visiting', in McLachlan, (ed), *Improving the Common Weal* , pp 459-479.

Mander R, 'Autonomy in midwifery and maternity care', *Midwives Chronicle*, October (1993), pp 369-374.

Mander R, 'Evidence-based practice', in Fraser, Cooper, (eds) *Myles' Textbook for Midwives*, pp 67-79.

Mander R, 'The midwife and the medical practitioner,' in Mander, Fleming (eds), *Failure to Progress*, pp170-188.

Mander R, 'Who needs midwifery?' *Nursing Times*, (1987), Vol 83 (26), pp 34-35.

Mander R, Fleming V, (eds), *Becoming a midwife*, (London: Routledge, 2009).

Mander R, Fleming V, (eds), *Failure to Progress: the contraction of the midwifery profession*, (London: Routledge, 2002), p170-188.

Mander R, Reid L, 'Midwifery power', in Mander, Fleming, (eds), *Failure to Progress,* pp 1-19.

Marland H, (ed), *The Art of Midwifery*, (London: Routledge, 1993).

Marland H, Rafferty, A M, (eds), *Midwives, Society and Childbirth*, (London: Routledge, 1997).

Milne G, (ed) *Aberdeen Medico-Chirurgical Society: A Bi-centennial History 1789-1989*, (Aberdeen: Aberdeen University Press, 1989).

Milne G, 'The history of midwifery in Aberdeen', in Milne, (ed) *Aberdeen Medico-Chirurgical Society*, pp 227-240.

Moir D, *Pain Relief in Labour*, (*5th ed*), (Edinburgh: Churchill Livingstone, 1986).

Mortimer J, *Tending to Care* (*2nd ed*), (Bedale: Blaisdon Publishing, 1999).

Moss L, 'Doctors: We're being cut out by empire-building midwives' *The Scotsman*, 12 March (2010), p 17.

Munro Kerr J M, *Maternal Mortality and Morbidity: A Study of their Problems*, (Edinburgh: E and S Livingstone, 1933).

Munro Kerr J M, 'The maternity services', in Munro Kerr, Johnstone, Phillips, (eds) *Historical Review,* p 3.

Munro Kerr J M, Haig Ferguson J, Young J, Hendry J, *A Combined Textbook of Obstetrics and Gynaecology*, (Edinburgh: E and S Livingstone, 1923).

Munro Kerr J M, Johnstone, R W, Phillips M H, (eds), *Historical Review of British Obstetrics and Gynaecology 1800-1950,* (Edinburgh: E and S Livingstone Ltd, 1954).

Murphy-Black T, 'Care in the Community during the Postnatal Period', in Robinson, Thomson, (eds), *Midwives, Research and Childbirth*, Vol 3, pp 120-146.

Murphy-Black T, 'Systems of midwifery care in use in Scotland', *Midwifery*, (1992), (8), pp 113-124.

Murray E F, 'Some observations on puerperal sepsis with special reference to its occurrence in maternity hospitals', *Transactions of Edinburgh Obstetrical Society*, Session LXXXIX, (1930), pp 145-153.

Myles M, *A Textbook for Midwives*, (1st, 2nd, 3rd, 4th, 6th, eds), (Edinburgh: E & S Livingstone 1955 (reprint), 1956 (reprint), 1958, 1962, 1968).

Myles, M, *A Textbook for Midwives*, (7th, 8th eds), (Edinburgh: Churchill Livingstone, 1971, 1975).

National Board for Nursing, Midwifery and Health Visiting for Scotland (NBS), *Supervision of Midwives in Scotland*, (Edinburgh: NBS, 1998).

Navarro V, The mode of state intervention in the health sector, in, Black N, Boswell D, Gray A, Murphy S, Popay J, (eds), *Health and disease, a reader*, (Milton Keynes, Open University Press, 1984) pp 163-169.

NHS Quality Improvement Scotland, KCND Programme, *Pathways for Maternity Care*, (Edinburgh, 2009).

NMC, *The code: standards of conduct, performance and ethics for nurses and midwives*, (London: NMC, 2008).

Nursing and Midwifery Order (SI2002/253), (London: NMC, 2001).

Oakley A, 'Doctor knows best', in Black, Boswell, Gray, et al, (eds), *Health and*

266

Disease, pp 170-175.

Oakley A, *The Captured Womb*, (Oxford: Basil Blackwell Ltd, 1984).

Page L, Jones B, Bentley P et al, One-to-one midwifery, *British Journal of Midwifery*, (1994), Vol 2 (9), pp 444-447.

Pallister M, 'Quest to deliver a mother's birth right', *The Herald*, 23 May, 1997, p 18.

Peters R, 'Nursing and Midwifery Services' in Peters Kinnaird (eds), *Health Services Administration*, pp 294-321.

Peters R, Kinnaird J, *Health Services Administration*, (Edinburgh: E& S Livingstone, 1965).

Pickstone J, Cooter R, *Medicine in the twentieth century* (Singapore, Harwood Academic Publishers, 2000).

Pitt S, 'Midwifery and Medicine', in Marland, Rafferty, (eds), *Midwives, Society and Childbirth*, pp 218-231.

Poxton I, Heffron A, 'Neonatal Tetanus on St Kilda and other tales of avian neurotoxigenic clostridia'; presentation to *Society for Anaerobic Microbiology (SAM)*, 2004, http:www.clostridia.net/SAM/Presentations/Presentations.html.

Raphael-Leff, J, *Psychological Processes of Childbearing*, (London: Chapman and Hall, 1991).

Reid L, 'A killer on St Kilda', *The Practising Midwife*, (2009),Vol 12 (1), p 50.

Reid L, 'Balfour, Elizabeth, (Betty)', in Ewan E, Innes S, Reynolds S, Pipes R, (eds) *Scottish Biographical Dictionary of Women*, (Edinburgh University Press: Edinburgh, 2006), p 24.

Reid L, 'Bearing the load for women', The Practising Midwife, (2008), Vol 11 (7), p 50.

Reid L, 'Best practice: aims and realities', in Reid, (ed) *Freedom to practise?* pp 9-29.

Reid L, 'Home births in the dunny', *The Practising Midwife*, (2008), Vol 11 (4), p 50.

Reid L, *Keeping Childbirth Natural and Dynamic: a Resource*, (Edinburgh: Scottish Multi-professional Maternity Development Group, 2008).

Reid L, (ed) *Midwifery: freedom to practise?* (Edinburgh: Elsevier, 2007).

Reid L, 'Midwifery in Scotland 1: the legislative background', *British Journal of Midwifery*, (2005), Vol 13 (5), 277-283.

Reid L, 'Midwifery in Scotland 2: developing antenatal care', British Journal of Midwifery, (2005),Vol 13 (6), pp 392-396.

Reid L, 'Midwifery in Scotland 3: intranatal practices', British Journal of Midwifery, (2005),   Vol 13 (7), pp 426-431.

Reid L, 'Midwifery in Scotland 4: postnatal care', *British Journal of Midwifery*, (2005), Vol 13 (8), pp 492-496.

Reid L, 'Normal birth in Scotland', in Reid, (ed), *Freedom to practise?* pp 240-260.

Reid L, 'Organisation of Health Services in the UK', in Fraser, Cooper, (eds), *Myles Textbook for Midwives* (*15th ed*), pp 1027-1038.

Reid L, *Scottish Midwives (1916-1983): the Central Midwives Board for Scotland and practising midwives*. Unpublished PhD thesis, University of Glasgow, 2003

Reid, L, *Scottish Midwives: Twentieth Century Voices (2nd ed)*, (Dunfermline: Black Devon Books, 2008).

Reid L, 'Shanks's pony to Council 'caur'', *The Practising Midwife* (2008), Vol 11 (5), p 74.

Reid L, 'Starting from scratch', *The Practising Midwife*, (2010), Vol 13 (4), p 42.

Reid L, 'The development of midwifery legislation in Scotland: a history to be proud of', (2003), *RCM Midwives Journal*, Vol 6 (4), pp 166-169.

Reid L, 'Two pips on your shoulder', *The Scots Magazine*, (2009), March, pp 302-306.

Reid L, 'Uncertified midwives in Scotland: the howdies', *The Practising Midwife,* (2009), Vol 12 (5), pp 40-43.

Reid L, 'Using oral history in midwifery research', *British Journal of Midwifery*, (2004), Vol 12) (4), pp 208-238.

Reid L, 'Wartime midwives', *The Practising Midwife*, (2009), Vol 12 (3), p 50,

Reid L, 'Where's your comfort zone?' *The Practising Midwife*, (2010), Vol 13 (3), p 42.

Reid L, 'Woman-centred care – midwives in Scotland', *Nursing Times*, (1997), July 2-8, pp 52-53.

Reid L, Hillan E, McGuire M, 'The challenge of negotiating the maze of woman-centred care in Scotland', *British Journal of Midwifery*, (1997), Vol 5 (10), pp 602-606.

Reid L, Hillan E, McGuire M, 'Woman-centred care: part-time midwives – are they getting a fair deal?' *The Practising Midwife*, (1999), Vol 2 (1), pp 27-29.

Reid L, Hillan E, McGuire M, 'Woman-centred care: midwives' need to be heard', *The Practising Midwife,* (1998) Vol 1 (12), pp 22-25.

Relyea, J, 'The Rebirth of Midwifery in Canada: An Historical Perspective', *Midwifery*, (1992), (8), pp 159-169.

Robinson S, 'Maintaining the independence of the midwifery profession: a continuing struggle', in Garcia, Kilpatrick, Richards, *The Politics of Maternity Care*, pp 61-91.

Robinson S, 'Midwives, obstetricians and general practitioners: the need for role clarification', *Midwifery*, (1985), (1), pp 102-113.

Robinson, S, Thomson, A M, (eds), *Midwives, Research and Childbirth*, Vol 3, (London and Glasgow: Chapman and Hall, 1994).

Robinson S, Thomson A M, (eds), in *Midwives, Research and Childbirth*, Vol 4, (London: Chapman and Hall, 1996), pp 33-59.

Rorie D, 'The howdie', in Rorie D, *The Lum Hat Wantin the Croon*, p 64.

Rorie, D, *The Lum Hat Wantin the Croon*, (Edinburgh: W & R Chambers, 1935).

Royal College of Midwives (RCM), The role and education of the future midwife in the United Kingdom, (London: RCM, 1987).

RCM Supplement, 'Woman-centred Care', 1, January (1996).

RCM Supplement, 'Woman-centred Care', 2, April, (1996).

RCM, *Towards a healthy nation*, (London: RCM, 1991).

RCM, *Vision 2000*, (London: RCM, 2000).

Sackett D, Rosenburg W, Gray J A et al, 'Evidence based medicine: what it is and what it isn't, *British Medical Journal* (1996),Vol 312 (7023), pp 71-72, quoted in Mander, R, *Evidence-based practice.*

Sandall J, 'Midwives, burnout and continuity of care', *British Journal of Midwifery*, (1997), Vol 5 (2), pp 105-111.

268

Sandall J, 'Promoting normal birth: weighing the evidence', in Downe S, (ed), *Normal Childbirth,* pp 161-171.

Scott P H, *Still in bed with an elephant,* (Edinburgh: The Saltire Society, 1998).

Scottish Programme for Clinical Effectiveness in Reproductive Health (SPCERH) and the Dugald Baird Centre for Research on Women's Health, *Maternity Care Matters: an audit of maternity services in Scotland 1998,* SPCERH Publication Number 9, (Aberdeen:, SPCERH, 1999).

Skinner G, Roch S, 'Creating confidence by building on experience', *British Journal of Midwifery* (1995), Vol 3 (4), pp 284-287.

Skinner J, 'Risk, let's look at the bigger picture', *Women and Birth* (2008) (21), pp 53-54.

Staines C, 'Moving forward in antenatal care: the Sighthill project, Edinburgh', RCM Professional Day Paper, *Midwives Chronicle Supplement,* (September 1983), pp 6-9.

Steel T, *Life and Death of St Kilda,* (Bungay: Fontana, 1975).

Stephens L, 'Midwifery-led care', in Reid L, *Midwifery: Freedom to Practise?* pp 144-163.

Stride P, 'St Kilda, the neonatal tetanus tragedy of the nineteenth century and some twenty-first century answers', *Journal of the Royal College of Physicians of Edinburgh,* (2008), (38), pp 70-77.

Stringer C, 'Review', Campbell, Macfarlane, *Where to be Born? Midwives,* (July 1995), p 226.

Sturrock J, 'Sir James Young Simpson and his Memorial Hospital', Scottish Society of the History of Medicine Symposium, *Edinburgh's Infirmary,* (Edinburgh: Lammerburn Press, Ltd, 1979).

Sturrock J, 'The Edinburgh Royal Maternity and Simpson Memorial Hospital', Reprinted from the *Journal of the Royal College of Surgeons of Edinburgh,* (May 1980), Vol 25, pp 173-187.

Sutherland H, *A Time to Keep,* (London: Geoffrey Bles, 1934).

Symon A, 'Midwives and professional status', in *British Journal of Midwifery,* (1996), Vol 4 (10), pp 543-550.

Tait H, 'Maternity and Child Welfare', in McLachlan (ed), *Improving the Common Weal,* pp 413-440.

van Teijlingen E, 'A critical analysis of the medical model as used in the study of pregnancy and childbirth', *Sociological Research Online* (2005) , www.socresonline.org.uk/10/2/teijlingen.html.

van Teijlingen E, *A social or medical model of childbirth? Comparing the arguments in Grampian (Scotland) and the Netherlands,* unpublished PhD thesis, (University of Aberdeen 1994).

van Teijlingen E, Lowis G, McCaffery P, Porter M, (eds) *Midwifery and the Medicalization of Childbirth: Comparative Perspectives,* (New York: Nova Science Publishers, Inc, 2000).

Tew M, *Safer Childbirth? A critical history of maternity care, (2nd ed),* (London: Chapman and Hall, 1995).

Thomson A, 'Is there evidence for the medicalisation of maternity care?' *MIDIRS Midwifery Digest,* (2000), Vol 10 (4), pp 416-420.

Towler J, Bramall J, *Midwives in History and Society* (London: Croom Helm 1986).
Transactions of the Edinburgh Obstetrical Society, Vol 20, Session 1894-95, (Edinburgh: Oliver and Boyd, 1895).

Tucker J, Hall M, Howie P et al, 'Should obstetricians see women with normal pregnancies? A multicentre randomised controlled trial of routine antenatal care by general practitioners and midwives compared to shared care', *British Medical Journal*, (1996) (312), pp 554-559

Turnbull D, Reid M, McGinley M, Sheilds N, 'Changes in midwives' attitudes to their professional role following the implementation of the midwifery development unit, *Midwifery*, (1995), (11), pp 110-119.

Uprichard M, 'The evolution of midwifery education', *Midwives' Chronicle,* (January 1987), pp 3-9.

Walsh D, *Evidence-based care for normal labour and birth*, (London: Routledge, 2007).

Walsh D, *Improving maternity services* (Oxford: Radcliffe Publishing, 2007).

Walsh D, 'Is woman-centred care becoming a pious platitude?' *British Journal of Midwifery*, (1996), Vol 4 (4), pp 173-174.

Walsh D, Newburn M, 'Towards a social model of childbirth: Part one', *British Journal of Midwifery*, (2002), Vol 10 (8), pp 476-481.

Watson J K, *A Complete Handbook of Midwifery for Midwives and Nurses, (3rd ed)*, (London: The Scientific Press, 1914).

Wilkinson J, *The Coogate Doctors: The History of the Edinburgh Medical Missionary Society 1841 to 1991*, (Edinburgh: The Edinburgh Medical Missionary Society, 1991).

Williams A S, *Women and Childbirth in the Twentieth Century*, (Stroud: Sutton Publishing, 1997).

Womersley J, 'The evolution of health information services', in McLachlan, G, *Improving the Common Weal,* pp 545-594.

Young J, 'A scheme of maternity Service co-ordinating antenatal Treatment, domiciliary and hospital treatment', *The Transactions of the EOS*, Session LXXXVIII, 1928-1929, pp 95-107.

Scottish Midwives
Twentieth-Century Voices
by Lindsay Reid

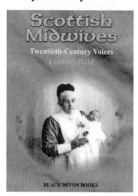

Lindsay Reid has interviewed midwifery practitioners from across Scotland in her quest to understand midwives and their practice in the twentieth century.

Scottish Midwives: Twentieth Century Voices brings together interweaving narratives, based on midwives' oral testimonies. These personal experiences and reminiscences of midwives trace the development of midwifery in Scotland in the twentieth century.

'I wis jist aboot eighteen when I delivered ma first baby... I'd never seen a bairn bein born afore. Doddie Davidson, 1930s, Aberdeenshire.

'Just before the child was born the sirens sounded and the blast blew out the sacking covering the windows, and soot blew into the room from the roofs. Under these conditions I delivered the baby.' Alice Porter, 1939-1940, wartime Aberdeen.

'We delivered babies in houses where there was real poverty with nothing ready for the baby. No cot, blankets or clothes. Ella Banks, 1940s, Glasgow.

'There appeared to be a general fascination with, "How does a man become a midwife?"' Stuart Hislop, 1981, Stirling.

'Another thing I remember – she wanted syntometrine, and the syntometrine ampoule cracked. You only get one ampoule [for a home birth] so she couldn't get her syntometrine. So she had a completely natural third stage. It was wonderful.' Ayleen Marshall, 1990s, Inverness.

Scottish Midwives: Twentieth Century Voices
ISBN: 978-0-9557999-0-7 UK £ 8.99 plus postage and packing.

Available from The Scottish History Press,
14 Flures Crescent, Erskine, Renfrewshire PA8 7DJ
Email: shp@keapub.fsnet.co.uk; www.keapublishing.com
and
Black Devon Books, North Lethans, By Saline, Dunfermline, Fife, KY12 9TE.
Tel: 01383 733144; Email:Lindsay.reid1@btinternet.com; www.lindsayreid.co.uk

Index